MW01204233

The Right Hemisphere
and Disorders of
Cognition and Communication

Theory and Clinical Practice

The Right Hemisphere and Disorders of Cognition and Communication

Theory and Clinical Practice

Margaret Lehman Blake, PhD

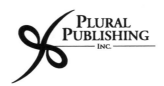

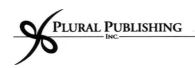

5521 Ruffin Road
San Diego, CA 92123

e-mail: info@pluralpublishing.com
Website: http://www.pluralpublishing.com

Copyright © 2018 by Plural Publishing, Inc.

Typeset in 10.5/14 Palatino by Flanagan's Publishing Services, Inc.
Printed in the United States of America by McNaughton & Gunn

All rights, including that of translation, reserved. No part of this publication may be reproduced, stored in a retrieval system, or transmitted in any form or by any means, electronic, mechanical, recording, or otherwise, including photocopying, recording, taping, Web distribution, or information storage and retrieval systems without the prior written consent of the publisher.

For permission to use material from this text, contact us by
Telephone: (866) 758-7251
Fax: (888) 758-7255
e-mail: permissions@pluralpublishing.com

Every attempt has been made to contact the copyright holders for material originally printed in another source. If any have been inadvertently overlooked, the publishers will gladly make the necessary arrangements at the first opportunity.

Library of Congress Cataloging-in-Publication Data:
Names: Blake, Margaret Lehman, author.
Title: The right hemisphere and disorders of cognition and communication :
   theory and clinical practice / Margaret Lehman Blake.
Description: San Diego, CA : Plural, [2018] | Includes bibliographical
   references and index.
Identifiers: LCCN 2017028234 | ISBN 9781597569620 (alk. paper) | ISBN
   1597569623 (alk. paper)
Subjects: | MESH: Communication Disorders | Cognition Disorders |
   Cerebrum--physiopathology | Brain Injuries--physiopathology
Classification: LCC RC423 | NLM WL 340.2 | DDC 616.85/5--dc23
LC record available at https://lccn.loc.gov/2017028234

Contents

Preface

This book covers decades of work by researchers in a variety of fields who all have been interested in what happens in the right side of the brain. It is designed for advanced graduate students and practicing clinicians interested in neurogenic disorders of cognition and communication. The perspective is from the field of speech-language pathology, but the knowledge should be useful for a broad range of professionals interested in cognition and communication.

The first chapter provides an introduction to right hemisphere brain damage (RHD) and some of the reasons why patients and clients with RHD often do not receive the same recognition or treatment as survivors of left hemisphere strokes. The second chapter provides a review of some fundamentals of clinical practice, including the World Health Organization's structure for viewing health and disability, cultural awareness, evidence-based practice, and practice-based research. While it may seem odd to have two introductory chapters, they serve very different purposes: one to introduce the population, and the second to set the stage for working with that population. It is important to approach assessment and treatment with consideration of clients' personal and environmental contexts, their cultural background, and plans to assess treatment effectiveness all firmly in the front of your mind. Thus, the review of these areas appears before the chapters on the disorders.

The remaining chapters all begin with an overview of the construct and how that construct is processed in the intact right hemisphere. This is followed by how the construct is affected by RHD and what we currently know about assessment and treatment. Given the current state of the art and science in the area of RHD, the assessment and treatment sections are relatively scarce in terms of concrete evidence-based practice. With this current reality, it is crucial to have a solid understanding of cognitive and communication processes and the theories of how they are affected by RHD to guide clinical decision making. The treatment sections build upon what we do know, and contain many suggestions based on evidence from the traumatic brain injury (TBI) literature and theoretically based expert opinion. For areas in which the research and the theories are solid enough to support treatment approaches, I provide specific suggestions for approaching treatment (e.g., language comprehension). For other areas (e.g., anosognosia), explicit approaches that go beyond the existing expert opinion or evidence from TBI are not provided because the theoretical support is not strong enough for me to feel comfortable doing so.

There are many possible ways in which the chapters could be organized, because the areas of cognition and communication overlap and interact. Indeed, communication *is* a cognitive process. They are divided here because in the field of speech-language pathology we tend to think of language and communication as separate from other cognitive processes. In this book, aspects of communication are presented first, followed by the other cognitive areas. The pragmatics chapter provides a model of social communication that sets the stage for all of the processes discussed in the book, thus it is the first "content area" following the introductory chapters. This is followed by language comprehension and prosody. The remaining chapters cover cognition: attention and neglect, executive function and anosognosia, and finally memory.

Foreword

About 23 years before I had the pleasure of reading the prepublication chapters of Margaret (Peggy) Blake's wonderful, informative new book, I had asked her to do the same thing for me. At that time I was a young(er) professor and was thoroughly delighted to have convinced Peggy to come work with me as a PhD student. Fast-forward several years, past her assiduous work on several of my grants, a number of our joint publications, and multiple research projects of her own, and Peggy had become the only PhD graduate I know whose dissertation committee required not even one change in her thesis document. The clarity of thought and style connoted by this fact continue to be evident in the current volume.

Peggy quickly developed into, and has remained, an influential sister-in-arms in the pursuit and evaluation of knowledge about the nature, assessment, and management of cognitive/language disorders in adults with damage to the right side of the brain. There weren't many investigators interested in the topic 23 years ago and there still aren't—a fact that makes me even prouder of Peggy's continued, substantive leadership through her research and publications, educational offerings, and professional service roles. It has been a joy to collaborate with her and to learn from her over the years, having watched her grow into the expert who, among other considerable contributions to the field, wrote the clear, engaging, and authoritative volume you have in your hands.

The entire book is terrific, but I particularly loved Chapter 1, in which Peggy astutely comments on how and why patients with right hemisphere disorders (RHD) often get "lost in the system." She elaborates on the discrepancy in detecting and intervening with the problems of right versus left brain stroke patients, beginning with the earliest medical contacts and proceeding through various clinical assessment and management processes. The rest of the chapter provides additional important introductory material about the population of adults with RHD. Peggy really connects with readers through fun thought experiments about vital right hemisphere contributions to communication. This chapter also emphasizes essential issues such as patient/symptom heterogeneity, thinking beyond the standard clinical stereotypes, and common research problems.

Chapter 2 helps to lay a strong foundation for clinical work with the people who have RHD. It is an extremely useful guide to viewing the existing evidence with an appropriately critical eye, and to helping readers understand how they can be involved in expanding this evidence. The chapter focuses in part on the nature of evidence and different sources of evidence, along with challenges to clinical assessment and evidence-based practice. It also offers some solutions to these challenges. For example, Peggy calls the lack of data and investigation "a golden opportunity" to apply a practice-based evidence model with the RHD population, by gathering evidence in typical clinical situations to influence management practices.

The remaining chapters each tackle cognitive/language areas that are often affected by RHD: pragmatics and social communication (including discourse production), discourse comprehension, prosody, attention, neglect, executive functions, awareness, and memory. In each chapter, Peggy begins by introducing relevant theories and models and reviewing evidence on normal right hemisphere functioning. Each chapter ends with coverage of RHD symptoms, assessment, and treatment considerations. The coverage is typically comprehensive and always clear and understandable. Periodic sidebars help to clarify difficult concepts, making the material even more engaging. Tables and figures provide useful summaries or illustrations, including, for example, the extremely helpful table that depicts manipulations that affect performance in the chapter on Neglect, and the excellent examples of the "contextualization process" for novel idioms in the chapter on Language Comprehension.

These chapters admirably bring together vast, complex, and often contradictory bodies of literature. In addition, they offer the best clinical solutions currently available, including borrowing from the evidence about other populations with similar disorders and theoretically based possibilities. Equally important, Peggy's approach provides clinicians with reminders and tools that will help them find the best solutions next week, next year, and many years from now.

This is a really opportune moment for Peggy's book. The literature on normal right hemisphere function has boomed— much of it after investigators who were interested in left brain functioning saw the right hemisphere activation in their investigations of the brain bases of normal language and cognitive processes. Theory and evidence about right hemisphere disorders and their clinical management have continued to grow since the last book of this sort. And the literatures on evidence-based practice and practice-based evidence have blossomed. Bringing these literatures together in a comprehensible and enlightening way does a real service for readers of all kinds. I enjoyed reading every word and can't wait to see what Peggy does next.

—Connie A. Tompkins, PhD, CCC-SLP, BC-ANCDS
Professor Emeritus
Communication Science and Disorders
Center for the Neural Basis of Cognition
University of Pittsburgh
Pittsburgh, PA

Acknowledgments

This book would not have been possible without the many very smart, dedicated, amazing people who influenced my educational journey through the "other side" of the brain. My first introduction to right hemisphere brain damage (RHD) came in my graduate program at Arizona State University when Dr. Leonard LaPointe suggested that I focus on RHD for my Master's thesis. I am forever indebted to him for that suggestion, as it was the launching point for my career researching, teaching, writing, and wondering about the right hemisphere. My path was solidified when I spent several years working with Connie Tompkins at the University of Pittsburgh. She began as my mentor, and became my colleague and friend. The year I spent at the Mayo Clinic working with Joe Duffy and Edy Strand strengthened not only my clinical skills, but also my appreciation for other parts of the brain, like the basal ganglia and the left hemi-sphere. It also allowed me the opportunity to collaborate with Penny Myers and add a more direct clinical component to my views on RHD. Thanks also to the many colleagues who have been supportive of my work throughout the years.

While working on this book I received valuable assistance with collecting, sorting, and reviewing information from several students at the University of Houston: Natalie Ewing, Dionne Dias, Aaron Rodriguez, Kelly Tobey, and especially Jessica Connors, who spent many hours poring over psychometric properties of cognitive and communication assessments. Thanks also to Jerry Hoepner and Rik Lemoncello who lent their expertise to the chapters on executive function and practice-based evidence. Finally, thanks to Kalie Koscielak at Plural, who was so helpful at every stage of this process, and to the reviewers who took the time to read the book draft and make smart, thoughtful suggestions for changes.

Reviewers

Plural Publishing, Inc. and the author would like to thank the following reviewers for taking the time to provide their valuable feedback during the development process:

Alfredo Ardila, PhD
Professor
Department of Communication
  Sciences and Disorders
Florida International University
Miami, Florida

Jill K. Fahy, MA, CCC-SLP
Associate Professor
Department of Communication
  Disorders and Sciences
Eastern Illinois University
Charleston, Illinois

Karen Hux, PhD
Professor
Department of Special Education and
  Communication Disorders
University of Nebraska–Lincoln
Lincoln, Nebraska

Amebu Seddoh, PhD
Associate Professor
Department of Communication
  Sciences and Disorders
University of North Dakota
Grand Forks, North Dakota

To the Lehman clan (Best. Family. Ever.)
and to Dave,
who knows my right hemispheric deficiencies better than anyone.

1

The Right Hemisphere

This chapter provides a broad overview of the current understanding of the functions of the right hemisphere (RH), highlighting the areas of practice and perception that have resulted in the general sense that the RH is less compelling or important than the left hemisphere (LH). The overview includes a history of deficits associated with right hemisphere brain damage as well as current medical and research practices in diagnosis and treatment. The chapter concludes with a review of general aspects of assessment and treatment for this population.

Introduction

The RH has long been considered the nondominant hemisphere for language processing, but the perception that it is less important and less compelling than the LH extends far beyond language processing. Vertosick (1996) in his book about life as a neurosurgery resident stated: "To a brain surgeon, there are two cerebral hemispheres: the left one, and the one that isn't the left one" (p. 213). While the critical role of language to the human experience should not be minimized, the functions of the RH play a profound role in communication. There is no question that the LH is essential for finding the right words and putting them into the right order to create sentences that convey thoughts and ideas, and understanding someone else's words and sentences. However, communication solely through words and sentences is extremely limiting, as illustrated through a few thought experiments.

■ Think about the last time you had to convey sensitive information through e-mail and had difficulty expressing your feelings or true convictions using only words and sentence structure (and occasional use of caps or punctuation). Think about the ensuing misunderstanding that took place when the recipient read your e-mail and, based only on the words and sentence organization, misinterpreted your intent.

▨ Imagine using an app to translate the phrase, "It's not you, it's me" into another language. While you may get the right words in the correct order, you probably cannot translate the underlying meaning of that phrase.

▨ Think about how many different intents you can convey through manipulating the prosody of the single word "really" (astonishment, confirmation, excited disbelief, expected disbelief, emphasis of importance); and then consider the extra text or explicit explanation you would need to express any of those intents if you were communicating only through writing.

Through production and interpretation of facial expression, body language, prosody and combining word connotations in different ways to generate novel meanings, the RH enhances communication. You end up with communication that can be nuanced, subtle, sarcastic, humorous, and much less apt to be misconstrued.

At a recent conference, a speaker was discussing recovery from and treatment of aphasia, and lamented the fact that the RH had "variously inept substrates" to support language processing that might be exploited in recovery from aphasia. While it is true that the RH has relatively limited linguistic abilities, it is also true that the LH has "variously inept substrates" for nonlinguistic aspects of communication. Loss of function of portions of either hemisphere can have significant consequences on the efficiency, quality, and depth of communication and can dramatically affect quality of life and participation in social and vocational activities.

The population of adults with RHD is heterogeneous. As with any subset of the population, they represent a variety of ages, cultures, ethnicities, personalities, educational backgrounds, and life experiences. Additionally, though, is the heterogeneity of the presentation of RHD. There are few clear patterns of deficits and as of the writing of this book there is no way to predict the constellation of deficits that any one person will present with following RHD. Added to that is the heterogeneity of the "normal" adult population regarding cognition and pragmatics. There are no clear cutoffs for cognitive function or pragmatic skills expected for successful daily functioning. While behaviors that lie on the extremes are relatively easy to identify, it may be impossible to determine where the demarcation between "normal" and "disordered" pragmatics should be. To emphasize this heterogeneity, the phrases "may be impaired" or "some adults with RHD" will be used abundantly in this book.

These phrases also should serve as a reminder to those who choose to explore the research literature and read the original articles. Critical reading is important because there are two pervasive problems in the RHD literature. The first is reporting only group data in research studies. In studies that do examine individual performance, approximately one-third to one-half of the RHD participants tend to perform similarly to the control group of adults without brain damage (e.g., Balaban, Friedmann, & Ariel, 2016; Balaban, Friedmann, & Ziv, 2016; Blake, 2009a, 2009b; Blake & Lesniewicz, 2005; Cheang & Pell, 2006), while the other half exhibits deficits. Unfortunately, in many studies there is no mention of individual performance, and only group data are reported. In these cases, it may be impossible to ascertain how many of the participants actually exhibited deficient performance.

The second problem occurs when researchers ignore individual variability and make pronouncements about the entire population based on impaired performance of only a subset of participants. One particularly striking example is from a study of nonliteral language (Cheang & Pell, 2006). The authors report that 4 of their 10 participants with RHD evidenced difficulties with joke completion and 5 participants had difficulty determining whether statements were jokes versus lies or sarcasm. A closer look at the individual results indicate that only 3 participants had difficulty on more than one task or condition, and only 1 of the 10 had difficulty on all four experimental conditions. In their conclusions, the authors acknowledge that there was heterogeneity of the group, yet state that "RHD participants are likely to have significant difficulties with respect to humor appreciation" (p. 458), and "use of pragmatic knowledge about interpersonal relationships in discourse was significantly reduced" (p. 447). Sweeping generalizations such as these have helped to perpetuate the stereotypical descriptions that pervade clinical thought and have hampered the development of a clear understanding of RHD.

Several years ago I stopped providing a stereotypical description of a person with RHD in my chapters and articles. I am concerned that the stereotyped picture of RHD may be biasing our diagnoses and treatment; we may be reading too much into behavioral characteristics because they fit with the pragmatic deficits that may be associated with RHD, and looking for infrequent but interesting behaviors that may not be important. As a consequence, there may be overdiagnosis of some problems that are "stereotypical RHD" and underdiagnosis of other deficits that are less typical but could significantly impact communication. I feel that reinforcing the stereotypes does a disservice to our patients and clients, who need to be treated as individuals and carefully examined to determine each person's pattern of strengths and weaknesses.

Another deliberate use of semantics in this book is the choice to explain deficits in terms of "reduced ability" as opposed to "lack of" or "loss of." For example, while "lack of awareness" is commonly used as a description of anosognosia, I use the more accurate phrase "reduction of awareness." It is rare that any brain lesion, but especially a focal lesion due to stroke, results in complete loss of any cognitive function. The phrase "loss of" also implicitly suggests the notion that deficits are all or none, either present or absent. Conversely, there is extensive evidence that performance can be facilitated by manipulation of tasks, stimuli, and context (see discussions of language comprehension in Chapter 4, attention in Chapter 6, and unilateral neglect in Chapter 7). Again, we do a disservice to our patients and clients by using imprecise language that hyperbolizes their deficits. This is particularly detrimental in educating patients and their families about RHD-associated disorders that seem bizarre and are relatively abstract to the general public.

RH Function

Lateralization of function and lateralized asymmetries are not unique to humans; they have been reported rather extensively in both vertebrates and invertebrates (Corballis, 2014). Most primates and marine mammals show LH dominance for action dynamics, and all primates studied thus far show RH dominance for emotion. Some species (e.g., frogs, mice) also show LH dominance for vocalization.

The RH has long been thought to have greater interconnectivity than the LH. Early work supported this idea based on the greater amount of white matter in the RH compared with the LH (Gur et al., 1980). More recent studies employing a variety of imaging techniques (magneto-encephalography, near infrared spectrometry) have provided additional evidence of differential white matter organization. The RH appears to have greater functional interconnectivity than the LH (Gootjes, Bouma, Van Strien, Scheltens, & Stam, 2006; Iturria-Medina et al., 2011; Li et al., 2014; Medvedev, 2014). The organizational patterns suggest that the RH is better at general information processing such as integration processes, in contrast to the LH, which is more efficient at specialized processing such as language and motor action (Iturria-Medina et al., 2011; Li et al., 2014).

It has been suggested that cognitive changes associated with aging reflect differential changes in the hemispheres. An early theory suggested that aging affected the RH more than the LH, resulting in RHD-like symptoms in older adults (Goldstein & Shelly, 1981). Neuroimaging evidence to support this theory is inconsistent (Rajah & D'Esposito, 2005); some studies do report asymmetrical changes related to aging (e.g., Dolcos, Rice, & Cabeza, 2002; Goldstein & Shelly, 1981; Miller, Myers, Prinzi, & Mittenberg, 2009), but others indicate that age-related changes in the size of structures are roughly equivalent across the hemispheres (Raz et al., 2005; Salat et al., 2004). While differential changes have been observed in regions within the prefrontal cortex, with greater changes in anterior and dorsal regions of the RH compared with the LH, these prefrontal changes occur in tandem with bilateral (and symmetrical) changes in the ventral regions (Rajah & D'Esposito, 2005). The RH may influence aging in other ways. Robertson (2014) suggests that the RH-biased networks for arousal, sustained attention, awareness, and response to novelty may underlie the construct of cognitive reserve, in which individuals with higher education, higher IQ, and more complex job responsibilities appear to have some "protection" against cognitive deficits related to brain injury and neurodegenerative disease.

History of Understanding RH Functions

Historically, discovery of localization of neurological function began with studying patients. This is true for RH functions. Much of our understanding of what the RH does comes from early studies of patients with focal lesions and an exploration of their deficits. While there were occasional descriptions of deficits attributed to RHD beginning in the late 1800s[1] (see review by Heilman, Bowers, Valenstein, & Watson, 1986), it was not until the mid-1900s that specific functions of the right hemisphere were explored in earnest (see reviews in Blake, 2016; Heilman et al., 1986; and Searleman, 1977).

Case studies and experiments involving visuoperceptual deficits, visuospatial agnosia, and unilateral neglect began appearing in the 1940s (McFie, Piercy, & Zangwill, 1950). While the early reports suggested that these disorders could not be unequivocally linked to RHD, it was not long before the RH was considered "dominant" for visuoperception. Language and communication were addressed in the 1960s, with the suggestion that RHD could affect abstract and complex language processing (Critchley, 1991; Eisenson, 1962).

In the 1970s there was a dramatic increase in the number of studies of emotion, prosody, visuoperception, and unilateral neglect (Blake, 2016; Ross, 1984) that led to the current understanding that the RH is dominant for these functions. During that same time frame, descriptive studies of language and communication supported ideas proposed by Critchley (1991) and Eisenson (1962) that RHD resulted in changes to "extra-linguistic" or complex language, including interpreting connotative meanings, story morals or gist, comprehending sarcasm and humor, and other forms of nonliteral language (Blake, 2016; Perecman, 1983; Wapner, Hamby, & Gardner, 1981). Development of theories to explain the language and communication deficits occurred in the

1990s, with Myers' (1990) inference failure hypothesis, Tompkins and colleagues' suppression deficit hypothesis (Tompkins, Lehman, & Baumgaertner, 1999; Tompkins, Baumgaertner, Lehman, & Fassbinder, 2000; Tompkins, Lehman-Blake, Baumgaertner, & Fassbinder, 2001), and Beeman's (1998) coarse coding hypothesis. These are discussed in more detail in Chapter 4, along with the first treatments for language deficits associated with RHD that were published in the 2000s. The clinical history of RHD thus is relatively new, beginning nearly a century after the dedicated interest in the LH.

Identification and Treatment of Right Hemisphere Stroke

RH and LH strokes occur at approximately the same frequency (RH 45%; LH 55%) (Foersch et al., 2005; Hedna et al., 2013). However, there are stark differences in the recognition and treatment of RH and LH strokes (Figures 1–1 and 1–2). To fully grasp the issues, it is important to understand stroke treatment. Currently, the most effective medical treatment for ischemic stroke is tissue plasminogen activator (tPA), a "clot-busting" drug. When administered within 4 hours after the onset of a stroke, it can dissolve the clot, restore blood flow, and substantially reduce the amount of tissue damage and resulting disability, thus significantly improving a patient's prognosis. Beyond

---

[1]Hughlings Jackson described visuoperceptual deficits in 1876; Babinski described anosognosia and changes to affect in 1914 (Langer & Levine, 2014).

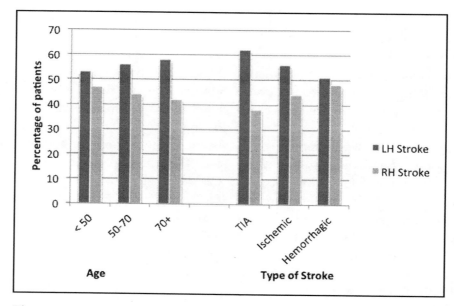

Figure 1–1. Differences in age of onset and stroke type based on side of lesion (based on Foersch et al., 2005).

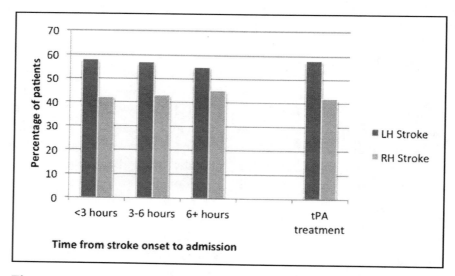

Figure 1–2. Timing of admission and pharmacological treatment based on side of lesion (based on Foersch et al., 2005). *Note.* tPA, the gold standard clot-busting treatment for ischemic strokes.

the 6-hour point, tPA has little effect. Thus, early identification of stroke is critical to receiving the best care.

Adults with LH stroke are more likely to get to an emergency department within the critical time frame, are more likely to get tPA, and tend to spend shorter amounts of time in acute care settings. In contrast, adults with RH stroke may not get to the hospital in time to receive the best medical treatment and typically have poorer outcomes (Fink et al., 2002; Foersch et al., 2005; Hedna et al., 2013; Wee & Hopman, 2005). This is particularly evident for transient ischemic attacks (TIAs): of TIAs diagnosed in the hospital, 63% are in the LH, and only 38% in the RH. The reason for this is not likely to be physiological, as RH strokes occur nearly as often as LH. Rather, it may be a difference in the rate of recognition of the mild signs or symptoms of LH versus RH TIAs (Foersch et al., 2005).

Characteristics associated with early arrival to a hospital are provided in Table 1–1. The physical and somatosensory signs (hemiparesis or hemisensory deficits) should occur equally as often from LH and RH strokes. However, in most cases aphasia probably is more obvious than the cognitive-communication deficits associated with RHD and is more likely to be recognized as a problem by patients or family members. Fink (2005) suggests that the presence of anosognosia, or reduced awareness of deficits, could be a major barrier to the recognition of RH stroke symptoms. Anosodiaphoria, or reduced concern for deficits, may also play a role. A person who appears to downplay any changes may be able to convince a spouse or family member not to seek medical attention for him/her. While these suppositions make logical sense, it is unknown how common anosognosia and anosodiaphoria are in initial presentation of stroke and if they are actual contributors to recognition of stroke signs and symptoms.

Table 1–1. Characteristics Influencing Timing of Arrival to an Emergency Department

Early Arrival
Good social network
Severe stroke
Hemorrhagic stroke (versus ischemic or TIA)
Signs/symptoms include:
sudden confusion
speech/language problems
hemiparesis
loss of consciousness
Late Arrival
Live alone
Mild stroke
Right hemisphere stroke
Female*

Note. *Females take 46% longer to get to an emergency department and wait 49% longer for treatment at hospitals than males.

Sources: Foersch et al., 2005; Jorgenson et al., 1999; Maze & Bakas, 2004; Turan et al., 2005.

The bias in diagnosis and treatment of stroke persists once an individual arrives at a hospital. Two of the most commonly used stroke scales are the National Institutes of Health Stroke Scale (NIHSS; Brott et al., 1989) and the Scandinavian Stroke Scale (SSS; Scandinavian Stroke Study Group, 1985). Both assess motor, sensory, and language functions and are used to assess severity of stroke. However, both are notably biased toward LH signs. Of the 42 points on the NIHSS, seven are related to language function to identify aphasia. Only two points are related to unilateral neglect, and those are based on observation of performance on a picture description task, not on a specific assessment of unilateral neglect. The SSS has 10 of 58 points related to language, but none for any deficit related to RHD. In a study examining the relationship between NIHSS scores and amount of tissue damage, for mild strokes (scores 0–5) individuals with RHD had twice as much tissue loss (8.8 cc) as those with left hemisphere brain damage (LHD) (3.9 cc), with comparable NIHSS scores (Fink et al., 2002). Additionally the NIHSS is relatively insensitive to cognitive deficits. In one recent study, approximately 40% of patients with an NIHSS score of 0 (extremely mild stroke) had at least one cognitive deficit (Kauranen et al., 2014).

Physicians and researchers from Johns Hopkins (Agis et al., 2010; Gottesman et al., 2010) have suggested several additions to the NIHSS to increase its sensitivity to RHD. One is to evaluate content units (CUs) produced in response to the Cookie Theft picture description task. A variety of measures of CUs (CU/minute, ratio of CU from left and right sides of the picture, number of interpretive CUs [see Chapter 4]) were related to tissue loss in various areas of the RH (Agis et al., 2010). The addition of visual extinction and line bisection tasks (see Chapter 7) also increased the sensitivity of the NIHSS to RH lesion size (Gottesman et al., 2010).

In addition to the stroke scales, neurologists and physicians have other ways to evaluate specific stroke-related deficits. While aphasia often is readily apparent after an LH stroke, it can be relatively objectively screened using a set of easy-to-administer tasks. The same is not true for cognitive-communication deficits associated with RHD. It is likely that aphasia, which occurs in about 50% of adults with LH strokes, is one of the primary concerns of neurologists. However, cognitive-communication deficits occur with about the same frequency—in about 50% of adults with RH strokes (Blake, Duffy, Myers, & Tompkins, 2002; Côté, Payer, Giroux, & Joanette, 2007)—but may not be considered at all.

Unilateral neglect is arguably the best-known deficit related to RHD. Indeed, the presence of neglect increases a patient's chance of receiving tPA by approximately 40% (Di Legge, Fang, Saposnik, & Hachinksi, 2005). It is commonly assessed by asking a patient to draw simple pictures such as a butterfly or an analog clock. Such representational drawing tasks are not very sensitive and may identify only a small percentage of individuals with unilateral neglect (Appelros, Nydevik, Karlsson, Thorwalls, & Seiger, 2003). Additionally, according to a recent study of acute stroke, unilateral neglect occurs in only about 25% of patients, and the presence of neglect alone identifies only 63% of RH strokes (Dara, Bang, Gottesman, & Hillis, 2014). Thus, even a sensitive measure of neglect will not fix the imbalance in the recognition of LH and RH stroke.

Beyond the initial diagnosis and medical treatment, the absence of clear patterns of deficits and a standard label for "right hemisphere cognitive-communication disorders" creates problems in both research and clinical practice. In research studies, often there are no a priori criteria to identify and exclude the potential participants who have no cognitive or communication disorder. This adds to the heterogeneity of participant samples, reducing the power of the experiments and the strength of the conclusions that can be drawn. Additionally, there are no standard clinical procedures for determining the presence of a cognitive-communication disorder. This is complicated by the limited options for valid, reliable, and sensitive assessment tools (see discussion in Chapter 2).

The disparities continue after a patient is sent home, in regard to available resources. General resources for stroke survivors obviously would be the same for RHD and LHD. However, an individual with aphasia has numerous resources for advocacy groups, support groups, and sources of education (Aphasia Access, National Aphasia Association, Aphasia Now, etc.). A patient with "cognitive-communication deficits" or some other vague diagnostic label will have a much harder time finding resources or education sources specific to his/her deficits.

Impact of Deficits Associated With RHD

A variety of studies have been conducted to identify predictors of stroke outcome. While there are many discrepancies across studies, some general patterns are apparent in relation to deficits associated with RHD (Table 1–2). The length of stay in a medical setting, either in acute care settings or acute and subacute settings combined, has been related to severity of stroke, the presence of unilateral neglect, and the presence of cognitive deficits (Appleros, 2007; Gillen, Tennen, & McKee, 2005; Jorgenson et al., 1999; Kong, Chua, & Tow, 1998; Pedersen et al., 1996). Functional status at discharge has been linked to stroke severity, age, unilateral neglect and anosognosia, depression, and presence of cognitive deficits (Meijer et al., 2005; Paolucci et al., 1996; Pedersen et al., 1996; Vossel, Weiss, Eschenbeck, & Fink, 2012; Wee & Hopman, 2005). The likelihood of being discharged to a dependent-living environment is related to older age, anosognosia for illness, unilateral neglect, and presence of cognitive deficits (Jehkonen et al., 2001; Kammersgaard et al., 2004; Paolucci et al., 1996; Wee & Hopman, 2005).

The presence of cognitive deficits impacts a variety of outcomes. However, what constitutes a "cognitive deficit" is not clear. While in speech-language pathology aphasia is generally considered in its own category and deficits such as attention, memory, and executive function are put into a "cognitive" category,[2] many other disciplines do not make this distinction. Thus, the outcomes linked to cognitive disorders described above are linked to problems in attention, memory, executive functions, and/or aphasia. A second issue is how cognition is measured. Often, general screenings such as the Mini Mental State Exam (Folstein, Folstein, & McHugh, 1975) are used as indicators of cognitive deficits. Such tools are designed only to screen for such deficits and are not sensitive measures of cognition (see discussion in Chapter 2).

---

[2]Language is a cognitive function, and thus aphasia is a cognitive disorder. However, there is a long-standing tradition in speech-language pathology to think of language separate from the "other cognitive disorders."

Table 1–2. Predictors of Stroke Outcomes

	Stroke Severity	Age	Depression or Anxiety	Cognitive Deficits	Unilateral Neglect	Anosognosia	Visuoperceptual Deficits
Length of stay (acute/subacute settings)	x			x	x		
Functional status upon discharge	x	x	x	x	x	x	
Discharge to dependent-living setting	x	x		x	x	x	
Long-term recovery	x	x		x			
Participation level outcomes	x	x		x	x		x
Quality of life	x	x	x				
Mortality	x	x		x			x
Independence in activities of daily living					x	x	x

Understanding RHD

As noted in the introduction, the heterogeneity of the RHD population and the absence of obvious subtypes or patterns of deficits continue to stymie our ability to understand "RH disorder." Martin and McDonald (2003, 2006) used theoretical explanations from autism and traumatic brain injury to explore the underlying source of pragmatic deficits related to RHD. Three possible explanations were poor theory of mind (ToM), "weak central coherence" (difficulty using context to determine intended meaning), and deficits in executive function (EF). Within their group of 21 participants with RHD, deficits in each of the areas were apparent for some tasks or participants but not others, and there were few meaningful correlations between the impaired processes. Thus, there was no one explanation that fit all of the pragmatic deficits for all of the participants. Given the heterogeneity in the RHD population, this is not surprising. RHD may indeed cause deficits in ToM, EF, and central coherence, but no one deficit is predominant in all patients.

The lack of a unitary explanation should not be unexpected. Imagine gathering a random sample of 21 individuals with LHD and testing them all to determine whether there was a single underlying deficit that explained a communication disorder common to all of them. Group results likely would be uninterpretable, with some participants evidencing difficulties primarily with semantics, others with phonology, and yet others with syntax. Some would have more difficulty with comprehension and others with expression, and a subset would have no deficits. We know that there are many components of the language system, and they can be impaired differentially based on what regions of the language network are damaged. To find patterns and discover the underlying deficit(s), one must look more closely than at just group results, and expect that there may not be one single explanation that will account for all of the behavioral deficits. Yet perhaps aphasia and the LH language system is not the appropriate comparison. Broca, Dax, Wernicke, and others were able to identify subtypes of language deficits in the late 1800s without the use of sophisticated language assessments or imaging techniques. The LH language network has a relatively modular organization that allows identification of subtypes and links to lesion locations through fairly rudimentary methods. The RH, in contrast, is more highly interconnected (Gootjes et al., 2006; Iturria-Medina et al., 2011; Li et al., 2014; Medvedev, 2014), and no obvious patterns have been identified over the past 50 years of research.

Conclusions and Implications

The understanding of the RH and its contribution to communication has come a long way in the past 60 years. While the phrase "nondominant hemisphere" still can be heard, it's often qualified as "nondominant for language." Still, the difference in early identification and medical treatment for RH strokes is troublesome. The work by Hillis and her colleagues at

Johns Hopkins to improve the recognition of RH strokes is important for improving the care and the outcomes for patients/clients. Additionally, projects are under way to identify patterns of deficits and propose criteria for determining which individuals are most appropriate for research and clinical intervention.

2

Fundamentals of Clinical Practice

This chapter will touch on a variety of aspects of clinical practice, including the World Health Organization's (WHO) framework for viewing health and disability, evidence-based practice and practice-based evidence, cultural awareness, and some fundamentals of assessment and treatment that are relevant for working with adults with right hemisphere brain damage (RHD). While the topics appear rather disparate on the surface, all are important to form a foundation from which to approach clinical practice with adults who have neurological disorders of communication and cognition.

Health and Disability: WHO ICF

In 2002 the WHO adapted its structure for thinking and communicating about health and disability and shifted the focus away from permanent disability to health and function. The resulting International Classification of Functioning, Disability and Health, known as the ICF, should be well known to health-related professionals, and thus will be reviewed only briefly here. As defined in Table 2–1 and illustrated in Figure 2–1, the ICF encourages attention not only to the bodily impairment (e.g., unilateral neglect caused by stroke) but also to the functional consequences on daily activities (reading the paper) and life participation (returning to work). The context in which a person lives is a critical component of assessing and treating a disorder. The context includes both environmental and personal factors. Environmental factors include the attitudes and level of support of people (family, friends, employers), technology, the natural environment, and services and systems such as transportation, education, and training. Personal factors include the person's level of education, prior employment, habits, and

Table 2–1. Definitions of the Components of the International Classification of Functioning, Disability and Health (ICF)

Body Functions are physiological functions of body systems (including psychological functions).

Body Structures are anatomical parts of the body such as organs, limbs, and their components.

Impairments are problems in body function or structure such as a significant deviation or loss.

Activity is the execution of a task or action by an individual.

Participation is involvement in a life situation.

Activity Limitations are difficulties an individual may have in executing activities.

Participation Restrictions are problems an individual may experience in involvement in life situations.

Environmental Factors make up the physical, social, and attitudinal environment in which people live and conduct their lives.

Source: Reprinted with permission from "Towards a Common Language for Functioning, Disability and Health," World Health Organization, p. 9, Copyright (2002), http://doi.org/WHO/EIP/GPE/CAS/01.3.

racial/ethnic background, among others. (For a full list of all of the components, see the ICF checklist, at http://www.who.int/classifications/icf/en/)

References to the WHO-ICF components are scattered throughout this book in relation to assessment and treatment of the various disorders associated with RHD. As experienced clinicians recognize, no two clients are the same. Each one has impairments that differentially affect activities and participation shaped by his or her specific personal characteristics and family/social/vocational environments. It is the responsibility of the clinician to explore these different components and select treatments that will enable the greatest success in activities and facilitate participation in the areas important to each client.

Evidence-Based Practice

Like the WHO-ICF, the concept of evidence-based practice (EBP) should be commonplace to clinicians. EBP involves the integration of the best available research evidence, the clinician's experience/expertise, and the client's values/needs/perspectives to inform assessment and treatment decisions.

There are two major sources for finding evidence to support decisions in clinical practice: original research articles

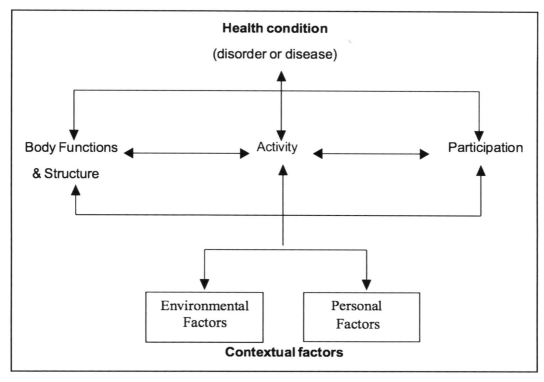

Figure 2–1. A diagram of the International Classification of Functioning, Disability and Health. Reprinted with permission from "Towards a Common Language for Functioning, Disability and Health," World Health Organization, p. 9, Copyright (2002), http://www. who.int/classifications/icf/icfbeginnersguide.pdf

and reviews. Original research provides information about a specific question, through a specific project. There are several systems for evaluating the quality of research (e.g., PeDRO, https://www.pedro.org.au/english/downloads/pedro-scale/) to aid readers in determining the level of control within the research, and by extension, how trustworthy the results might be.

Reviews include systematic reviews and meta-analyses. Systematic reviews are relatively comprehensive reviews of the existing literature. The "systematic" component involves a priori specifica-

tion of the types of research studies to be included (e.g., only randomized control trials [RCTs] or all studies with a specified level of experimental control) and the outcomes to be assessed (e.g., immediate impairment-level gains or long-term functional gains). Due to the differences in review criteria, very different results may be reported from reviews of the same topic area. For example, Cicerone and colleagues (2011) suggest that several treatments for attention and executive function should be considered practice standards or practice guidelines, while the review compiled by the Agency for Healthcare

Research and Quality (Brasure et al., 2012) concluded that there is not enough evidence to conclusively support any of the current treatments for attention or executive function. Because of the different inclusion criteria, different research studies were included in the two reviews, thus resulting in conflicting conclusions (see Chapters 6 and 8 for further discussion of these reviews and treatments for attention and executive function deficits). Meta-analyses are studies in which data from a set of previously published studies are compiled and statistical analyses are conducted on the larger data set. By combining data from multiple studies with limited numbers of participants, stronger and broader conclusions can be drawn about a particular form of assessment or treatment. Just as for systematic reviews, the inclusion and exclusion criteria influence the results and conclusions.

There are several ways of classifying levels of evidence to aid clinicians in making judgments about the strength of the evidence supporting a treatment. The Center for Evidence-Based Medicine at Oxford University (Howick et al., 2011; http://www.cebm.net/index.aspx?o=5653) proposes the following classification from strongest to weakest: systematic reviews, randomized trials, cohort studies, and case series. Expert opinion and mechanistic reasoning would be at the lower end. The authors emphasize that critical thinking and clinical judgment are needed in reviewing evidence, and for a given client, evidence from a case series might be more relevant than evidence from a randomized trial.

The prospect of EBP is not as daunting as it once was, as there are a variety of organizations and agencies that have reviewed original sources, conducted systematic reviews and meta-analyses, and evaluated the resulting knowledge to generate clinical recommendations (such as practice guidelines). A list of such resources for EBP related to disorders associated with RHD is provided in Table 2–2.

Given the current state of practice in the area of RHD, it can be challenging to conduct EBP. One obstacle is the limited number of reliable, valid tools for assessing disorders related to RHD. Without good assessment tools it is difficult to diagnose a deficit and measure outcomes of a treatment. Of the assessments available, the majority focus on the impairment level and provide little insight into the consequences of the deficits on activity and participation levels. A second obstacle is the small number of treatments. With the exception of unilateral neglect, there are few studies of treatments specifically for adults with RHD. Thus, there is heavy reliance on expert opinion, clinician experiences, and client values/perspectives. In the absence of solid evidence-based treatments, one recommendation is to use evidence gathered from other populations in which the deficits are similar to those associated with RHD (Blake, 2007). Cicerone (2005) and Sackett and colleagues (2000) provide an outline for evaluating whether or not evidence in the research literature might be applied to clinical practice (Table 2–3). The process begins with finding a treatment supported by well-controlled research studies in which

Table 2–2. Resources for Evidence-Based Practice

ASHA Practice Portal	http://www.asha.org/Evidence-Maps/
Academy of Neurologic Communication Disorders and Sciences (ANCDS) Practice Guidelines	https://ancds.memberclicks.net/evidence-based-clinical-research
American Speech-Language Hearing Association (ASHA)	http://www.asha.org/members/ebp/
Evidence Maps for assessment and treatment of communication disorders	http://www.ncepmaps.org/
The Evidence-Based Review of Moderate to Severe Acquired Brain Injury	http://www.abiebr.com/
Psychological Database for Brain Injury Treatment Efficacy (PsycBITE)	http://www.psycbite.com
Speech Pathology Database for Best Interventions and Treatment Efficacy (SpeechBITE)	http://www.speechbite.com

the disorder/impairment targeted in the treatment study is similar to that exhibited by the client, and the client is similar to the participants in the study in terms of important clinical (e.g., etiology, disease progression, co-occurring deficits) and demographic factors (e.g., age, education). If there are enough similarities, and if the benefits outweigh the potential costs, then that treatment might be appropriate. Importantly, this series of steps should be used to determine the use of any treatment for any client. For example, in order to determine whether a motoric-imitative treatment for expressive aprosodia (see Chapter 5) might be useful for one's own client, clinicians should compare the client's characteristics with those of the participants in the

research studies, evaluate the feasibility and potential costs versus benefits, and then use all of the information to determine whether the treatment might be a good choice.

Beyond EBP

There are a variety of barriers to EBP and the translation of new knowledge to clinical practice. Wilkinson, Sakel, and Milberg (2011) describe some of the problems with conducting RCTs, which include many restrictive rules and regulations governing research processes. These affect the ease of recruiting enough participants from a variety of sites to ensure

Table 2–3. Process for Selecting Treatments for Use in Clinical Practice

(1) Find well-controlled treatment study for disorder X with promising results.

(2) Compare current client with participants in the research study:
   a. demographics: age, race/ethnicity, gender
   b. clinical presentation: etiology, severity of deficit to be treated; co-occuring deficits that may impact treatment.

(3) Examine cost/benefit and feasibility:
   a. potential for gains versus potential costs (time, effort)
   b. feasibility for implementation in existing environment.

(4) Compare nature of treatment and potential gains to client's preferences and goals.
(5) If the client is deemed similar enough to those in the study, the potential benefits outweigh the costs, it is feasible to implement the treatment, and the nature of the treatment and potential gains conform with the client's preferences and goals, then implement the treatment.

Source: Based on suggestions by Cicerone (2005) and Sackett et al. (2000).

adequate external validity[1] of the studies. In many cases there is limited infrastructure and cooperation at the necessary levels to facilitate the process of approval through human-subjects committees and multiple institutional review boards. Thus, the emphasis on RCTs slows the research process.

A second critical weakness in the process of EBP is that there is a large and lengthy gap between when research results are published and when the knowledge about more efficient or effective treatments is put into practice. One estimate suggested that it takes 17 years for 14% of research to be put into practice (Weingarten et al., 2000). Research findings often do not get published due to negative results, small sample sizes, or weaknesses in research design (real

or perceived). Inclusion criteria for systematic reviews often include RCTs or other experimental group designs, resulting in exclusion of case studies or nonrandomized group studies. The result is that knowledge gained from the latter studies are not widely reviewed or distributed. Additionally, the research that is funded and published tends to have strong internal validity (tight experimental control) but relatively weak external validity (generalizability or clinical applicability), so that the results are not immediately applicable to clinical practice.

One approach to closing the research–practice gap is to broaden and speed up the transfer of information from researchers to clinicians. All of the resources listed in Table 2–2 are designed to make

---

[1]External validity affects how well the results of a study can be generalized to larger populations and different settings.

the information more accessible to clinicians. However, this one-way street from researcher to clinician may not be the most effective means of improving practice. Two other approaches are implementation science and practice-based research.

Implementation Science

Implementation science (also called translational research, knowledge transfer, and implementation research) is involved with exploration of (a) the barriers that impede the flow of research knowledge to clinical practice and (b) ways to overcome the barriers. This involves identifying and understanding the context of clinical practice, including the key stakeholders and the physical settings in which the clients are seen. The various barriers then must be identified and systematically prioritized before addressing them.

Damschroeder and colleagues (2009) created a framework for implementation research based on models and components from a variety of fields. The resulting Consolidated Framework for Implementation Research (CFIR) includes five domains. The first four encompass characteristics of the context: (1) the type, complexity, and specifics of the intervention; (2) the broad economic, political, and social structures in which an institution exists; (3) the institutional structure, culture, and available resources; and (4) characteristics of the stakeholders (clients, clinicians, managers, families), including not only demographic, educational, and clinical factors, but also attitudes. The fifth domain is the

process of implementation, from initial exploration and planning through education, installation, full implementation, and sustainability (see Olswang & Prelock, 2015 for a more detailed description and an example of implementation of communication treatment).

Practice-Based Evidence and Practice-Based Research[2]

EBP, as described above, tends to be a one-way street, with researchers providing information to clinicians. Practice-based research (e.g., Crooke & Olswang, 2015; Green, 2008; Horn & Gassaway, 2010) opens the street to two-way traffic, with clinicians and researchers working together and sharing information in both directions. The systematic use of data collected in natural settings to directly inform clinical practices is referred to as practice-based evidence (PBE). PBE offers a framework for evaluating one's own clinical practice with individual or small groups of clients by systematic analysis of treatment, generalization, maintenance, and control data to answer questions about treatment effects when there is a paucity of evidence or when your client does not match the participants in published research studies (Lemoncello & Ness, 2013; Olswang & Bain, 1994). Ideally, clinicians should be constantly engaged in PBE to guide their daily clinical decision making. PBE should not be considered a replacement for EBP; instead they should be considered complementary processes that, together, aid clinicians in providing the most efficient,

---

[2]This section was written in collaboration with Rik Lemoncello.

effective treatment for their individual clients (Lemoncello & Ness, 2013).

Olswang and Bain (1994) provided a thorough review of data types and colletion methods that can support PBE. In their tutorial article, they explain how collecting and analyzing treatment responses, treatment probe data, generalization probes, and control data can help answer clinical questions such as: Is my client responding to treatment? Is significant and important change happening? Is the treatment responsible for the observed change(s)? Has sufficient generalization occurred? While many clinicians will be familiar with the concepts of treatment data and generalization probes, introduction of control data can enhance one's own PBE and data-driven decision making (Lemoncello & Ness, 2013). Control data represent behaviors that are not expected to change as a direct result of the intervention (e.g., aprosodia should not improve when training visual scanning for unilateral neglect). If treatment data show improvement (i.e., improved reading comprehension) with stable control data (i.e., no change in aprosodia), then the clinician can confidently conclude that the treatment (i.e., visual scanning) is effective. On the other hand, if control data also show improvement during treatment (i.e., both reading comprehension and expressive prosody improved), then spontaneous recovery or general cognitive stimulation may be more responsible for the observed effects.

Another method to systematically collect and analyze individual treatment data utilizes single-case experimental research design (Wambaugh, 2007). Single-case designs provide a strong experimental framework for demonstrating treatment effects with individual or small groups of clients. Examples of single-case designs include multiple baseline, reversal, and alternating treatment studies. While implementation of a single-case design initially will require time and effort to learn, benefits of such implementation can include increased knowledge of treatment effectiveness, identification of treatment components that are more or less effective for specific clients, and objective data to support justification for treatment. Detailed discussions and examples of single-case designs are beyond the scope of this book and can be found elsewhere (e.g., Barnett et al., 2012; Beeson & Robey, 2006; Rassafiani & Sahaf, 2010; Thompson, 2006).

Cultural Awareness

An important part of all clinical practice is awareness of cultural backgrounds, characteristics, and influences. Clinicians should be aware of influences and traditions of their own culture as well as those of their clients. While cultural awareness should be used to inform and direct interactions with all clients and patients, it is particularly important for those with potential disorders of pragmatics, such as adults with RHD. Understanding the cultural "rules" or traditions regarding pragmatic aspects of communication such as eye contact, level of formality in conversation, and amount of self-disclosure is critical for distinguishing deficits versus differences, and for determining treatment goals. It is critical to remember that while individuals are influenced by their culture, most people do not ascribe to all of the aspects of that culture or tradition. Additionally, while there are broad features of a culture (e.g., the American culture), there are many subtypes within a larger culture. Within the United States, for example, there are ethnic, racial, gender, religious, geographical, and other subcultures that can create vast diversity across individuals who were all brought up in the USA.

A variety of resources are available to aid clinicians in increasing their cultural awareness and cultural competence. A small sample of sites with information and resources is provided in Table 2–4. One good place

Table 2–4. Resources for Exploring and Increasing Cultural Awareness

Resource	*Description of Select Content*
ASHA Practice Portal http://www.asha.org/Practice-Portal/Professional-Issues/Cultural-Competence/	Cultural awareness self-assessment. Recommendations for reducing potential cultural biases in assessment and treatment.
Center for International Rehabilitation Research Information and Exchange (CIRRIE) at the University of Buffalo http://cirrie.buffalo.edu/	Information about rehabilitation research from around the world. Informational descriptions of over 20 different cultures, including beliefs about health, disability, and rehabilitation.
National Center for Cultural Competence at Georgetown University http://nccc.georgetown.edu/	Publications and other information about cultural competency for medical professionals, including self-assessments and distance learning materials. Information regarding religious and spiritual aspects of cultural competence.
National Library of Medicine of the National Institutes of Health: Outreach Activities & Resources https://sis.nlm.nih.gov/outreach/multicultural.html	Wealth of materials and links to multicultural resources for health information.
US Department of Health and Human Services Health Resources and Services Administration: Culture, Language & Health Literacy Resources http://www.hrsa.gov/cultural competence/race.html	Information regarding increasing health literacy and providing respectful, ethical care for various racial/ethnic groups, as well as gender, disability, and age-related materials.
US Department of Health and Human Services Office of Minority Health http://minorityhealth.hhs.gov/	Materials to increase awareness of and solutions for health disparities related to race and ethnicity.

SIDEBAR: Cultural Awareness

Several years ago I gave an assignment in my Acquired Cognitive Disorders class in which students had to find a website or blog created by someone with a cognitive disorder (or her/his caregiver/spouse) and describe (a) the cognitive and communication deficits, (b) social, psychological, and emotional effects of the disorder, and (c) cultural influences. More than one student stated something akin to: "The author of the blog was American, so she had no cultural influences." The students were so immersed in their own culture that they saw the world only through that lens, considering the American way of life as the standard, with only non-Americans having cultural differences. (Perhaps the ethnocentrism was part of their American culture!)

---

to start is to complete a self-awareness questionnaire to identify one's own cultural understanding and biases, either conscious or unconscious (see side bar). After that, it may be easier to identify similarities and differences across cultures.

Assessment of Adults With RHD

An ideal assessment should include both standardized and nonstandardized measures, observations of the client in a variety of settings and interacting with a variety of other people, and conversations with both the client and his/her family or caregivers about the kinds of changes that have occurred and how important or concerning those changes are given the client's lifestyle, personality, and goals for recovery. A thorough assessment should cover body structure/function, activity and participation levels,

as well as contextual factors. The assessment also should be dynamic, exploring where breakdowns occur and what kinds of cues and supports are most beneficial. Clearly, such an ideal assessment is not possible in most areas of clinical practice, in part due to time restrictions but also because of the paucity of valid, reliable measures of the various deficits associated with RHD.

Domain- or disorder-specific assessments are addressed in each of the following chapters; thus, the present discussion will cover only broad-based assessments. There are several batteries designed for assessment of adults with RHD, and a few others that commonly are used for this population (Table 2–5). With the exception of the Montreal Evaluation of Communication (Joanette et al., 2016), most of them were developed many years ago and do not reflect current understanding of the deficits. Additionally, nearly all have weaknesses in validity and reliability

Table 2–5. Select Assessment Batteries for RHD

Test	Authors	Areas Assessed	Reliability*	Validity*
Burns Brief Inventory	Burns, 1997	RH Inventory: visuospatial skills, prosody, abstract language. Complex Neuropathology inventory: orientation, memory, attention.	Good	Weak
Mini Inventory of Right Brain Injury 2	Pimental & Knight, 2000	Visual processing, unilateral neglect, reading/writing, nonliteral language, emotion/affect, conversation, general behavior	Good	OK
Montreal Evaluation of Communication– English version	Joanette et al., 2015	Prosody, nonliteral language, conversation, pragmatic inference, discourse, lexico-semantics, awareness of deficits	OK	Weak
Rehab Institute of Chicago (RIC) Evaluation of Communication Problems in RH Dysfunction 3	Halper et al., 2010	Behavioral observation, pragmatic communication, visual scanning & tracking, writing, metaphorical writing	Weak–OK; depends on training and subtest	Weak
Right Hemisphere Language Battery, 2nd ed.	Bryan, 1994	Lexical semantics, nonliteral language, humor, inferences, prosody	OK	Weak
Ross Information Processing Assessment (Revised)	Ross-Swain, 1996	Memory, problem solving, auditory processing	Weak	Weak

Note. *Good = moderate–strong estimates of 2 or more types of reliability/validity; OK = moderate–strong estimates of 1 type of reliability/validity; weak = below adequate estimates of 1 or more types of reliability/validity; none = no estimates reported. See Appendix for detailed information about reliability and validity.

and were developed with relatively small samples.

In addition to the limitations of the available test batteries, there are three other factors that make RHD assessment particularly challenging. First, as described in more detail in Chapters 3 and 8, there are no clear definitions of what should constitute "normal" versus "impaired" functional pragmatics and cognition in adulthood. Thus, it is extremely difficult to determine clear cutoff points. Second, most of the assessments have substantial metacognitive demands. As described in Chapter 4 in relation to language processing, such demands affect performance, leaving clinicians to figure out whether or not poor test scores are due to a deficit in the construct being assessed (e.g., language or executive function) or the demands of the task itself. Third, many of the participation-level and quality of life measures rely on self-report. Responses from individuals with anosognosia (reduced awareness of deficits; see Chapter 9) may not accurately reflect the deficits or difficulties that are present.

Screenings

In some situations, clinicians may need to conduct a screening to determine whether a full assessment is warranted. More often, results of a screening are reported in a medical chart and must be interpreted by a clinician. There are no specific screenings for adults with RHD. There are several cognitive screenings that have been used with stroke survivors (Table 2–6). The most well known is the Mini Mental State Examination (MMSE; Folstein, Folstein, & McHugh, 1975). A more recent addition is the Montreal Cognitive Assessment (MoCA; Nasreddine et al., 2005). Results from several recent studies suggest that the MoCA is more sensitive than the MMSE for identification of cognitive deficits following stroke (Dong et al., 2010; Toglia, Fitzgerald, O'Dell, Mastrogiovanni, & Lin, 2011). However, screenings provide only a gross assessment of cognitive abilities and do not cover all areas of cognition. Results from some studies indicate that patients with screening scores within the normal range often have cognitive deficits diagnosed by more sensitive, in-depth measures (e.g., Duffin et al., 2012). Thus, screening tools should never be used in isolation to make diagnoses (e.g., Chan et al., 2014). Just as with the global stroke scales such as the NIHSS (Brott et al., 1989) or the SSS (Scandinavian Stroke Group, 1985) reviewed in Chapter 1, these cognitive screening tools have limited sensitivity to identify unilateral neglect and do not assess other deficits common after RHD such as aprosodia or pragmatic disorders. Thus, clinicians should not rely on screening tools to unequivocally rule out disorders of cognition and communication.

Environmental and Partner Assessment

Given the importance of context in the World Health Organization's structure for health and disability and on communication and pragmatics (see Figure 3–1 and the discussion of pragmatics in Chapter 3), evaluation of the environmental context

Table 2–6. Select Cognitive Screening Tools

Name	Authors	Scope of Test	Reliability*	Validity*
Cognistat: The Neurobehavioral Cognitive Status Examination	Kiernan et al., 1987	Memory, language, construction, calculations, and reasoning	None	None
Cognitive-Linguistic Quick Test	Helm-Estabrooks, 2001	Attention, memory, language, executive functions, visuospatial skills	Weak	OK
Mini Mental State Exam	Folstein et al., 1975	Orientation, memory, attention, language, visuoperception	Good	Good
Montreal Cognitive Assessment (MoCA)	Nasreddine et al., 2005	Orientation, memory, attention, language, visuoperception	Good	Good
Neuropsychological Assessment Battery (NAB)	Stern & White, 2003	Attention, memory, language, visuoperception, executive function	Good	Good
The Oxford Cognitive Screen	Demeyere et al., 2015	Apraxia, unilateral neglect, memory, language, exec function, and number abilities	OK	Good
Scales of Cognitive & Communicative Ability for Neurorehabilitation	Milman & Holland, 2012	Problem solving, language, memory	Good	Good

Note. *Good = moderate–strong estimates of 2 or more types of reliability/validity; OK = moderate–strong estimates of 1 type of reliability/validity or mix of weak and strong estimates; weak = weak estimates of 1 or more types of reliability/validity; none = no estimates reported. See Appendix for detailed information about reliability and validity.

can provide valuable information for clinicians, clients, and families. Such assessments provide insights into what kinds of environments and settings are easier or more difficult to navigate and what kinds of factors can facilitate or impede cognitive and communicative functioning. Assessment of communication partners also can be used to identify how different behaviors impact a client's communicative performance.

Environmental assessments have not been considered specifically for adults with RHD, with the exception of modifying the physical environment for individuals with unilateral neglect. Fortunately, the work related to adults with aphasia, dementia, and traumatic brain injury (TBI) provides a good starting point for thinking about how the environment and communication partners can be assessed and manipulated to aid clients with other cognitive and communication deficits. Some environmental manipulations are discussed in later chapters in reference to specific deficits.

Brush and colleagues (Brush, Calkins, Bruce, & Sanford, 2012; Brush, Sanford, Fleder, Bruce, & Calkins, 2011) developed the Environment and Communication Assessment Toolkit for Dementia Care (ECAT) to facilitate environmental and partner assessments. As with much of the research in this area, it is based on the environmental press model (Nahemow & Lawton, 2016). First developed in the 1970s, this model proposes that a person's capability for any particular activity (person) and his/her performance on that activity (performance), including the person's ability to adapt, are influenced by the social and physical environment (press). The ECAT (Brush et al., 2012) is based on a three-stage process of investigation, interpretation, and then intervention. Aspects of person, performance, and press should be considered at each of the three stages.

The Measure of Skill in Supported Conversation (MSC) and the Measure of Participation in Conversation (MPC) were developed by Kagan and colleagues as global measures of communication that included not only adults with aphasia, but also their communication partners, who could either exacerbate or minimize the effects of aphasia based on their behaviors. Togher, Power, Tate, McDonald, and Rietdijk (2010) adapted the scales for adults with TBI. These adapted scales could be an important addition to the assessment of communication by adults with RHD.

Treatment of Adults With RHD

Treatment of disorders associated with RHD is based primarily on expert opinion and tasks selected to address the symptoms rather than the underlying deficits. The reason for this is the relative paucity of treatment studies. A recent systematic review found a total of six treatments for communication disorders (language processing, pragmatics, and aprosodia) for which there was any evidence (Blake, Frymark, & Venedictov, 2013). More evidence is available for cognitive deficits such as memory and attention, and there are more than 18 different treatments for unilateral neglect that have been systematically evaluated. Due to the limited options related to treatment of communication disorders, it is doubly important that clinicians have a solid understanding of the underlying impairments and theories so that they can critically evaluate treatments designed for other populations or develop their own treatment approaches that are solidly based on theory instead of simply treating symptoms. In each of the subsequent chapters, the relevant treatment research will be reviewed, and suggestions for theoretically based treatment in the absence of evidence will be provided.

Emerging Trends in Treatment

Treatment for communication disorders goes far beyond the traditional behavioral therapy and includes neuroimaging, neuromodulation, and pharmacological treatments. As with much of the work around RHD, there is little research directly on adults with RHD with the exception of unilateral neglect.

There have been a variety of studies of pharmacological treatments for cognitive deficits associated with TBI. However, there is no strong, consistent evidence showing benefits of such treatments (Dougall, Poole, & Agrawal, 2015; Warden et al., 2006). Additionally, there is extremely limited evidence related to pharmacological treatments for attention deficits, including unilateral visuospatial neglect (Luvizutto et al., 2015; Sivan, Neumann, Kent, Stroud, & Bhakta, 2010).

Neuromodulation is a relatively new form of treatment. Methods such as transcranial direct current stimulation (tDCS) and repetitive transcranial magnetic stimulation (rTMS) are designed to elicit long-term changes in the firing rate of cortical neurons. The stimulation can be set to increase either excitation or inhibition of regions of the cortex in order to facilitate performance. Results from neuromodulation studies on individuals with aphasia show enhanced gains from language treatment (e.g., anomia treatment), primarily when it is paired with excitatory stimulation of perilesional areas of the left hemisphere (LH). Changes in both language performance and neurophysiology have been documented, although few long-term, functional changes in language or quality of life have been assessed or reported (Crinion, 2016; de Aguiar, Paolazzi, & Miceli, 2015; Elsner, Kugler, Pohl, & Mehrholz, 2013; Fridriksson, Hubbard, & Hudspeth, 2012; Holland & Crinion, 2012).

Some studies of tDCS treatment for aphasia have explored the benefits of stimulation of the RH. This can be done through anodal stimulation, which facilitates excitation in the RH components of the language networks that could potentially facilitate language despite the LH lesions. Alternatively, cathodal stimulation, which facilitates inhibition, also could result in improved language performance. This is based on the idea that inefficient processing in language-homologous areas of the RH impedes language processing of the preserved areas of the LH. Basically, the RH tries to conduct language processing, but it is not good at it, and this RH activation prevents the healthy areas of the LH from executing the language processing. A critical concern with this type of research is the potential for changes to RH processing that could occur with repeated stimulation. If stimulation of the LH results in changes to neurophysiology and long-lasting change to behavior, then RH stimulation may create similar changes to RH processing. While this may result in reduction of aphasic symptoms, the studies that have used this technique thus far have failed to evaluate RH functions (Kang, Kim, Sohn, Cohen, & Paik, 2011; Monti et al., 2013; Shah-Basak et al., 2015; Sparing, Dafotakis, Meister, Thirugnanasambandam, & Fink, 2008; You, Kim, Chun, Jung, & Park, 2011). Crinion (2016) reported that while no negative effects on cognition have been reported from rTMS, few studies monitor or assess cognitive function. Thus, it is not clear whether the same neuromodulation that improves language processing might negatively affect pragmatic, attention, or prosodic processing.

Regarding cognitive functions relevant to RHD, tDCS has been used for treatment of unilateral neglect, working memory (WM), and executive function (EF) (see review in Convento, Russo, Zigiotto, & Bolognini, 2016). Results for parietal lobe stimulation for unilateral neglect are mixed, with improvement on some but not other visuospatial tasks (see also Chapter 7). There is more consistency in the positive results obtained from stimulation to prefrontal cortical areas to target WM and EF, although the number of studies is quite small.

There are many questions yet to be answered regarding neuromodulation as a therapy technique for cognitive disorders, including the optimal location of stimulation, the best timing of treatment (e.g., as a supplement to spontaneous recovery or during chronic phases of recovery), the effect (both positive and negative) on cognitive functions not targeted, the long-term effects of modulation, and perhaps most importantly, the generalization of gains to activity- and participation-level activities (Convento et al., 2016; Crinion, 2016).

Conclusions and Implications

Various frameworks and models have been developed to increase the awareness of, and focus on, effective treatment for individual clients that take into account each client as a unique individual. The limited number of psychometrically sound RHD assessment tools often requires clinicians to explore domain-specific tools that may provide more reliable and valid assessments than any one standardized battery. The paucity of RHD treatment research creates a unique opportunity for researchers and practitioners to drive the field forward with a focus on practice-based research. While the relative lack of treatment research typically is highlighted as a significant weakness, it may be more useful to view this as a golden opportunity to push the envelope and lead the development of treatment informed by PBE instead of having to shift from an efficacy-based EBP model to a PBE model. This opportunity should be seized with both hands so that our clients with RHD can receive the best treatment possible.

3

Pragmatic Aspects of Communication

Pragmatics refers to the interactional and social use of language. As such, it overlaps extensively with language, particularly discourse production and comprehension, as well as nonlinguistic components of communication (e.g., prosody) and nonverbal communication (body language, facial expression, etc.). This chapter will be organized in relation to a model of social communication that includes the cognitive, limbic, and executive control processes that are integrated within a communicative context. The primary areas addressed here include theory of mind, emotion, empathy, humor, and language production. The other cognitive processes (attention, memory) and executive control will be covered in later chapters. Language comprehension will be addressed in Chapter 4.

A Model of Social Communication

Communication is a highly complex process that involves much more than just language and linguistics. The environment or context of the exchange, the people involved, executive function and other cognitive processes, and nonverbal exchange of cues or information all play a role.

For communication to be successful, the speaker must be able to convey meaning that is correctly interpreted by the listener. According to Speech Act Theory (Searle, 1969), there are three aspects of communication. The locutionary act is the literal meaning. The illocutionary act is the intended meaning. The third aspect of communication is the perlocutionary act, which is the impact or effect the speaker attempts to have on the listener. In some cases these are the same thing, but oftentimes the intended meaning must be derived from the context in which the communication is occurring. Table 3–1 provides examples.

Interpreting intended meaning (illocutionary act) is an intricate process that relies on perception, interpretation, and integration of words, sentence structures, tone of voice, vocal quality, facial expression, and the social and physical context

Table 3–1. Examples of Locutionary, Illocutionary, and Perlocutionary Acts

"I want cereal for breakfast"			
Communicative Context	Locutionary	Illocutionary	Perlocutionary
At a restaurant	I want cereal	Please bring me cereal	Ordering
Looking at options in pantry	I want cereal	I want cereal	Informing
Just given a plate of undercooked eggs	I want cereal	I don't want to eat what you just gave me; I would rather eat something else.	Hurt feelings; informed of substandard cooking; requesting new food
In the grocery store	I want cereal	Buy cereal	Buy cereal

surrounding the exchange (Krauss & Chiu, 1998; Levelt, 1989; Schober, 1998). Hartley's (1995) model of social communication included cognitive factors and executive control as well as influences from the environment and limbic inputs. A variation of her model is provided in Figure 3–1. In this adapted model, all of the components that impact communication (cognitive processes, executive control, and limbic inputs) occur within a context or environment. Each component will be discussed below.

Cognitive processes that impact communication include attention, perception, and memory, as well as the visuospatial and linguistic capabilities of each communication partner (Table 3–2). Communication may be inefficient or unsuccessful if either partner is not attending to the conversation, does not perceive facial expression or tone of voice, or is unable to decode the linguistic message. Another component, theory of mind (ToM), refers to one's understanding that other people

have views, purposes, and levels of knowledge and understanding that might differ from one's own. Successful communication requires manipulation of the level of explanation and background information based on the level of knowledge that the partner has (or is assumed to have). For example, for an avid sports fan, conversations about a recent tournament are likely quite different when that person is talking to other sports fans than when he is talking to people who do not follow sports.

The limbic system, which plays a critical role in arousal, emotion, and motivation, impacts communicative effectiveness and efficiency. Decreased arousal or motivation will reduce the likelihood that a person will initiate or seek out communication opportunities. Increased motivation may lead to inappropriate communication interactions, such as initiating conversations with strangers or continuing a conversation once the partner has signaled she has to leave. Communication adequacy decreases when either the

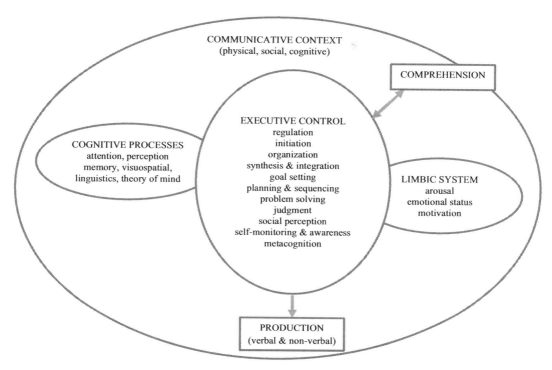

Figure 3–1. Model of social communication. Adapted from Hartley, *Cognitive-Communicative Abilities Following Brain Injury*, 1E. © 1995 Delmar Learning, a part of Cengage Learning, Inc. Reproduced by permission. http://www.cengage.com/permissions

speaker or the listener is in a highly emotional state (very angry, sad, frustrated, or happy). Emotional lability is characterized by increased emotional reactions to external or internal stimuli. It occurs more often when a person is in a heightened state of stress or fatigue but also is not uncommon following a stroke (Chemerinski & Robinson, 2000; Robinson, 1997). Some patients may have pseudobulbar palsy, in which the emotional reactions are not related to the person's emotional state (e.g., Duffy, 2013). Emotional lability or pathological emotional responses may be incorrectly interpreted by a communication partner as reflecting a person's actual emotional state, and in turn may affect the communication exchange.

The influences of cognitive processes and the limbic system all interact with the executive control systems. Reasoning, problem solving, and judgment can be impacted by deficits in attention and memory as well as changes in emotional status and motivation. Executive control also affects the cognitive processes. As described in Chapters 6 and 10, top-down executive control can be used to more efficiently allocate attention based on knowledge of patterns to make predictions, and retrieval of memories can be facilitated by organization.

As depicted in the model (see Figure 3–1), all of these systems and processes occur within a communicative context. This context encompasses the physical

Table 3–2. Influence of Cognitive Processes on Communication

Attention	An attentional lapse can cause a listener to miss some information, which results in incorrect comprehension or inferences.
	Reduced attention decreases the likelihood that information will be encoded and stored in memory for later retrieval.
	Distractibility on the part of a speaker can result in disorganized or tangential discourse production.
Perception	Aids in recognition of nonverbal cues such as facial expression and prosody.
Memory	Working memory is important for comprehension, for holding on to the linguistic message while further information is being processed; for revising interpretations within and across sentences, holding on to the details of the story you want to tell, and getting all the information out in the right order.
	Long-term memory is accessed for stores of knowledge, both episodic memories that are the basis for stories you tell as well as declarative, world knowledge used to verify the truth of what you hear.
Visuospatial processes	Along with perception, aids in recognition of facial expression and body language.
	Critical for reading and writing.
Linguistic processes	Deficits or inefficiencies in processes to activate meanings (coarse coding) or suppress inappropriate interpretations can affect general discourse and narrative comprehension.
	Rapid, accurate word finding, particularly for abstract words, facilitates expression of ideas and emotions.

environment in which the exchange takes place, the social aspects of the exchange, and the cognitive status of the people involved.

The physical environment can influence communication behaviors. The content and degree of self-disclosure may change if the conversation occurs in a public versus a private place. Proximity of objects or people can affect word choice—for example, pointing or referring to "that" or "her" as opposed to labeling an object or person. Noisy environments affect auditory perception of spoken language, which

in turn affects synthesis, integration, and comprehension of the information that is conveyed. Communication in a noisy place may increase the importance of nonverbal cues such as facial expressions and gestures, which in turn requires a shift in regulation and attention to such cues.

The social aspects of communication include social roles. These are determined in part by social status (e.g., authority, age, social relationship). The social roles of communication partners, especially when there are large differences in status, can influence style, formality, topic choice, and the degree of self-disclosure. Cultural norms and differences also are part of the social context (see Chapter 2 for a discussion of cultural awareness). Awareness and understanding of the other person's (a) level of knowledge, (b) communicative purpose or goal, and (c) perspective are also part of the communicative exchange.

Cognitive Processes: Theory of Mind

Most of the cognitive processes and their impact on pragmatics and communication are covered in other chapters. Theory of mind is discussed here because of its extensive overlap with the concept of pragmatics. ToM is a complex concept. It refers to one's ability to understand that others have knowledge, thoughts, ideas, intents, and feelings that might be different from one's own. These are then taken into account during interactions; a speaker must provide enough information but not too much given what he thinks the listener knows. There are several types of beliefs that are tested in assessing ToM. The most common are first- and second-order beliefs (see examples in Table 3–3). First-order beliefs are what a protagonist knows. Second-order beliefs are what a protagonist knows about another character's knowledge or beliefs. These are particularly important for understanding persuasion, sarcasm, and deception, such as white lies and double-bluffs. In order to persuade someone, for example, it helps to know what the other person thinks or feels about the item in question. Trying to convince her husband to replace the furniture, a wife can select a persuasive tack

by knowing what his main concern is: the expense (I found a new place that has reasonable prices), the inconvenience (I can go after work this week and see what is available), or sentimentality (I know this is the first couch we bought after we got married, but . . .).

Making the construct of ToM even more complicated is the distinction between cognitive and affective ToM. Cognitive ToM comprises one's beliefs about another person's beliefs, while affective ToM comprises beliefs about another person's feelings (Shamay-Tsoory, Tomer, Berger, Goldsher, & Aharon-Peretz, 2005). Most studies do not make a distinction between these. In the few that do, differential performances by adults with right hemisphere brain damage (RHD) are not readily apparent (Balaban, Friedmann, & Ziv, 2016a)

There are several traditional ways to assess ToM: (a) written vignettes and questions designed to test first- and second-order beliefs, irony/sarcasm interpretation or identification of social faux pas, (b) cartoon interpretation, and (c) descriptions of the movements of animated shapes. Vignettes typically describe interactions between at least two characters followed by comprehension and interpretation questions (see Table 3–3). The faux pas test involves one character who accidentally does or says something that is socially inappropriate. An individual with good ToM will be able to identify what the person did not know about the situation or communicative context that led to the faux pas. Cartoon interpretation circumvents the language demands of vignettes but requires good visuoperceptual processes to aid in interpretation of

Table 3–3. Sample Theory of Mind Stimuli and Tasks

First- and Second-Order Beliefs	Questions
It was a hot summer day and John and Katie were busy cleaning the garage. John carefully set his pink flamingo beside the door so that he would remember to put it in the yard when they were done. He then went inside to get a cold drink. Katie kept working. She spied the flamingo by the door and moved it onto the shelf she had just cleared. As John finished his drink he decided to put the flamingo in the front yard so it would be out of the way.	
• First-order belief: John knows the flamingo is by the door. • First-order belief: Katie knows the flamingo is on the shelf.	Where does John think the flamingo is? Does John think the flamingo is by the door? (TRUE belief) Does John think the flamingo is on the shelf? (FALSE belief)
• Second-order belief: Katie moved the flamingo when John was gone; she knows it is on the shelf and that John thinks it is still by the door.	Where will John look for the flamingo?

Indirect Speech	Questions
Scott had to do some errands on the south end of town. He wasn't familiar with the area, so he called his friend Sandy. Scott asked, "Do you know where the bookstore is in the south end?" Sandy replied, "Sure I do."	Did Sandy answer Scott's question? What did Scott want Sandy to tell him?

Faux Pas	Questions
Jessica had just bought her first car. She sent a picture of the lime green VW bug to her cousin Francis and said she would be driving it when they met their friend Lily for dinner later that night. Jessica arrived early and was waiting in front of the restaurant. As Francis and Lily walked up, Jessica heard Lily say, "Can you believe that people actually buy those VW bugs? They are terrible cars!" Francis saw Jessica and said, "Jessica, I'm glad you're here already. I'm starving!"	Did someone say something he or she shouldn't have? Who said something he or she shouldn't have? Why did he or she say it? Did Lily know that the car was Jessica's? How do you know? How did Jessica feel when she heard what Lily said?

the stimulus. A final task is the description of animated shapes. Individuals describe shapes as they move around either randomly or with apparent interaction. ToM is inferred as being present if the individual describes social interactions (e.g., the square is knocking on the door; the square is a bully and won't leave the circle alone) or ascribes emotions to the shapes (e.g., the triangle was angry at the square).

ToM and the Intact RH

The neural network underlying ToM processes (also called the "mentalizing" network) extends bilaterally and across several lobes (Figure 3–2). Cognitive ToM is linked to several dorsal regions, including the dorsal anterior cingulate, dorsolateral and dorsomedial prefrontal cortices, and the superior temporal sulcus and temporoparietal junction. Frontal regions, including the inferior frontal gyri, orbitofrontal cortices, and ventromedial prefrontal cortex, have been linked to affective ToM (Bohrn et al., 2012; Dvash & Shamay-Tsoory, 2014; Hillis, 2014). RH structures have been suggested by some to be more involved in affective ToM, while cognitive ToM is mediated bilaterally by the frontal lobes, perhaps with a slight left hemisphere (LH) bias (Hillis, 2014; Shamay-Tsoory, Tomer, Goldsher, Berger, & Ahron-Peretz, 2004).

ToM After RHD

Investigations of pragmatic interpretation and the idea that impairments of ToM could be a consequence of RHD were first published around 1990 (Kaplan, Brownell, Jacobs, & Gardner, 1990; Weylman & Brownell, 1989). Brownell's group suggested that an inability to understand another person's thoughts and knowledge might underlie misinterpretations

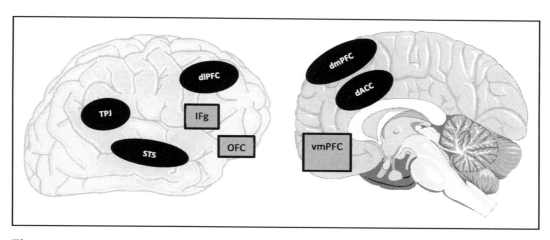

Figure 3–2. Regions involved in cognitive (*black ovals*) and affective (*gray rectangles*) theory of mind. *Notes.* dACC= dorsal anterior cingulate cortex; dlPFC= dorsolateral prefrontal cortex; dmPFC = dorsomedial prefrontal cortex; IFg = inferior frontal gyrus; OFC = orbitofrontal cortex; TPJ = temporoparietal junction; vmPFC = ventromedial prefrontal cortex. Theory of mind networks are bilateral, but are shown here only in the right hemisphere.

of intended meaning. Since then, only a handful of studies has focused specifically on RHD stroke survivors. Not surprisingly, the results are inconsistent and may be related to the cognitive demands of the tasks used.

Martín-Rodríguez and León-Carrión (2010) systematically evaluated a set of 26 studies of ToM in adults with acquired brain injury that encompassed over 600 participants. The vast majority of studies primarily included adults with traumatic brain injury (TBI). The results indicated that impairments were most often observed on tests of irony/sarcasm and faux pas, followed by second-order beliefs. Impairments of first-order beliefs were the least common. Studies with a greater proportion of participants with lesions in the frontal lobes or in the RH showed greater impairments on the irony/sarcasm and faux pas tasks. Given the nature of this systematic review, the authors were unable to determine the potential effects of executive function, empathy, or other deficits on performance. To better understand the specific contribution of the RH to ToM, and the possible ToM impairments related to RH stroke, a review of the studies specific to RHD is needed.

Happé, Brownell, and Winner (1999) conducted the first study of ToM after RHD. Three different tasks were employed, including cartoon interpretation, first- and second-order beliefs, and comparison of cartoon pairs. In half of the items there was a "nonmental" inference that relied on physical causality. In the other half there was a "mental" inference that tested ToM. Their results indicated that adults with RHD had a ToM deficit.

The problem was not with inferencing itself, as the participants were accurate on the causal inferencing questions. The results were replicated in a later study (Griffin et al., 2006).

Results from a study of ToM using shape animations (Weed, McGregor, Feldbaek Nielsen, Roepstorff, & Frith, 2010) are difficult to interpret. The authors suggested that the group with RHD evidenced a ToM deficit apparent in their descriptions. They described actions (e.g., "they just flew around on the screen") but were less likely to ascribe mental states (e.g., "the red tried to capture the blue one"; p. 71). The RHD group as a whole also was less accurate at discriminating between animations that depicted random movements versus those that appeared to show intention. However, there was substantial variability in performance across RHD participants, and raters had a fairly large proportion of disagreement in interpretation of the descriptions. Thus, it is difficult to determine whether the results actually reflect a ToM deficit related to RHD.

The ToM deficits observed after RHD may be related to the complexity of the stimuli. Surian and Seigal (2001) reported accurate responses to first-order false beliefs when visual aids were provided to lessen the demands on working memory. Additionally, Tompkins, Scharp, Fassbinder, Meigh, and Armstrong (2008) examined the stimuli used in Happé's study and found that the causal inference stories were less complex than the ToM stories. After revising the stimuli to be more equivalent in terms of length, lexical complexity, number of characters, and number of shifts in perspective, they found that adults with RHD performed similarly on the ToM and the causal inference stories.

Balaban and colleagues (2016a) constructed a set of tasks for assessing ToM that includes a variety of methods including questions about first- and second-order beliefs, level of empathy, faux pas identification and cartoon interpretation, among others. Out of their 25 participants with RHD, 8 performed within normal limits on nearly all tasks; the other 17 exhibited impaired performance on the majority of the tasks. This included poor performance (less than 70% accuracy compared with a group without brain injury) on both multiple-choice questions and open-ended explanations. There was no obvious difference between the subgroups on demographic (age, education) or clinical (location of lesion, presence of attentional or linguistic deficits, unilateral neglect) factors.

In a second study, the researchers examined the use of referential language in the adults with ToM impairments (Balaban, Friedmann, & Ziv, 2016b). The tasks involved situations in which there was the potential for ambiguity based on a listener's knowledge or the similarity between objects. For example, in a story that referenced multiple shopping bags, ambiguity could occur if a character was asked to pick up "the shopping bag" as opposed to "the blue shopping bag." Participants' responses were analyzed to identify whether they avoided ambiguity by using a full noun phrase or name instead of a pronoun, whether a relevant feature was selected to distinguish two similar characters, or whether they took into account the listener's knowledge in crafting their responses. The participants with ToM impairments consistently made errors on the majority of the referential language tasks. They failed to adjust their responses based on what the listener knew. The same participants had no difficulty on a range of complex syntactic tasks, indicating that the deficits were not with complex language processing, but rather seemed to be specific to ToM processing.

Several studies have been conducted to determine other processes that may impact ToM performance, such as executive function or other pragmatic abilities (e.g., empathy). No clear relationships have been observed. ToM is not strongly or consistently related to executive function (Champagne-Lavau & Joanette, 2009; Griffen et al., 2006; Martin & McDonald, 2006), attention, or unilateral neglect (Balaban et al., 2016a)

Limbic System: Affect and Emotion

Extensive research on emotion production and interpretation has resulted in the conclusion that there are six universal emotions (joy, sadness, fear, anger, surprise, disgust). These are represented in nearly all countries and cultures and are expressed through similar facial expressions and prosodic characteristics. Recognition of these emotions is cross-cultural, although easier within a shared culture or among people with similar languages (e.g., Latin-based languages; Elfenbein & Ambady, 2002; Pell, Monetta, Paulmann, & Kotz, 2009). Emotion can be expressed through a single modality, but in social interactions there are usually multiple cues. In verbal interactions, for example, both semantics and prosody are used to determine emotional content, and in many cases they can provide equivalent amounts of information (Pell, Jaywant, Monetta, & Kotz, 2011).

Affect and Emotion and the Intact RH

There are several theories that suggest that the two hemispheres have distinct roles in emotional processing (see summary in Table 3–4). According to the Right Hemisphere Hypothesis, the RH is dominant for all emotional processing. Early support for this hypothesis came from research that showed adults with RHD had defi-

cits in emotion comprehension compared with adults with LHD (Borod, 1993; Borod et al., 2000). Additional research findings contradict the predictions of the strong version of this hypothesis, as adults with LHD often have some deficits in emotional processing even if they perform better than adults with RHD (e.g., Braun, Traue, Frisch, Deighton, & Kessler, 2005; Kucharska-Pietura, Phillips, Gernand, & David, 2003; Pell, 2006; Schirmer, Alter, Kotz, & Friederichi, 2001; for a meta-analysis, see Witteman, van Ijzendoorn, van de Velde, van Heuven, & Schiller, 2011). Imaging studies of healthy adults consistently identify an extensive, bilateral network for emotional processing (Ethofer et al., 2012; Kotz et al., 2003; Rymarczyk & Grabowska, 2007; Wildgruber, Ethofer, Grandjean, & Kreifelts, 2009). A weaker

Table 3–4. Emotional Processing Hypotheses

Hypothesis	Explanation	Summary of Evidence
Right Hemisphere Hypothesis	RH dominant for all emotions. Strong version: all emotions are processed in the RH.	Strong version not supported.
	Weak version: emotional processing is bilateral, with greater RH contributions.	Weak version supported by a variety of studies.
Valence Hypothesis	RH dominant for negative emotions; LH dominant for positive emotions.	Some studies find the dissociation, but most do not.
Emotion Type Hypothesis	RH dominant for basic emotions (joy, fear, sadness, etc. LH dominant for cultural or learned emotions (pity, boredom, etc.)	Based on studies of normal aging; no evidence from imaging or patient studies.
Differential processing	RH holistic processing; LH feature-level processing.	Supported by at least two studies of affective facial expression.

version of the hypothesis, in which there is bilateral processing but greater activation in the RH compared with LH in most tasks, is consistent with current findings (e.g., Witteman et al., 2011).

Other hypotheses have been developed to explain the different roles of the RH and LH in emotional processing. The Valence Hypothesis suggests that positive and negative emotions are processed in different hemispheres: negative emotions in the RH and positive in the LH (Davidson, 1984). Some studies of neural activation support this hypothesis: in healthy adults the LH is more active during positive emotional processing and the RH is more active for negative emotions (e.g., Iredale, Rushby, McDonald, Dimoska-DeMarco, & Swift, 2013; see also a review by Demaree, Everhart, Youngstrom, & Harrison, 2005). Other research, however, has not replicated these patterns (Braun et al., 2005; Etofer et al., 2012). The Valence Hypothesis has been used as partial support for the notion that adults with RHD generally tend to be happy (because of the intact LH's processing positive emotions), while those with LHD are prone to develop depression. Research has failed to support this latter assumption: depression is not related to side of lesion in stroke survivors (Bour, Rasquin, Limburg, & Verhey, 2011).

According to the Emotion Type Hypothesis (Ross & Monnot, 2011), the RH is dominant for processing primary emotions (fear, sadness, happiness), while social or culturally learned emotions such as embarrassment, pity, pride, and boredom are processed in the LH. This hypothesis is based on changes that occur with normal aging and reported similarities among behaviors typical of RHD and normal aging that mimic patterns of impaired affective prosody recognition seen in RHD (Orbelo, Testa, & Ross, 2003). Carefully controlled studies of stroke survivors are needed to provide evidence for or against this hypothesis.

Finally, some results suggest general processing differences across the hemispheres. One hypothesis is that the RH is more adept at automatic, unconscious processing, while the LH has a greater role in conscious, controlled processing that extends to emotional processing (Gainotti, 2012). A second, more widely accepted account is that the RH processes stimuli holistically, while the LH conducts feature-level processing (Abbott, Wijerante, Hughes, Perre, & Lindell, 2014; Calvo & Beltrán, 2014; Thomas, Wignall, Loetscher, & Nicholls, 2014). According to this proposal, the LH is more accurate at determining emotion when only certain features or a partial stimulus is present (e.g., only eyes or the mouth is shown), whereas the RH is better at holistic (e.g., whole face) processing.

There are a variety of factors that likely contribute to the inconsistent results of emotional processing studies: the types of emotions, modality, stimulus characteristics, and task demands. In relation to the type(s) of emotions, some studies evaluate only a single positive (happy) and negative (sad) emotion. Others average responses to multiple emotions of different valences (happy and surprised versus sad, fearful, disgusted, and angry). The averaged responses may not be comparable to performance on a single emotion and thus make comparisons across studies difficult. Indeed, many researchers have examined individual emotions and found that not all positive emotions are processed similarly or even in the same location within the brain (Adolphs, Damasio, & Tranel, 2002; Charbonneau, Scherzer, Aspirot, & Cohen, 2003; Dara, Bang, Gottesman, & Hillis, 2014; Orbelo et al., 2003; Paulmann, Seifert, & Kotz, 2010; Ross & Monnot, 2008; Rymarczyk & Grabowska, 2007; Wildegruber et al., 2009). Finally, several studies report that overall responses to positive emotions are faster and more accurate, suggesting that they are somehow "easier" (Abbott et al., 2014; Kucharska-Pietura et al., 2003; Pell, 2005; but see Harciarek, Heilman, & Jodzio, 2006 and Iredale et al., 2013 for conflicting results). Given the differences in methods, it is difficult to combine all of the results and obtain a single conclusion about emotion processing.

A second factor is the modality. Facial expression and emotional prosody are most commonly studied. However, results from one modality may not be generalizable to the other. Several researchers have reported differences in performance on recognition or discrimination of emotional prosody compared with facial expressions (Charbonneau et al., 2003; Harciarek et al., 2006; Kucharska-Pietura et al., 2003).

Characteristics of the stimuli also may play a role. Citron, Gray, Critchley, Weekes, and Ferstl (2014) suggest that both the valence and the intensity of the stimuli affect processing. Specifically, intense or negative stimuli create a withdrawal tendency, while mild or positive stimuli create an approach tendency. Mixing these two, such as creating a mild negative or an intense positive, may result in different processing because of the inconsistency in the "signals" that the brain receives.

Finally, different tasks are used across studies. Comprehension of emotional processing is evaluated through discrimination, identification, and recognition tasks. It seems logical that determining whether two syllables are produced with the same emotional prosody would require different cognitive processes compared with hearing one syllable and identifying the emotion conveyed. Additionally, production is assessed through repetition or imitation, as well as cued and spontaneous production tasks. Careful attention to the type of task (e.g., repeat this sentence in the same tone of voice versus say this sentence in a sad tone of voice) is needed to fully understand the scope or pattern of emotional prosody production deficits that might occur after RHD.

A variety of RH regions have been implicated in emotional processing. Key among these are the inferior frontal gyrus, orbitofrontal cortex, frontal operculum, dorsolateral frontal areas, and the anterior insula (Paulmann et al., 2010; Schirmer & Kotz, 2006; Wildgruber et al., 2004). Subcortical areas also have been linked to emotional processing (Karow, Marquardt, & Levitt, 2013), specifically the basal ganglia and regions of the thalamus and amygdala (Paulmann, Pell, & Kotz, 2008). Paulmann and colleagues (2010) suggest that the early perceptual processing in which implicit and unconscious reactions to emotions are triggered occur subcortically. Conscious recognition and labeling of emotions occurs later in the process, in the orbitofrontal cortex.

Affect and Emotion After RHD

Clinically, adults with RHD can be hyper-affective, with exaggerated emotional responses, or hypoaffective, exhibiting little emotional response. In one study, hyper- and hypoaffective behaviors were reported to occur at approximately the same rate, each in about 40% of patients with RHD admitted to an inpatient rehabilitation unit (Blake, Duffy, Myers, & Tompkins, 2002).

A review of emotionality studies with stroke survivors (Borod, Bloom, Brickman, Nakhutina, & Curko, 2002) indicated that the majority of results supported a selective deficit in emotional processing in adults with RHD compared with LHD or no brain damage. The majority of studies focus on recognition or production of a specific subset of emotions, but these findings shed little light on emotional experiences. In a recent study of emotional experiences, participants were asked to indicate the presence and intensity of emotional responses (joy and sadness) to either an external stimulus (film clip) or an internal stimulus (personal story). The results indicated that adults with RHD exhibited the same pattern of emotional responses as did a control group: both had more intense emotional responses to their personal sto-

ries than to the film clips (Salas Riquelme, Radovic, Castro, & Turnbull, 2015).

The presence and awareness of emotional changes was examined by Visser-Keizer, Meyboom-deJong, Deelman, Berg, and Gerritsen (2002). They provided self-report questionnaires to stroke survivors (LHD and RHD) and their partners to assess the presence of a variety of emotional and cognitive deficits. The RHD group reported several changes in emotions, including hyperemotionality (reported by 55% of participants), feeling sad or depressed (31%), being more irritable (28%), and having increased anxiety (28%). Interestingly but not surprising was that the partners reported more, and more severe, deficits than the stroke survivors reported (Table 3–5). These findings suggest that the stroke survivors were aware of emotional changes, yet still underestimated the changes or the impact of the changes in their daily interactions.

As with most processes affected by RHD, emotional processing is not abolished. As described in other chapters, emotional stimuli can facilitate performance on memory and attention tasks, even in

Table 3–5. Reports of Emotional Changes by 36 RH Stroke Survivors and Their Partners

Emotional Changes	Percentages of Individuals Reporting Changes	
	RHD Participants	Partners
Hyperemotionality	50%	66%
Sad/depressed	31%	46%
More irritated	28%	61%
More anxious	28%	40%

Source: Based on Visser-Keizer et al., 2002.

the presence of unilateral neglect (e.g., Berrin-Wasserman, Winnick, & Borod, 2003; Grabowska et al., 2011; Grandjean, Sander, Lucas, Scherer, & Vuilleumier, 2008; Lucas & Vuilleumier, 2008).

Linguistic/Lexical Emotional Processing. One method of expressing emotion is through word choice. Having a bad day is different from having a "terrible, horrible, no-good, very bad" day (Viorst, 1972). Being angry is different from being infuriated. The expression of emotion through word choice/lexical selection may be affected in some adults after RHD. Across a variety of studies, the overall results suggest that they tend to use fewer emotional words and less expressive emotional words (e.g., angry versus infuriated; see review in Blake, 2003). Stories about emotional events are less concise, relevant, and specific compared with stories about nonemotional topics (Borod et al., 2000). Sherratt (2007) reported that, as a group, adults with RHD tended to provide more evaluations than actual emotions in stories about funny or frightening experiences. She did note, however, that there was extensive variability across the RHD participants, as well as across the participants without brain damage. The expression of emotion in experimental tasks may be affected by the presence of visuospatial, comprehension, or cognitive deficits or by co-occurring depression, none of which is carefully evaluated or controlled in most studies (Blake, 2003).

Interpretation of emotions conveyed semantically also can be affected (Borod, Andelman, Obler, Tweedy, & Welkowitz, 1992). In judging the intended meaning of statements (e.g., jokes versus sarcasm), adults with RHD were less likely to take into account descriptions of a speaker's mood than were control participants (Brownell, Carroll, Rehak, & Wingfield, 1992). In contrast, Tompkins (1991a, 1991b) reported that semantic cues increased RHD adults' ability to accurately interpret emotion conveyed either linguistically or through prosody. Difficulties arose when there were conflicting cues (e.g., the words did not match the prosody).

Facial Expression and Emotion. In studies of production of facial expression, adults with RHD are rated as using fewer, and less expressive, spontaneous facial expressions (see review in Borod et al., 2002). Additionally, they exhibit poorer performance on tasks requiring imitation or prompted responses (Charbonneau et al., 2003). Identification or discrimination of emotional facial expressions also can be affected (Borod et al., 2002; Harciarek et al., 2006; Nijboer & Jellema, 2013). Generally, deficits are observed for both positive and negative emotions. Several studies have examined discrimination of whole faces versus partial faces (e.g., only eyes or only a mouth; Abbott et al., 2014; Calvo & Beltrán, 2014; Thomas et al., 2014). Abbot and colleagues (2014) examined whether participants with RHD or LHD could accurately judge whether two faces showed the same emotion. Some photos showed only the mouth or eyes, while others included a whole face. Both groups had difficulty when only partial faces were shown, but only the RHD group was impaired on whole faces. The authors suggested that the RH is better at holistic processing, while the LH can process individual features.

Prosody and Emotion. RHD has been shown to affect both identification and production of emotional prosody (Borod et al., 2002; Charbonneau et al., 2003; Guranski & Podemski, 2015; Harciarek et al., 2006; Pell, 2006). Negative emotions are not consistently affected more than positive emotions, and there is heterogeneity among groups of adults with RHD in terms of prosodic deficits (e.g., Pell, 2006). Prosody will be considered in detail in Chapter 5.

Executive Control and Pragmatics

It seems logical that deficits in executive functions (EFs) would have obvious and direct effects on communication and pragmatics. However, most studies fail to show meaningful correlations between pragmatics and EF. For example, Martin and McDonald (2003, 2006) failed to find strong or consistent relationships between EF and ToM. Another report indicated that ToM was not related to executive flexibility (Griffin et al., 2006). Champagne-Lavau and Joanette (2009) also failed to find consistent patterns. Six of their 15 RHD participants had EF deficits (inhibition and flexibility) with no co-occurring problems with ToM or nonliteral language interpretations. Three other participants were impaired on nonliteral language and inhibition, and another five exhibited deficits on nonliteral tasks as well as flexibility. Treatment for ToM created no improvement in EF, and a restorative attention treatment showed no generalization to ToM (Brownell & Lundgren, 2015).

In one of the few studies to report relationships, Zimmerman, Gindri, deOliveira, and Fonseca (2011) compared executive and pragmatic deficits in two small groups of adults with TBI versus RH stroke. They found, not surprisingly, that the TBI group tended to have more, and more varied, impairments across pragmatic and EF abilities, while the RHD group had more focused impairments restricted primarily to conversational discourse and narrative comprehension. For all participants together, significant correlations were obtained between performance on a variety of pragmatic and EF tasks, with processing speed being related to multiple pragmatic abilities.

Other Pragmatic Aspects of Communication

There are several aspects of pragmatics that arise from a combination of the factors depicted in the model. Two will be discussed here. Empathy is a combination of ToM, social perception, and emotion. Humor involves all of those as well as other components of executive control, such as planning, judgment, and self-monitoring.

Empathy

Empathy is an extension of both emotion and ToM. It is the ability to "recognize, share in, and make inferences about another person's emotional state" (Hillis, 2014, p. 981). Empathy is important for prosocial behavior as well as predicting others' actions (Gonzalez-Liencres, Shamay-Tsoory, & Brüne, 2013).

While affective ToM involves beliefs about another person's emotions, sharing those emotions are part of empathy. Like ToM, empathy has both a cognitive and an affective component. Understanding someone else's emotions is part of cognitive empathy, while actually sharing in feeling someone else's emotion is affective empathy (Dvash & Shamay-Tsoory, 2014). For example, understanding that your sister is happy when she gets a new job is cognitive empathy; experiencing happiness yourself in response to her happiness is affective empathy. Affective empathy can further be subdivided into emotional contagion and perspective taking. Emotional contagion is a more basic process that develops early in childhood and involves recognizing and sharing emotions. Later, perspective taking develops, which allows one to make inferences about the other person's emotions.

Empathy and the Intact RH

Empathy is controlled by an extensive bilateral network. Core structures identified across imaging studies of healthy adults include the dorsal anterior cingulate and anterior medial cingulate, supplementary motor area, and insula (Fan, Duncan, DeGreck, & Northoff, 2011). The RH tends to be more active in affective empathy and the LH in cognitive empathy (Fan et al., 2011; Hillis, 2014).

Combining results from studies of healthy adults as well as lesion studies, the right inferior frontal cortex and orbitofrontal cortex appear to be critical for emotional contagion (Hillis, 2014). The right prefrontal region is involved in affective perspective-taking, along with other fron-

tal regions involved in cognitive processes such as attention, working memory, flexibility, and abstraction (Leigh et al., 2013). Several other areas are related to both emotional contagion and perspective taking, including the right anterior insula, anterior cingulate, amygdala, and temporal pole. The temporoparietal junction, bilaterally, is involved in "mentalizing" that likely contributes to empathy but also to other processes such as ToM. The other aspect of affective empathy, perspective-taking, appears to be frontally mediated (Hillis, 2014).

Empathy After RHD

Deficits in the various components of empathy—emotional contagion, perspective taking, and cognitive empathy—have been reported in adults with RHD (Hillis, 2014; Leigh et al., 2013; Yeh & Tsai, 2014). Empathy deficits can co-occur with impaired comprehension of emotional prosody, but the deficits also can be dissociated. For example, Leigh and colleagues (2013) reported that approximately half of their participants had deficits in prosodic comprehension but normal affective empathy.

Lesions within the network described above can result in deficits in empathy, including damage to the right anterior insula, temporal pole, and anterior thalamus (Leigh et al., 2013). Both RH and LH prefrontal lesions can cause deficits in empathy, but only RH parietal lesions cause such deficits (Shamay-Tsoory et al., 2005). Damage to white matter tracts that connect regions of the empathy network, particularly the right uncinate fasciculus, also can cause deficits in affective empathy (Oishi et al., 2015). As suggested by the cognitive/affective pattern of lateralization described above, RHD usually impacts affective empathy and LHD cognitive empathy, but the reverse also has been reported (Yeh & Tsai, 2014).

Few studies have investigated the impact of deficits of empathy on outcomes or quality of life. However, the limited data that are present are striking. Hillis and Tippett (2014) surveyed a small group ($N = 14$) of stroke survivors and their caregivers to examine the importance of a broad range of stroke-related deficits. Two years after the stroke, a reduction in empathy was identified by 50% of caregivers as very important; no other deficit was identified by 50% or more of caregivers. Only two (14%) of the stroke survivors identified empathy as very important. Given the form of the questions on the survey, it was not possible to determine whether the stroke survivors were not bothered by reduced empathy or were not aware of the deficit.

Humor

Humor is an important part of social interaction. Appropriate use and interpretation of humor relies on good ToM (to understand what the other person does and does not know), emotional processing (to want to share in positive emotions), and good language processing, particularly for puns or other forms of humor that rely on ambiguities or revision of interpretations.

Humor and the Intact RH

The RH has been suggested to play a role in verbal humor due to its coarse coding processing style (see following chapter on language comprehension) and its importance for ambiguity resolution. Joke processing generally is divided into two stages: recognition of an incongruity and reinterpretation for resolution of the incongruity. Regions of both hemispheres and the cerebellum are involved in interpretation of both linguistic and visual humor, including the superior and middle temporal gyri bilaterally, and the right inferior frontal gyrus (e.g., Bartolo, Benuzzi, Nocetti, Baraldi, & Nichelli, 2006; Wild, Rodden, Grodd, & Ruch, 2003).

Marinkovic et al. (2011) observed three phases of neural activation during joke comprehension. First there is activation within the LH, followed by bilateral prefrontal activation. These are thought to reflect initial semantic activation and then activation and evaluation of plausible interpretations. The third phase is selection of one interpretation and resolution which occurs bilaterally in frontotemporal regions. Coulson and Williams (2005) examined differential activation in the LH and RH during comprehension of jokes (statements with unexpected endings) and nonjokes (statements with expected endings). Activation of the LH in the joke version was much greater than the nonjoke condition, representing the incongruity of the unexpected ending. In the RH, however, activation was similar across joke and nonjoke conditions. The authors interpreted the findings to mean that the RH was able to accept an unexpected ending as coherent rather than incongruous, because it was able to consider multiple possible interpretations (similar to predictions of the coarse coding hypothesis; Beeman, 1998; see also Chapter 4).

Humor After RHD

Early reports of changes in humor appreciation after RHD suggested that these individuals were less able to appreciate nuanced, verbal humor, tended to display an atypical sense of humor, and were drawn to physical stunts, also known as "black" or "gallows" humor (LaPointe, 1991; Wapner, Hamby, & Gardner, 1981). Shammi and Stuss (1999) reported that deficits in humor appreciation were most often related to damage in the right frontal lobes compared with LHD and right parietal lesions.

Interpretation of humor after RHD has been directly examined in a small handful of studies (Brownell, Michelow, Powelson, & Gardner, 1983; Bihrle, Brownell, & Powelson, 1986; Cheang & Pell, 2006; Winner, Brownell, Happe, Blum, & Pincus, 1998). Comprehension typically is measured by presenting cartoons or jokes and asking participants to select a funny ending. In both verbal and visual formats, Brownell and colleagues (1983; Bihrle et al., 1986) found that, as a group, participants with RHD were less accurate at selecting a funny ending. The errors tended to be selection of a *non sequitur*, which provided a surprising but incoherent ending. The authors concluded that adults with RHD are sensitive to the key aspect of a joke—that it ends with a surprising conclusion—but were unable to select an ending that was both surprising and coherent with an alternate interpretation of the situation.

One important factor about these two studies (Brownell et al., 1983; Bihrle et al., 1986) was the working memory demands of the task: the stories were read aloud, after which the participants had to select one of five possible endings. The researchers included a second condition, in which the stories were not humorous, and the task was to select an appropriate ending. The RHD group performed poorly on both the joke and the story-completion conditions, suggesting that the deficit was perhaps not with joke interpretation itself. In order to control for the memory demands, Cheang and Pell (2006) adapted the stimuli used in the previous studies by providing both written and auditory presentations and reducing the number of possible endings from five to four. With these adaptations, only 4 of the 10 participants evidenced difficulty with interpreting humor.

Winner and colleagues (1998) examined joke comprehension from the perspective of ToM. Jokes, they asserted, require second-order true beliefs: they are based on situations in which the speaker (joke-teller) knows what the other person knows. In contrast, lies require second-order false beliefs, in which the speaker does not know that the other person knows a specific piece of information (Table 3–6). The complex results were interpreted to indicate that while adults with RHD have difficulty with second-order beliefs in general, they are better at interpreting the true beliefs (jokes) than the false beliefs (lies).

Both generation and response to humor were examined in a naturalistic study conducted by Heath and Blonder (2003, 2005). They videorecorded conversations between participants and their spouses. Participant groups included 11 adults with RHD, 10 adults with LHD, and 7 individu-

Table 3–6. True and False Second-Order Beliefs

	Second-Order Belief	Interpretation
Paul and June were getting ready to host the bridge club at their house. June was arranging cookies and fruit on a tray. She asked Paul to take the tray to the living room but not to eat any cookies. Paul picked up the tray and once he was in the other room, he popped a cookie into his mouth.		
ENDING #1		
As he chewed, he saw that June had followed him into the living room and watched him take the cookie. "AHA! I knew I couldn't trust you not to eat a cookie!" June said. "No," said Paul. "I didn't eat a cookie. It was a grape."	TRUE: Paul knows that June knows he ate a cookie.	JOKE—Paul realizes he's been caught, so makes a joke of the situation.
ENDING #2		
As he chewed, he didn't see June follow him into the living room and watch him take the cookie. "AHA! I knew I couldn't trust you not to eat a cookie!" June said. "No," said Paul. "I didn't eat a cookie. It was a grape."	FALSE: Paul does not know that June knows he ate a cookie.	LIE—Paul doesn't realize he's been caught, so he lies about eating the cookie.

als who had recently been hospitalized for orthopedic problems. The video recordings were then analyzed by two college students who had been trained to identify humor events. The raters identified the events as well as the responses to the events. There were no group differences in either the number of humor attempts or the responses to those attempts. The only observable difference was in disagreements between the raters. For the RHD group, there were more events for which only one of the two raters thought there was an attempt at humor. One can only guess at the reason for this, but it could be that the RHD stroke survivors had more unsuccessful attempts at humor.

Heath and Blonder (2003, 2005) also asked participants and their spouses to complete a scale of humor use and appreciation. Stroke survivors, based on self-responses and ratings of their spouses, evidenced a decline in the use and appreciation of humor following their stroke. When interpreted in combination with the conversational rating results, these findings suggest that changes in humor can be subtle enough that they are not necessarily recognized by naïve raters but are noticed by survivors and their families.

Discourse Production and Conversational Exchange

The output of social communication processes discussed above includes language production and conversational exchange. Production involves language processes such as the selection of words, syntactic structures, and the organization of ideas. In a communication exchange, it also includes consideration of the setting and the conversation partner(s), as well as the use of nonverbal cues. The production deficits associated with RHD often are subtle and nuanced. One may come away from a conversation with an adult with RHD with a sense that it was awkward or somehow not quite right without a clear sense of exactly what it was that was "abnormal." In some cases the topic, the word choice, the give and take, or the flow of the conversation may have been subtly affected, but none really standing out as clearly impaired. In contrast, in other cases the production may clearly be outside the realm of "normal." The discussion below will begin with linguistics and then continue into aspects of conversational exchange.

Aspects of discourse production can be divided into two general areas: microlinguistics and macrolinguistics. Microlinguistic components include syntax, phonology, lexical semantics, and morphology. These processes are controlled primarily by the left hemisphere, and usually are not affected by RHD, with the exception of mild semantic deficits that will be discussed later. Macrolinguistics include content and structure beyond the word and sentence level, and are more likely to be impaired after RHD.

Aspects of macrolinguistics include the following:

- Cohesion refers to connectors that tie together pieces of information within or across sentences. Cohesive ties include referents and their antecedents, pronouns, and conjunctions.

- Coherence is the connectedness of semantics and pragmatics and is judged by whether or not all the sentences in a paragraph fit the same topic. The presence of tangential statements decreases coherence (see sidebar).
  - ☐ Global coherence refers to a story as a whole.
  - ☐ Local coherence refers to ideas conveyed in adjacent sentences.

- Structure refers to the logical relationships between people and events. If the person is relating a story, the critical elements (beginning, middle, and end) and episode structure (initiating event, action, and consequence) should be present.

- Content includes the main ideas and essential concepts. It can be assessed in terms of number or accuracy of ideas or concepts.

- Appropriateness can be measured in terms of topic, word choice, and style or tone. All are dependent on the communicative situation and partner. For example, topics and styles appropriate for conversing with one's family often may not be appropriate for formal interactions with a person of a higher social status.

SIDEBAR

The following is an example of local but not global coherence, in which each sentence is related to the previous one but together they do not all fit a single topic.

Kristy went grocery shopping on Thursday morning. She saw that the grocery carts were strewn around the front entrance. The carts had been blown around by a major windstorm. The wind speed had exceeded 50 miles an hour. The severity of the storm made it the worst weather event in the past 25 years in the small town. The town was known for its beautiful weather and mild climate. Summer was the most profitable time in the town for the tourism industry. The easy access to boating and water activities as well as the tradition of good food were a huge draw.

■ Productivity and efficiency refer to the amount of discourse or content provided. They can be measured in units of time, such as words per minute or correct information units (CIUs) per minute.

Production in the Intact RH

The RH traditionally has been thought to have a minimal role in speech and language production. Such a role has been examined in only a handful of studies. In cortical stimulation studies of patients undergoing cortical resections for epilepsy, Andy and Bhatnagar (1984) reported some language production abilities in the RH. Electrical stimulation to specific areas of the RH was applied during a variety of language tasks: picture naming, phrase completion, and answering simple questions (e.g., what do we drive?). In the three patients tested, errors and omissions were elicited during cortical stimulation of temporal and parietal regions of the RH. The authors concluded that the RH has some latent language production abilities.

More recently, RH activation in frontal and temporal lobes has been observed during language generation tasks, such as thinking of verbs related to a target noun or thinking of words to complete a sentence (Kircher, Brammer, Andreu, Williams, & McGuire, 2001; Price, 1998). Such activation could be related to contextual processing and generation of multiple meanings (see discussion of these processes later in this chapter). In other studies, RH activation during production tasks (e.g., verbal fluency) has been linked to decision making and attentional processes (van Ettinger-Veenstra et al., 2010) rather than to language production.

Discourse Production After RHD

Following RHD, discourse or narrative production can be affected in terms of both quantity and quality. Some individuals develop paucity of speech, in which responses are short and unelaborated and may be incomplete. Others exhibit verbosity, with long, sometimes tangential or disorganized responses that may or may not be relevant for the communicative context (Blake, Duffy, Myers, & Tompkins, 2002; Trupe & Hillis, 1985).

The stereotypical description of an adult with RHD includes disruptions of any number of the macrostructural components. Many studies have been conducted to identify core deficits or patterns. However, no consistent deficits or clear patterns have been identified. One problem is the wide variety of variables measured. Over 34 different aspects of discourse production encompassing both micro- and macrolinguistic features have been reported across 24 studies. A second problem is that different elicitation tasks have different cognitive demands and levels of naturalness that may affect performance. Conversation is arguably the most natural form of discourse, but it includes pragmatic components such as turn-taking and establishing a common frame of reference that are not relevant for tasks such as picture description or procedural discourse. Storytelling involves a memory component that increases cognitive demand while providing organizational structure that does not have to be generated by the client.

Ferré, Fonseca, Ska, and Joanette (2012) have suggested that impaired conversation is a key component of RHD communication deficits. In a series of cross-linguistic studies, they report that of the four clinical profiles that arise from the Montreal Evaluation of Communication (Ferreres et al., 2007; Fonseca et al., 2007; Joanette, Ska, & Côté, 2004), disordered

conversation is present in three of them (the fourth includes patients without substantial communication deficits) (Ferré et al., 2012). Conversation is evaluated on a broad-based, 17-item checklist. While summary scores from such a checklist are useful for broadly identifying disordered language production, they do not provide information about *how* conversation is affected.

A compilation of results from several other studies of conversation fail to identify areas that are consistently problematic after RHD (Brady, Mackenzie, & Armstrong, 2003; Hird & Kirsner, 2003; Kennedy, 2000; Mackenzie, Begg, Brady, & Lees, 1997; Mackenzie, Begg, Lees, & Brady, 1999). Across these studies, groups of adults with RHD were no different from adults without brain damage in terms of discourse production variables such as number of words, amount of information conveyed, organization, and topic maintenance. Mixed results were found for main topic structuring and referencing. Differences in pragmatic and paralinguistic aspects of conversation, such as turn-taking and eye contact, will be discussed below.

Cohesion and coherence specifically were assessed in several studies of storytelling (Marini et al., 2005; Sherrat & Bryan, 2012). In these studies, participants generated a story based on a series of six pictures. When the pictures were arranged for the participants, no deficits in coherence or cohesion were noted. However, when participants had to first arrange the six pictures and then generate a story, both coherence and cohesion were affected. The authors did not differentiate between local and global coherence, but other studies have suggested that global coherence is more cognitively demanding than local coherence (Rogalski et al., 2010).

Discourse structure, story grammar, and organization have been examined in studies of structured conversations, storytelling, and picture description. Only one study (Hird & Kirsner, 2003) identified deficits in participants with RHD. In all of the others, the structure or organization was comparable to that of adults without brain injury (Brady et al., 2003; Brady, Armstrong, & Mackenzie, 2005; Mackenzie et al., 1997, 1999; Sherratt & Bryan, 2012).

Deficits in accuracy and scope of content have been reported in studies employing storytelling and picture description (Bartels-Tobin & Hinckley, 2005; Cherney, Drimmer, & Halper, 1997; Mackenzie et al., 1997, 1999; Marini et al., 2005). The problems include fewer main ideas, deficient content or thematic units, and fewer inferential or interpretive concepts. The inferential complexity of the picture stimuli has been shown to impact the adequacy of production (Myers & Brookshire, 1994).

Content can also be judged by the inclusion of irrelevant or inappropriate information. Tangential information, overpersonalization, and value judgments have been reported in RHD studies. Blake (2006) reported rather large effects of tangentiality and overpersonalization in a thinking out loud task in which participants talked about a story as they read it, commenting on what was happening and making predictions about outcomes. Individual variation in tangentiality was reported in a story retelling task (Cherney et al., 1997) and in picture description (Mackenzie et al., 1999). In contrast, no excessive tangentiality or overpersonalization was reported in personal narratives, story retelling, or procedural discourse (Mackisack, Myers, & Duffy, 1987; Sherratt & Bryan, 2012; Tompkins et al., 1992).

Reports of changes in productivity are quite variable. During conversation and procedural discourse, productivity seems to generally be within normal limits (Brady et al., 2005; Sherratt & Bryan, 2012). The results from picture description and storytelling tasks are quite variable, both across studies and across participants (Bartels-Tobin & Hinckley, 2005; Cherney et al., 1997; Marini et al., 2005; Sherratt & Bryan, 2012; Tompkins et al., 1992).

Appropriateness of style, tone, or word choice has been evaluated primarily in relation to the use of emotional words (see Blake, 2003 for a review). As a whole, adults with RHD are less likely than adults without brain injury to use emotional words when describing pictures, telling a story from picture sequences, and describing personal experiences (Bloom, Borod, Obler, & Gerstman, 1992; Bloom, Borod, Obler, & Koff, 1990; Borod, Koff, Lorch, & Nicholas, 1985; Borod et al., 1996; Borod et al., 2000; Cimino, Verfallie, Bowers, & Heilman, 1991).

Production of inferential versus literal concepts has been examined in relation to the Cookie Theft picture description task (Table 3–7). Myers (1979) reported that adults with RHD produced fewer interpretive concepts than adults with LHD or without brain injury. Tompkins and colleagues (1992) failed to replicate this result. Differences in the presence and severity of neglect and visuospatial processing deficits across the studies may have contributed to the conflicting results.

Table 3–7. Literal and Interpretive Concepts From the Cookie Theft (Interpretive concepts are italicized)

Two	Little	*Mother*	*In the kitchen (indoors)*
Children	Girl	Woman (lady)	*General statement about disaster*
Little	*Sister*	Children behind her	Lawn
Brother	Standing	Standing	Sidewalk
Standing	By boy	By sink	House next door
On stool	Reaching up	*Washing (doing)*	Open window
Wobbling (off balance)	*Asking for cookie*	Dishes	Curtains
3-legged	Has finger to mouth	Drying	
Falling over	*Saying shhh (keeping him quiet)*	Faucet on	
On the floor	*Trying to help (not trying to help)*	*Full blast*	
Hurt himself	*Laughing*	*Ignoring (daydreaming)*	
Reaching up		Water	
Taking (stealing)		Overflowing	
Cookies		Onto floor	
For himself		*Feet getting wet*	
For his sister		Dirty dishes left	
From the jar		Puddle	
On the high shelf			
In the cupboard			
With the open door			
Handing to sister			

Source: Republished with permission of ASHA, from Yorkston, K. M., & Beukelman, D. R. (1980). An analysis of connected speech samples of aphasic and normal speakers. *Journal of Speech and Hearing Disorders, 45,* 27–36. Permission conveyed through Copyright Clearance Center, Inc.

A recent study of acute stroke patients indicate that measures such as the number of content units, the number of content units from the left versus right side of the picture, and percent of interpretive concepts were related to the size of the lesion but not side of lesion (Agis et al., 2016).

Difficulties with nonliteral or figurative language are commonly reported after RHD. Nearly all of the literature on nonliteral language focuses on comprehension (which is covered extensively in Chapter 4). Van Lancker-Sidtis and Postman (2006) examined the use of formulaic language in conversational speech produced by 15 adults: 5 each with RHD, LHD, or no brain injury. Their definition of formulaic language included familiar idioms, conventionalized phrases (e.g., "as a matter of fact"), conversational speech formulas (e.g. "first of all . . . "), pause fillers, and sentence stems (e.g., "I guess") among others. Their results indicated that about 25% of words produced by adults without brain damage were part of formulaic phrases, while for the RHD group the proportion was only 17%. Group comparisons conducted on the combined average of idioms, conventional expressions, and conversational speech indicated no significant differences between the non–brain damaged and RHD groups. Future studies with larger numbers of participants are needed before valid generalizations about nonliteral language production after RHD can be made, including whether changes in the use of figurative language have a meaningful impact on the client's activity or participation.

Conversational Exchange After RHD. Just as with findings related to discourse production, a compilation of results from studies of conversation fails to reveal areas that are consistently problematic after RHD (Brady et al., 2003; Hird & Kirsner, 2002; Kennedy, 2000; Mackenzie et al., 1997; 1999). Across these studies, groups of adults with RHD were no different from groups without brain damage in terms of number of words, amount of speaker time, amount of information conveyed, organization, initiation, turn-taking, topic maintenance, or presupposition. Mixed results were found for main topic structuring and referencing, and difficulties with termination of conversation were reported in one study (Kennedy, 2000). The deficits that were observed in multiple studies were related to use of nonverbal cues such as intonation, facial expression, and eye contact (Mackenzie et al., 1997, 1999, 2007).

Chantraine and colleagues (Chantraine, Joanette, & Ska, 1998) used a referential barrier task to assess exchange of information. Participants had to describe abstract tangram shapes to someone who could

---

SIDEBAR

A highly educated man with RHD expressed frustration with conversations. He often wanted to contribute to conversations, but had difficulty identifying the natural gaps or pauses in which he could speak. As a result, he frequently would interrupt or join in at inappropriate times. The problem was not with understanding the "rules" of conversation, but with identification and timing.

Another highly educated man with RHD was quite aware of some of his deficits in conversation. He knew that he tended to interrupt—sometimes with unrelated or tangential thoughts, and other times with questions related to the task. His strategy was to ask for feedback ("tell me if I'm asking too many questions") or tell his communication partner to let him know if he was interrupting too much. This strategy did provide the communication partner with liberty to stop him; however, he tended to overuse it, repeatedly asking if he was interrupting too much. The frequent requests for feedback often were more distracting than the initial interruptions.

not see them. Some of the adults with RHD produced conversational exchanges that were rated "better" than the control participants, while others tended to use irrelevant or ambiguous references. Still others had idiosyncratic communication behaviors that decreased the efficiency or effectiveness of their communication. Yet, across the seven RHD participants there were no consistent problems with cooperation or the use of self-corrections, interruptions, clarification questions, or digressions from the goal.

Clinically, the heterogeneity of conversational competence can be striking. Some clients may have no difficulties, some may be aware that they have deficits but are not able to anticipate or avoid them, and some may be unaware of their inappropriate conversational behaviors.

Assessment

Assessment of pragmatics is complex and difficult for several reasons. First is the broad range of what is accepted as "normal" social interaction. Second is the influence of cultural differences in socially acceptable or normative interaction. Third is the problem in objectively assessing social interactions in a way that preserves the spontaneity, naturalness, and complexity of interactions while providing a structure in which assessment can be objective and replicable. A final concern is the need for family input. As was demonstrated in Heath and Blonder's (2003) study of humor, family input is critical for identifying aspects of pragmatics that have changed, even if the change is not striking enough to be obvious to outsid-

ers. The value of the contribution of family input needs to be empirically studied.

The time course or evolution of pragmatic deficits is unknown. It is possible that some pragmatic deficits may not be observed or recognized early in recovery. For example, changes in empathy may not be noted acutely, when self-absorption or focus on the self at the expense of others may be accepted as a part of the response to a traumatic event. By the time the stroke survivor is discharged home and resumes a more normal activity pattern, families may have exhausted funding for rehabilitation.

There are several broad measures of pragmatics developed for adults with TBI (Table 3–8). These include rating scales (e.g., Pragmatic Protocol [Prutting & Kirchner, 1987]; Profile of Pragmatic Communication Impairment [Linscott, Knight, & Godfrey, 1996]) and structured questionnaires (LaTrobe Communication Questionnaire [Douglas, O'Flaherty, & Snow, 2000]). As discussed in Chapter 2, the use of environmental assessments (Brush et al., 2012) and conversational skills (Togher et al., 2010) may add important insights into the pragmatic deficits and the positive and negative influences of specific settings or partner behaviors.

The following discussion will cover just a few specific pragmatic deficits: ToM, empathy, discourse production, and conversation. Assessment of other cognitive areas is covered in other chapters (e.g., attention in Chapter 6; executive function in Chapter 8).

Assessment of Theory of Mind

For the assessment of ToM, there are a variety of stimuli and tasks that have

Table 3–8. Select Assessment Measures of Pragmatics

Test	Authors	Scope of Test	Reliability*	Validity*
Behaviorally Referenced Rating System of Intermediate Social Skills (BRISS)	Wallander et al., 1985	Verbal (e.g., conversation content, style, speech characteristics). Nonverbal (eye contact, body language)	Good	Good
Communication Performance Scale	Ehrlich & Barry, 1989	Conversational interaction behaviors (e.g., eye contact, initiation, coherence, intelligibility)	OK	Weak
LaTrobe Communication Questionnaire	Douglas et al., 2000, 2007	Perceived communication ability in relation to quantity, quality, relation, and manner	Good	OK
Pragmatic Protocol	Prutting & Kirchner, 1987	Linguistic, paralinguistic, and nonverbal communication	Weak	None
Profile of Pragmatic Impairment in Communication (PPIC)**	Linscott et al., 1996; Hays et al., 2004	Conversational interactions; content, style, organization, etc.	Good	Good
Social Communication Skills Questionnaire	McGann et al., 1997	Conversation, including expressing and responding to opinions	None	None

Notes. **Formerly known as the Profile of Functional Impairment in Communication (PFIC).

*Good = moderate–strong estimates of two or more types of reliability/validity; OK = moderate–strong estimates of one type of reliability/validity or mix of weak and strong estimates; weak = weak estimates of one or more types of reliability/validity; none = no estimates reported. See Appendix for detailed information about reliability and validity.

been used in the literature. Balaban and colleagues (2016a) recently constructed a battery for assessing ToM. It includes tasks to assess a variety of components of ToM, including first- and second-order beliefs, empathy, and cartoon interpretation. Although details about the reliability and validity are needed, the initial results appear promising. With this and other measures of ToM, stimulus complexity is an important factor. Tompkins et al. (2008) caution that the standard, complex verbal materials used for ToM assessments may prevent the differentiation of problems in

ToM from deficits in executive functions (abstraction/mental flexibility), working memory, and/or language comprehension. Balaban et al. (2016b), in response, suggest that ToM is a complex process and that using complex stimuli is the only way to assess it.

Assessment of Empathy

Empathy can be assessed with the Interpersonal Reactivity Index (IRI; Davis, 1980a, b). It is a 25-question self-report measure. It has reasonable validity (Davis, 1983), but reliability has not been reported. The IRI contains four subscales that address different components of empathy: Perspective Taking ("the tendency to adopt the psychological point of view of others" [Davis, 1980a, p. 1]), Fantasy (understanding or feeling emotions of characters in books or movies), Empathic Concern (feelings of concern or sympathy for others), and Personal Distress (personal anxiety in interpersonal interactions). Hillis (2014) cautions that using a self-report measure can be problematic for adults with RHD who may have deficits of self-awareness (see Chapter 9).

Assessment of Discourse Production

Assessment of discourse production should include evaluation of performance on a variety of tasks, genres, communication situations, and partners. It should also include discussions with family members or others who know the patient well to identify what aspects of communication have changed from pre-stroke behaviors.

Speech-language pathologists (SLPs) are adept at evaluating communication and identifying communicative behaviors that are not solidly within the range of "normal." However, this may result in over-diagnosis in which SLPs identify aspects of communication as impaired while family members report that those same behaviors were present prior to the stroke (Baron, Goldsmith, & Beatty, 1999). Most judgments of discourse production deficits are subjective, and may be based on one or two characteristics that an individual clinician feels are indicative of RHD (Tompkins et al., 1992). Clinicians must be aware of their internal biases in judging "normalcy" of conversation or discourse production. Some may be rather generous in their conception of what is "normal" for older adults, and judge productions of adults with RHD to be within normal limits, while others have a more strict sense of what is "normal" and classify adults without brain damage as having discourse production deficits (Blake, 2006). These biases may not be directly related to clinical experience or knowledge of RHD communication disorders. This is another reason that it is very important to talk to families who can provide insight into whether or not a client's language production differs from pre-stroke behaviors.

Assessment of production generally involves obtaining and evaluating language samples to analyze efficiency and accuracy. Such samples can be elicited through a variety of methods. The most common include picture description, generating or retelling narratives, procedural discourse (e.g., how to make a sandwich or change a lightbulb), and conversation.

Discourse analysis can be used to evaluate both micro- and macrolinguistics

(Coelho et al., 2005). For adults with RHD, the focus should be on the macrolinguistics, but it is also important to determine whether there are deficits in basic language functions that are present (either a co-occurring aphasia or other microlinguistic deficit). Discourse analysis requires obtaining a language sample of about 200 words and then systematically examining the structure and content (coherence, cohesion, organization, etc.). Comparison of performance on a variety of tasks and genres can illuminate deficits that may be associated with other cognitive processes. For example, a patient may have no difficulty with a picture description, because the stimulus is present throughout the task to provide a visual structure for the language production. The same patient may have more difficulty retelling a story in which memory is a key component and there is no visual cue to aid in organization of ideas. Discourse analyses can be time-consuming and may not be practical in most clinical settings.

The review of the literature illustrates that there are no clear patterns of performance or core discourse characteristic(s) that occur after RHD. Additionally, clinicians are not necessarily accurate in classification of discourse production from adults with and without stroke. Thus, a critical piece of the assessment is to talk to the families and identify what changes have occurred since the stroke and what characteristics are premorbid.

Alternative Methods for Obtaining and Analyzing Language Samples

The absence of a clear deficit or pattern of deficits in the discourse production of adults with RHD may be in part a reflection of the tasks. Deficits were more often observed on complex tasks, such as story arrangement and retelling, than on simple retelling or picture description (Marini et al., 2005; Sherratt & Bryan, 2012). The use of complex elicitation tasks may be needed to draw out the subtle deficits associated with RHD. A task such as the New York Trip (Fleming & Harris, 2008; Harris, Kiran, Marquardt, & Fleming, 2008), in which clients have to describe the plans for a trip, including dates, budgets, and scheduled activities, may be more sensitive to mild language production deficits. This task has been shown to be sensitive to changes related to normal aging and mild cognitive impairment even in the presence of normal performance on the Mini Mental State Examination (Folstein, Folstein, & McHugh, 1975) and the Boston Naming Test (Kaplan, Goodglass, & Weintraub, 2001). While some differences were found on linguistic variables such as the proportion of pronouns or mazed words, the number of core thematic concepts included in the narrative was a strong discriminating factor. The need for imagination, abstract thinking, planning, and problem solving increases the cognitive demands which may in turn affect language production and lead to the identification of mild impairments that are not apparent on more simplistic production tasks.

The methods used for analyzing discourse also may contribute to the lack of differences between adults with and without RHD. Most studies use quantitative assessments such as the number of deviations of specific macrolinguistic features. It may be that no one feature is consistently affected but that combinations of features may interact. Lê, Coelho, Mozeiko, and Grafman (2011) examined storytelling by adults with TBI by rating both the completeness and the organization. Neither feature on its own consistently separated the participants with TBI from those without brain injury. When the two features were combined into a measure of "story goodness," a fairly clear distinction was apparent. Those with TBI tended to produce stories that were both less complete and more poorly organized. It may be that the discourse analyses typically used in RHD research parse the material too selectively and miss the forest for the trees.

Assessment of Conversational Exchange

Barnes and Armstrong (2010) suggest that particularly for conversation, quantitative analysis (e.g., discourse analysis) on its own may be misleading, and a corresponding qualitative analysis is critical for evaluating the discourse within a communicative context. The familiarity and roles of conversational partners can have a substantial effect on the form of conversation. Interactions with a new acquaintance should differ from those with a family member. Interactions in which the client is in a "patient" role interacting with a doctor or clinician should differ from an interaction with peers. Short, factual responses may be appropriate in the patient–doctor situation but not necessarily in a familial interaction. Another factor to consider in conversations is the role of the communication partner, and what she is bringing to the interaction. A partner may be able to provide a link for a comment that may at first appear to be tangential or off-topic,

thus making it relevant to the conversation. Or she may acknowledge it as off-topic and steer the conversation back. A careful analysis of the interactional context is necessary to appropriately classify each partner's contributions.

Findings by Jorgensen and Togher (2009) support the potential positive effects of communication partners on narrative production by adults with TBI. When the participants told a story about a picture sequence, impairments in cohesion, story grammar, productivity, informational content, and exchange structure were evident. In a second task, the same participants watched a video clip with a friend and jointly related the story. In this joint storytelling condition, the performance of adults with TBI was on par with a control group. Thus, the structure added by a familiar partner facilitated their storytelling ability.

The impact of partners on communicative competency can be considered through the lens of distributed cognition. Distributed cognition is a theoretical framework for understanding higher-level cognitive processes such as language (Duff, Mutlu, Byom, & Turkstra, 2012). It is based on the conception that these processes are not specific to an individual but are distributed (a) across people in a social interaction, (b) across internal and external environments, and (c) across time. Thus, language is not only what a client produces, but is affected by the responses of the communication partners, the interaction of cognitive states and processes (e.g., memory, world knowledge, emotional state), and the events that transpire throughout the time course of the task. Duff and colleagues (Duff, Hengst, Tranel, & Cohen, 2008; Duff et al., 2012) have demonstrated the phenomenon of distributed cognition across social interactions in their studies of adults with amnesia. In a barrier task in which partners must describe how to organize tangram pictures, adults with amnesia are less likely than those without to use specific referents. However, the partners of adults with amnesia also are less likely to use such referents (Duff et al., 2008). Thus, the partners in social interactions both were affected by, and affected, the communication of the person with amnesia.

Examination of communicative interactions using the distributed cognition framework illuminates communication strengths and weaknesses that are not apparent in quantitative analyses. For example, Turkstra, Brehm, and Montgomery (2006) analyzed the communication behaviors of two adults with TBI. During the semi-structured interactions, both made eye contact with their partner about 50% of the time. However, the patterns differed dramatically. One individual used eye contact to signal turn-taking and to relinquish the floor to the other person. The other individual had a relatively random pattern of eye contact. Thus, although the quantitative data suggested that the two individuals were similar, the functional use of eye contact was vastly different and resulted in different perceptions of communicative competency.

As suggested above, to obtain a more complete picture of communicative effectiveness at the participation level, evaluation and analysis of conversation should include not only the client's production, but also the role of the communication partner and the environment to identify how those factors affect the client's language (Barnes & Armstrong, 2010; Duff et al., 2012; Jorgensen & Togher, 2009). It is also important to assess different communicative contexts. Different aspects of conversation (e.g., turn-taking, collaborative sharing) may occur in interactions with familiar partners or peers, while other skills (e.g., asking questions) might be facilitated by interactions with a clinician (Togher, Taylor, Aird, & Grant, 2006). Finally, it is important to remember that discourse and conversation are not static processes, but evolve and change within an interaction (Turkstra et al., 2006). Identifying patterns of performance may be more informative than simply counting behaviors.

Discourse and conversational analyses can be time-consuming and may not be practical in most clinical settings. Thus, many evaluations are based on conversation or stories elicited during a broader evaluation, with subjective judgments of whether or not, as a whole, the client's language production seems "normal" or not. Several checklists (see Table 3–8) are available for assessing discourse and conversation to provide some structure to the diagnostic process. They are useful primarily as guides for what aspects of production might be affected by stroke or other brain injury, as they generally do not have good interrater reliability without extensive practice.

Treatment for Pragmatic Disorders

Only one study directly addresses treatment of pragmatics specifically for adults with RHD. Lundgren and Brownell (2010) describe a treatment for ToM in which participants are led through scenarios in which they must identify different characters' knowledge and beliefs, compare knowledge and beliefs across characters (e.g., what beliefs are the same and what beliefs differ), and inhibit their own beliefs to predict or explain the actions of the characters. Limited data from one participant with RHD are available. Additional data from two individuals with TBI (Brownell & Lundgren, 2015) suggest that both participants were able to complete the treatment protocol and improve interpretation of cartoons that required understanding of first- and second-order beliefs. Generalization of treatment gains to functional communication was not assessed.

Language production has not been a focus of treatment for adults with RHD. One pilot study was conducted for an adult with TBI with damage restricted primarily to the right hemisphere (Cannizzaro & Coelho, 2002). The story grammar treatment was unsuccessful at improving the quality of story production. The focus of TBI treatment research has been on social communication among adolescents/adults with moderate to severe brain injury (Helffenstein & Wechsler, 1982; Togher, Power, Rietdijk, McDonald, & Tate, 2012).

There is evidence to support social communication treatment for adults with TBI. In a randomized control trial, Dahlberg and colleagues (2007) reported the effectiveness of a 12-week group treatment program. The program targeted pragmatics, behaviors, and the cognitive skills underlying them. Areas addressed included communicating needs and thoughts; listening, using, and interpreting nonverbal communication; regulat-

ing emotions; respecting social boundaries and rules; working with others; and being assertive. Key components of the treatment program included: (a) leaders representing two clinical professions (SLP and social work) to provide different perspectives, feedback, and role models; (b) an emphasis on self-awareness, self-assessment, and goal setting; (c) a group setting to facilitate interaction, feedback, social support, and problem solving; and (d) a focus on generalization through involvement of family or significant others, homework, and community activities.

The treatment resulted in positive effects on nearly all subtests of the Profile of Functional Impairment in Communication (PFIC; Linscott, Knight, & Godfrey, 1996), with gains maintained up to six months following treatment. The treatment program is manualized, and thus can be replicated. The success of the program was replicated in a later study (Braden et al., 2010) that included participants more typical of the general population of adults with TBI who had concomitant psychiatric, substance abuse, or additional neurological conditions (e.g., stroke, multiple sclerosis).

Another treatment with promising results is Cognitive Pragmatic Treatment (Gabbatore et al., 2014). Also a group treatment, it covers awareness and use of linguistic, paralinguistic, and extralinguistic communication modes, conversation, ToM, and planning activities.

It is important that the efficacy and effectiveness of pragmatic treatment programs are assessed in adults with RHD. While the pragmatic deficits associated with TBI and RHD appear similar on the surface, there are substantial differences in the ages of the typical survivor of stroke versus TBI, and different social and vocational outcome goals. Additionally, the severity of brain injury and the number of concomitant deficits likely differ across these populations. Despite these cautions, the treatment research for TBI provides guidance for developing and implementing treatment for adults with pragmatic deficits resulting from RHD.

Conclusions and Implications

The impact of pragmatic deficits on functional outcomes is not well studied, but there are strong suggestions that there can be important consequences. A deficit in empathy, as mentioned above, is an important concern for caregivers (Hillis & Tippett, 2014), and marital satisfaction is weakly related to facial affect discrimination (Blonder, Pettigrew, & Kryscio, 2012). More broadly, social participation may be related to emotional processing (as measured by facial expression and prosody recognition; Cooper et al., 2014).

Pragmatic deficits have been reported to be at the core of RHD, yet there are no identifiable patterns of deficits. Part of the problem may be that no two people are affected in exactly the same way. There may be various interactions between intact and impaired components within the broad model of social communication resulting in heterogeneous presentations. Positive results have been obtained from group treatments that broadly address a variety of pragmatic deficits in adults with TBI. These approaches should be useful for adults with RHD who exhibit many of the same problems.

4

Language Comprehension

The label "nondominant" or "minor hemisphere" was ascribed to the right hemisphere (RH) based on its apparent lack of language processing abilities compared with the language-rich left hemisphere (LH). The RH appears to have little syntactic or phonological processing abilities; however, it is important for semantic and pragmatic processing, particularly when multiple meanings or interpretations are possible. This includes interpreting meaning within a specific context.

This chapter will begin with a model of comprehension and descriptions of the semantic processes within the intact RH. The two most studied hypotheses of RH semantic processing, the coarse coding and suppression deficit hypotheses, will be covered along with the predictions they make about language comprehension deficits associated with RH brain damage (RHD). Related aspects of language processing, including inferencing, using context, and interpreting nonliteral language, will then be described. Assessment and treatment of the deficits will be discussed in relation to the theories and suspected underlying impairments.

A Model of Language Comprehension

There are a variety of comprehension processes attributed to the intact RH and comprehension deficits that have been linked to RHD. These include inefficiencies of word-, sentence-, and discourse-level semantic processes (e.g., coarse coding, suppression) as well as broader sentence- and discourse-level difficulties such as generating inferences, resolving competing interpretations, interpreting nonliteral language, understanding the gist of a text, and using contextual cues. Knowledge of intact RH language processing and deficits associated with RHD will be described for four forms of comprehension processes: semantic activation, inferencing, use of context, and nonliteral language.

To understand the underlying deficits and inefficiencies in language processes associated with RHD, a brief review of normal comprehension processes is needed. There are a variety of models of normal comprehension processing, but most share features with, or are elaborations upon, the construction-integration model proposed by Kintsch (1988). As the name suggests, comprehension proceeds in two repeating phases: construction and integration. During the construction phase, multiple meanings and features of words are activated. In the integration phase, words are integrated into the surrounding context; meanings or features that become contextually irrelevant are inhibited or suppressed while activation is enhanced for those that are relevant (Gernsbacher, 1990, 1996). The process is depicted in Figure 4–1. Upon hearing the word "spring," the three meanings are activated: a metal coil, a small stream of water, and the season. If the word occurs in a context, such as "he went fishing in the spring," the "coil" meaning of the word is suppressed, because it is not relevant for the context. The other two meanings are both still plausible: the person could be fishing in the stream or in the springtime. If new context is provided, such as "it was the first warm day of the season," then the "stream" meaning becomes less plausible and would be suppressed.

Semantic Processes

Semantic Processing in the Intact RH

There is extensive research on the semantic processing abilities of the RH. The evidence suggests that both the LH and RH have independent semantic networks, but the organization and function differ across hemispheres. The following discus-

sion will begin with a review of the organization and activation of the RH network related to the construction phase of comprehension. These characteristics are summarized in the coarse coding hypothesis, which in turn is used to predict deficits associated with RHD. Suppression processes, which occur during the integration phase of comprehension, also will be described.

Semantic Networks and Activation

Conclusions from a variety of studies and methodologies (e.g., divided visual field, neuroimaging, event-related potential [ERP]) indicate that the RH and LH both process semantic information independently, albeit in different ways (Collins, 1999; Kahlaoui, Scherer, & Joanette, 2008; Kiefer, Weisbrod, Kern, Maier, & Spitzer, 1998; Koivisto, 1998; Lovseth & Atchley, 2010; Reilly, Machado, & Blumstein, 2015; Turner & Kellogg, 2016; Yochim, Kender, Abeare, Gustafson, & Whitman, 2005).

The RH appears to activate larger, broader semantic networks. This means that the LH strongly activates dominant meanings or common features of words. In contrast, activation within the RH network occurs more slowly and results in a broader activation that includes not only the dominant meanings and common features, but also subordinate and more distantly related features. Thus, subordinate or less-common word meanings (e.g., "bug" as a type of listening device) are more likely to be activated in the RH than the LH. Similarly, atypical category members, such as "penguin" as a type of bird, are more likely to be activated in the

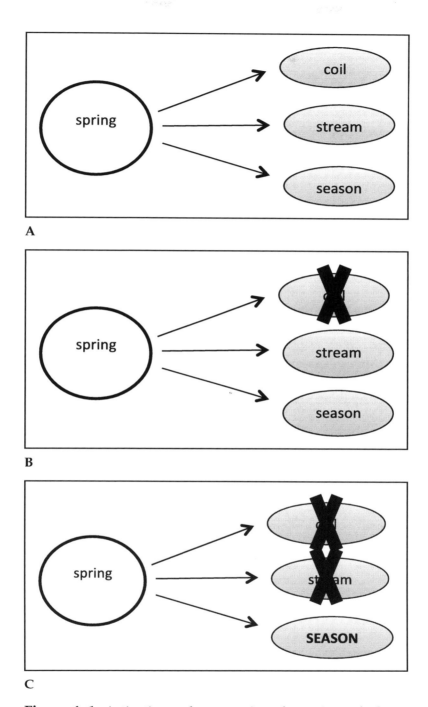

Figure 4–1. Activation and suppression of meanings of a homonym. **A.** "SPRING" **B.** "He went fishing in the spring." **C.** "It was the first warm day of the season."

RH than the LH (Passeri, Capotosto, & Di Matteo, 2015). The organization of the networks also appears to differ across hemispheres. Results from priming studies suggest that the RH responds more efficiently to semantically associated words (e.g., bed and sheet) than to categorically related words (e.g., bed and couch) (Bouaffre & Faita-Ainseba, 2007). The major characteristics of hemispheric processing are captured in Beeman's (1998) fine/coarse coding hypothesis described below.

Peleg and Eviatar (2017) suggest that orthographic-semantic connections exist in both the LH and RH, but orthographic-phonological connections are found only in the LH. Thus, the RH cannot sound out words, but can recognize the meaning of words. This hypothesis may explain why the RH is faster and more accurate than the LH at recognizing irregular word forms (Dickson & Federmeier, 2014) and interpreting text-message–like word abbreviations (e.g., SOCR for SOCCER) embedded in context (Head, Neumann, Helton, & Shears, 2013).

Vigneau and colleagues (2011) conducted a meta-analysis of imaging studies that reported RH activation during language tasks. Results suggested that several areas of the RH were involved in language processing. The pars opercularis and triangularis, Broca's area homologs, were active in interpretation of syntactic and semantic plausibility, along with the anterior insula. Regions within the temporal lobe were involved with sentence and text comprehension. Other reports suggest that the RH semantic network includes the inferior parietal lobule as part of a prefrontal-temporal-parietal network (Donnelly, Allendorfer, & Szaflarski, 2011)

and that both medial and dorsolateral prefrontal regions contribute to semantic processing (McDonald et al., 2005).

Coarse Coding

Beeman (1993, 1998) proposed the fine/coarse coding model of hemispheric processing based on the characteristics of semantic networks described above. The LH, he asserted, uses "fine coding," by which it activates the dominant or most frequent or familiar meanings/features of a word and quickly selects the most appropriate. The RH, in contrast, uses "coarse coding." Activation includes a wide range of potential meanings and features, including distantly related features (such as "rotten" as a feature of apples). The activation is broader and is maintained for a longer period of time, allowing for overlap between meanings and features (Table 4–1). Coarse coding can be considered part of the construction phase of comprehension in which multiple meanings are activated. A variety of findings have been interpreted within the coarse coding framework, including generation of nonliteral language, generation of inferences, and some forms of semantic priming.

Suppression

Suppression refers to the inhibition of meanings or features that become contextually less relevant in the integration phase (Gernsbacher, 1990, 1996). Reduced activation of these features or meanings allows the most related or relevant meanings to be selected for integration into the sentence. Suppression thus is a compo-

Table 4–1. Fine and Coarse Coding

	Left Hemisphere/fine coding (activation of small group of closely related or dominant features/ meanings)	*Right Hemisphere/coarse coding* (broad activation of many features/ meanings, both closely and distantly related)
Shirt	Clothing, sleeves	Clothing, sleeves, buttons, collar, fabric, wrinkled
Apple	Fruit, crunchy, red	Fruit, crunchy, red, green, tree, pie, rotten

nent of the integration phase. As will be discussed below, adults with RHD have been reported to have inefficiencies in suppression (Tompkins, Baumgaertner, Lehman, & Fassbinder, 2000; Tompkins, Lehman-Blake, Baumgaertner, & Fassbinder, 2001). This does not mean that suppression is specifically an RH function, but that the RH contributions to suppression can be affected after RHD.

Semantic Processing After RHD

Deficits in semantic processing after RHD are most commonly described in terms of the coarse coding and suppression hypotheses. RHD can result in deficits in both coarse coding and suppression, thus affecting both the construction and integration phases of comprehension (Tompkins et al., 2000, 2001; Tompkins, Fassbinder, Scharp, & Meigh, 2008). As part of the coarse coding hypothesis, Beeman (1993, 1998) proposed that adults with RHD were less able to activate multiple meanings or more distantly related features of words, and this deficit was the underlying source of the reported

RHD deficits in inferencing. If distantly related features of words such as barefoot (walk, tender, cut), glass (sharp, cut), and cry (pain, cut) overlap, then the inference "cut" can be generated from a story about a man walking barefoot on the beach, who did not see broken glass, then cried out in pain.

A rigorous test of the RH coarse coding hypothesis suggested that the coarse coding deficits are restricted to particularly distantly related features (Tompkins et al., 2004, 2008; Tompkins, Scharp, Meigh, & Fassbinder, 2008). Activation of features that are more closely related was not affected after RHD. For example, given the word SHIRT, the features "sleeves," "collar," and "buttons" would be activated in most adults with RHD because they are either core or closely related features. However, the feature "wrinkled" is more distantly related, and thus may not be activated as quickly by those with a coarse coding deficit.

One reason why coarse coding deficits are important is that they can be related to narrative comprehension (Tompkins et al., 2004; Tompkins, Fassbinder, et al., 2008; Tompkins, Scharp, et al., 2008). During comprehension, if distantly related features are important for understanding a context (e.g., the woman was late leaving for work because she had to iron her wrinkled shirt), then inefficient activation of such features will slow down the comprehension process (Table 4–2). This may be particularly problematic for auditory comprehension (versus reading) when the listener cannot stop the flow of information in order to fully process intended meanings.

Tompkins and colleagues (1999, 2000, 2001, 2004) conducted a series of studies on suppression. They found that adults with RHD were slower to suppress the meanings of ambiguous words (lexical ambiguities), even when those words were presented in biasing contexts (Tompkins et al., 2000). For example, they were slower to indicate that "oars" was not related to the sentence, "He sat in the front row" compared with the sentence, "He sat in the front seat." Importantly, they were accurate; thus, they could suppress the inappropriate meaning, but the suppression process was inefficient.

Suppression was also inefficient for inferential ambiguities: sentences that could be interpreted in more than one way. In these studies, Tompkins et al. (2001, 2004) created two-sentence contexts in which the first sentence could have more than one meaning. For example, in the sentence, "Lila began running in the park," Lila could either be exercising or escaping. A second sentence, "The snarling dog

Table 4–2. Examples of How Coarse Coding and Suppression Affect Comprehension

Coarse coding	Violet grabbed a shirt from her closet. She grumbled as she took it off the hanger. She looked at the clock and plugged in the iron. As she smoothed out the wrinkles, she realized she was going to be late for work again.	If "wrinkled"—a distantly related feature of SHIRT—is activated in the first sentence, then comprehension of the later sentences about ironing will be facilitated.
Suppression: Lexical ambiguity	He sat in the front row—oars He sat in the front seat—oars	Relatedness judgment (i.e., is "oars" related to the sentence?) is slower to the sentence ending in "row" than "seat."
Inferential ambiguity	Rosanne asked Christopher to trim carefully in the back. She wanted her yard to look perfect.	Initial activation of "hairdresser" and "gardener" occurs after the first sentence. Rapid, efficient suppression of the contextually inappropriate meanings will lead to better comprehension of the text as a whole.

had frightened her," disambiguated the meaning. In this example, after hearing both sentences, adults with RHD were slower to indicate that "exercise" was not related to the meaning of the context when compared with an unambiguous context such as: "Abbie ran screaming down the alley. The snarling dog had frightened her." Just as with the lexical ambiguities, the responses by adults with RHD were accurate but slow compared with adults without brain damage. Results from all of these studies indicated that inefficient suppression is related to narrative comprehension; a slight slowing in this process affects general comprehension.

Further work by Tompkins and colleagues (Tompkins, Blake, Wambaugh, & Meigh, 2011; Tompkins, Scharp, Meigh, Blake, & Wambaugh, 2012) established that coarse coding and suppression deficits can co-occur. Because the coarse coding deficits tend to affect activation of distantly related features or meanings, clients with such deficits still can activate multiple core features or closely related meanings. If a co-occurring suppression deficit is present, there is inefficient suppression of those features/meanings that are contextually inappropriate. Treatment for coarse coding and suppression deficits will be discussed below.

Inferencing and Use of Context

Inferencing and Use of Context in the Intact RH

As suggested above, the different processing styles of the two hemispheres contribute to the comprehension process. This is true also for interpreting meaning within context. Federmeier (2007) proposed the Production Affects Reception in Left Only, or PARLO, model (see also Federmeier & Kutas, 1999, 2002 and Kandhadai & Federmeier, 2008) to explain how the hemispheres use context. She suggested that the LH engages in predictive processing, with preactivation of words or meanings that are most likely to occur. This includes dominant meanings of ambiguous words or the most likely sentence ending given a strongly predictive context (e.g., The day was breezy so the boy went outside to fly a KITE). In contrast, the RH engages a "wait and see" integrative approach, in which each new word or piece of information is compared with the growing context with no preconceived predictions or expectations. As a result, the RH is more adept at accepting unexpected yet plausible words (e.g., The day was breezy so the boy went outside to fly a DRONE) and integrating subordinate meanings. Similarly, the RH is important for learning novel word meanings from context (Borovsky, Kutas, & Elman, 2013).

Additional insight into the typical functions of the LH and RH during language comprehension can be found in other imaging studies of adults without brain damage. Several researchers have suggested that the RH has an important role in "integrating semantic information into the context as a whole" (Bookheimer, 2002, p. 178; see also Coulson, Federmeier, Van Petten, & Kutas, 2005; Giora, Zaidel, Soroker, Batori, & Kasher, 2000; Menenti, Petersson, Scheeringa, & Hagoort, 2008). The intact RH appears to be more influenced by sentence-level contexts than the LH, particularly strongly biasing sentence contexts (Coulson et al., 2005; Goldthourp & Coney, 2009a, 2009b; Long & Baynes, 2002). During reading comprehension, activation in the RH occurs at the sentence level and is even greater at the discourse level, in which broader coherence and inferencing processes are required (Xu, Kemeny, Park, Frattali, & Braun, 2005). The greatest RH activation occurs during the story resolution and conclusion. There are two possible explanations for this pattern. One is that activation in the RH is delayed or is slower to "ramp up," resulting in full activation only near the end of a text. The other explanation is that the RH activation facilitates integration of the textual information and generation of overall meaning. The latter explanation fits well with the deficits ascribed to RHD in terms of integrating contextual cues, drawing inferences, and interpreting the main idea or gist of a passage.

The RH's role in interpreting meaning based on context has also been examined using stimuli in which there is a contradiction between the text and world knowledge (Hald, Steenbeek-Planting, & Hagoort, 2007; Menenti et al., 2008). In these studies, the key is the interpretation of a sentence that appears to be anomalous, such as "with lights on you can see less at night." In isolation, this statement would be false. However, when embedded in a context that describes an astronomer trying to see the night sky, it is true—you do see fewer stars at night when there are lights on. In the study, activation of the LH and RH was measured for sentences in isolation as well as embedded in context. In both hemispheres, activation indicated that the contradiction was noted. Once the sentence was embedded into the context,

only the LH continued to respond to the anomaly. This result suggests that the RH used the surrounding context to interpret the target sentence and no longer identified it as being anomalous.

The intact RH has been reported to be important for detecting other conflicts or contradictions, such as semantic illusions (Ericson & Mattson, 1981). This occurs when one key, but de-emphasized, component of a question is erroneous. The phenomenon is often called "the Moses effect," stemming from the stimulus question, "How many of each kind of animal did Moses put on the ark?" The answer is none, because in the biblical story, it was Noah who put animals on the ark, not Moses. However, since the focus of the question is the number of animals, many people do not notice that the name of the person is incorrect. Detection of such subtle contradictions or conflicts has been ascribed to the RH (Raposo, 2013).

Inferencing and Use of Context After RHD

Inferencing is the process of drawing conclusions based on known information or cues. We generate inferences to fill in gaps where information is not explicitly provided. Seeing a woman holding the hand of a child, we may infer that the woman is the child's mother. Noticing that a coworker arrives late to work and overhearing him say that there was an accident on the freeway, we may infer that he was stuck in the traffic jam caused by the accident.

Difficulties with inferencing have been part of the RHD stereotype since the late

1970s. However, we now know that only *some* adults with RHD have difficulty with *some* types of inferencing processes. In language contexts, there are various types of inferences that require different amounts of time and cognitive processing to generate (see Table 4–3 for examples). On the continuum of inferences, the two bookends are *bridging* and *elaborative* inferences. Bridging inferences, also called local inferences, are necessary to link adjacent sentences or ideas together. Such inferences are routinely generated very quickly by adult comprehenders and require few if any additional cognitive resources (McKoon & Ratcliff, 1990; Singer, 1994; van den Broek, 1994).

Elaborative inferences are on the other end of the continuum. They are not necessary for comprehension, and they require

more time and cognitive resources to be generated. They are not routinely generated by comprehenders. The likelihood of generating an elaborative inference depends in part on the strength of the contextual cues that suggest the inference (Calvo & Castillo, 1996; Fincher-Keifer, 1996; Garrod, O'Brien, Morris, & Rayner, 1990). There are several types of elaborative inferences. Predictive inferences are those that involve predictions about what will happen next. If a correct predictive inference is generated (e.g., inferring that Jennifer will sweep the floors after hearing that she took out a broom and dustpan), then subsequent sentences that confirm that prediction will be comprehended faster than if the inference had not been generated. Tool inferences are those in which comprehenders infer that a specific

Table 4–3. Types of Inferences

Bridging/local inferences: Link adjacent sentences or ideas. Typically necessary for comprehension and generated quickly or automatically by most comprehenders.		
Bridging inference	*Julie and Nathan went to the grocery store. The cashier cooed over him.*	The cashier works at the grocery store.
Causal inference	*Gavin poured water onto the flames. All that was left was smoking wood.*	The water extinguished the fire.
Elaborative inferences: Elaborate upon or enhance the meaning of text. Not necessary for comprehension, but if accurately generated, might facilitate comprehension of subsequent information. Generation requires additional cognitive resources; likelihood of generating elaborative inferences depends in part on the strength of the contextual cues.		
World knowledge inference	*Julie and Nathan went to the grocery store. The cashier cooed over him.*	Julie is Nathan's mother. Nathan is a baby. Julie is finished shopping.
Predictive inference	*Jen took the broom and dustpan out of the closet.*	Jen will sweep the floor.
Tool inference	*Chuck pounded the nail into the wall.*	Chuck used a hammer.

tool was used to complete a task. Hearing the sentence, "Chuck pounded the nail into the wall," most comprehenders infer that Chuck used a hammer. As with predictive inferences, a correctly generated tool inference will facilitate comprehension of subsequent material that involves the tool.

Many studies from the 1980s and 1990s suggested that RHD resulted in deficits in inference generation (Brownell, Potter, Bihrle, & Gardner, 1986; Moya, Benowitz, Levine, & Finklestein, 1986; Myers & Brookshire, 1994; Wapner, Hamby, & Gardner). However, few of these studies defined the type(s) of inferences tested, and may have included combinations of bridging and elaborative inferences (Lehman & Tompkins, 2000). Further research found that adults with RHD can generate bridging inferences (Brownell et al., 1986; Lehman-Blake & Tompkins, 2001; Tompkins, Bloise, Timko, & Baumgaertner, 1994; Tompkins, Fassbinder, Lehman-Blake, Baumgaertner, & Jarayam, 2004; Tompkins et al., 2001). Thus, the basic inferences needed to link adjacent sentences that are quickly and reliably generated by most comprehenders are also generated by most adults with RHD. Difficulties arise with elaborative inferences. However, it is not an all-or-none deficit. If there are strong contextual cues that suggest a specific predictive inference, then most adults with RHD can still generate them similar to adults without brain damage (Blake, 2009a, 2009b; Blake & Lesniewicz, 2005; Lehman & Tompkins, 2000).

Inferencing requires integration of contextual cues, and questions about the ability to use context to determine meaning have been infused throughout the RHD literature since the 1980s. Frequently it

was used as a conclusion: they cannot make inferences, so it must be because they do not use context. Myers (1991) suggested that a deficit in the ability to interpret and integrate cues within a context, termed "inference failure," might be at the core of RHD cognitive-communication disorders. According to this hypothesis, inference failures could be the source of problems with the ability to interpret a degraded figure using visuospatial cues, to use pictorial contextual cues to reinterpret an item in a picture that initially did not make sense, or to understand the intended meaning of a joke, sarcastic comment, idiom, or metaphor. Unfortunately, the inference failure hypothesis was never empirically tested. Additionally, the name suggested that inferences were not generated, although evidence on which the hypothesis was developed clearly indicated that inferencing occurred but was not always complete or accurate.

There is some research designed to systematically and incrementally identify whether adults with RHD can use contextual cues. Leonard, Waters, and Caplan (1997a, 1997b) explored whether adults with RHD could use semantic cues during comprehension. In one study, they used a word monitoring task, in which participants had to push a button as soon as they heard a target word (in this example, store). The word was then embedded into either a semantically appropriate sentence such as: "They were relieved to find that a store was near" or a sentence that was semantically anomalous such as, "They were impressed to feel that a store was gradual." The group with RHD exhibited the same pattern as a control group in that they were faster to respond in semantically plausible sentences than in nonsense sentences. This indicated that the adults with RHD were processing the semantics of the sentence and thus were able to predict the location of the target word in the plausible sentences.

Several other studies have convincingly demonstrated that adults with RHD can use semantic cues and world knowledge to determine the referent for ambiguous pronouns (Leonard et al., 1997a, 1997b). Examples are provided in Table 4–4. Brownell, Carroll, Rehak, and Wingfield (1992) also reported that adults with RHD use pronouns as links to determine the intent of statements within conversational vignettes and that they tend to use this relatively preserved linguistic skill to aid in interpretation.

Blake and colleagues (Blake, 2009a, 2009b; Blake & Lesniewicz, 2005; Lehman-Blake & Tompkins, 2001) examined use of contextual cues in the generation of predictive inferences. Results from a series of studies suggested that adults with RHD can generate predictive inferences when strong contextual cues are present that all support a single prediction. For example, reading, "Steven put his rod in the car and drove to the lake," they infer that he is going fishing. These inferences are also maintained over time until they are confirmed or disconfirmed in the story. However, problems arise when there are multiple cues that must be integrated to select a single, most plausible prediction.

When there are multiple, strong contextual cues that all suggest the same predictive inference or outcome, adults without brain damage tend to quickly generate and select a single most plausible inference. When the cues are not as strongly biasing

Table 4–4. Use of Semantic Cues to Assign Ambiguous Pronouns*

Use of Semantic Cues and Syntactic Preferences		*RHD Results*
Max lost to Ben because he was a *poor player*.	With the verb phrase "lost to," the syntactic preference is to link the pronoun to the subject (Max).	Accurately link "he" to Max
Max lost to Ben because he was a *great player*.	The semantics (great player) suggest that "he" refers to the object (Ben) despite the syntactic preference.	Accurately link "he" to Ben
Use of Semantic Cues and World Knowledge		*RHD Results*
Aiden performed at the theater while Bobby went to the office. He *performed Shakespeare*.	World knowledge suggests "he" refers to Aiden.	Accurately link "he" to Aiden
Aiden performed at the theater while Bobby went to the office. He *brought along a briefcase*.	World knowledge suggests "he" refers to Bobby.	Accurately link "he" to Bobby

Note. *Examples based on Leonard et al. (1997a, 1997b).

and more than one outcome is plausible, they generate multiple outcomes. Most adults with RHD also can generate multiple predictive inferences suggested by contextual cues (Blake & Lesniewicz, 2005). However, as a group they seem to be less able to use the cues to determine the most likely outcome. In stories with multiple contextual cues that suggest one most plausible outcome, adults with RHD generate that inference, but also generate additional possible outcomes.

Deficits also have been found in inference revision, in which comprehenders must revise an initial interpretation in light of new information (Brownell et al., 1986; Tompkins et al., 2001). Hearing the sentence, "Barbara became bored with the history book," most people infer that Barbara is reading the book. If the following sentence, though, is, "She had already spent five years writing it," then the initial inference must be revised based on the new information and the listener concludes that Barbara was an aspiring author who was bored of writing her book. As with other language processes, adults with RHD can revise their initial inferences, but they are not as quick or efficient as adults without brain damage (Tompkins et al., 2001).

To summarize the work on inferencing and context, adults with RHD generally do not have difficulties with basic, bridging inferences. They can use strong contextual cues to generate some elaborative inferences. Difficulties or inefficiencies arise when initial interpretations must be revised based on new information or when there are multiple cues that must be integrated to generate or select the most plausible interpretation. It is unclear whether these inferencing inefficiencies are related to general comprehension. These deficits associated with RHD are consistent with the intact RH's role in contextual integration and interpretation.

Nonliteral Language

Nonliteral language is just that: words or phrases that convey meaning that is not the literal meaning. They are extensively used in everyday life to make communication more interesting, humorous, or poetic. Indirect requests, metaphors, idioms, and sarcasm/irony are the most commonly studied forms in the RHD literature.

Indirect requests such as "can you hand me a pencil?" or "the dog looks hungry" can be used to make a request that is polite or less direct. In the former case of an indirect request that centers on a single word, such as "can" versus "would," the literal interpretation is "are you able to," whereas the intended meaning is "would you."

Sometimes indirect requests are used to hint that something should be done. These can be used to avoid directly asking or to be more polite. In these cases, the indirect request could be interpreted either as a statement or as a request based on the surrounding communicative context. For example, saying, "The dog is hungry" in the morning while the dog is standing near his food bowl could be an indirect request for someone to feed the dog. However, the same statement while the dog is wolfing down his food would be an observation about the dog. World knowledge about when the dog eats and visual cues regarding the dog's behavior would help disambiguate the meaning of the statement.

Metaphors typically take the form of comparisons in which two disparate items are equated to highlight a feature of one of them (e.g., pigeons are flying rats; "art washes away from the soul the dust of everyday life"—Picasso). Some metaphors are single words that have both a literal and a figurative meaning (e.g., warm can refer to temperature [literal] or a caring individual [metaphoric]). Within the category of metaphors are many subtypes that vary by familiarity, imageability, semantic similarity of the comparators, and the appropriateness of the comparison (e.g., Marschark, Katz, & Paivio, 1983).

Idioms are phrases for which the intended meaning is not directly linked to the words in the phrase. They often are culturally and geographically specific. Just as with metaphors, there are a variety of types of idioms, classified across three different dimensions: literality, decomposability, and transparency (e.g., Titone & Connine, 1994; see Table 4–5 for examples). Familiarity is a crucial aspect of idiom interpretation. Familiar idioms generally are processed and comprehended quickly and easily. Interpretation of unfamiliar idioms is affected by the type of idiom and the presence and extent of supportive context.

Literal idioms, also known as ambiguous idioms, are those that have both a literal and an idiomatic meaning. *There's more than one way to skin a cat*, meaning that there's more than one solution to a problem, has a literal interpretation—that there are multiple methods of removing the fur from a feline. Nonliteral idioms, such as *she's on cloud nine*, do not have a rational or logical literal meaning, given that there are no numbered clouds upon which people can perch.

Decomposability refers to whether or not the meaning of an idiom can be determined (at least partially) by the words in the phrase. *There's more than one way to*

Table 4–5. Types of Idioms

	Literality (a plausible literal interpretation)	*Decomposability* (meaning can be partially derived from words in the phrase)	*Transparency* (figurative meaning can be partially derived from semantic relationships)
There's more than one way to skin a cat: there's another way to achieve the goal	Yes (can actually skin a cat)	Yes ("more than one way" to do something)	No
He kicked the bucket: he died suddenly	Yes (physically kicking)	No	No
She's on cloud nine: she's elated	No	No	Yes (on a cloud ~ elevated ~ elated)

skin a cat is a decomposable idiom because "more than one way" is the key to the idiomatic meaning. The idiom *to kick the bucket*, meaning to die suddenly, is nondecomposable. There is no way to parse or interpret the words in that phrase that would lead to the idiomatic meaning.

The third factor is transparency. This refers to whether or not the meaning of the idiom can be derived (at least partially) from semantic cues. The idiom *to saw logs*, meaning to snore, is transparent because of the similarity between the sound of sawing and the sound of snoring. *She's on cloud nine* also is transparent, because the image of someone up in the clouds can be likened to someone who is elated.

These factors influence how easy it may be to determine the meaning of an unfamiliar idiom. Unfamiliar idioms that are transparent or decomposable are easier to interpret, because decomposing language and determining meaning based on semantics and syntax are basic linguistic processes. Literal idioms are more difficult than nonliteral ones, because there is more than one possible interpretation. Comprehenders must consider the surrounding context to determine whether the literal meaning is plausible, and if not, then to seek a nonliteral meaning.

A final factor important for interpretation of unfamiliar idioms is the presence of context. Novel decomposable or transparent idioms presented in isolation (without any context) might be correctly interpreted. For example, people not familiar with the German idiom *he understands only the train station* may be able to deduce that it refers to someone who has difficulty with comprehending complex ideas, or who seems to think on a rather

basic level. This interpretation is based on one's knowledge of train stations and that the trains follow a schedule, can only come in or depart from one of two directions, etc. In contrast, the Italian idiom *to attach a button* is opaque and nondecomposable. It is highly unlikely that without any supporting context, one would come up with the actual meaning, which is to talk too much. Without any context, the literal interpretation of sewing on a button is plausible. When such idioms are presented in isolation, comprehenders use decomposition and transparency to guess at a meaning. For this particular idiom, comprehenders suggested meanings such as: to make a simple fix to something, to sew something up, or put something together (Blake & Freeland, 2014).

Sarcasm or irony is a form of language in which the literal meaning is the opposite of the intended meaning. The intended (opposite) meaning can be inferred through the recognition of the direct contradiction. Saying "the weather is perfect for our picnic today" might be intended as sarcasm if it is pouring rain outside, indicating an obvious contradiction between the reality and the statement. The tone of voice or the prosodic characteristics used to emphasize components of the statement also signal that the intended meaning is not literal (Shamay-Tsoory, Tomer, & Aharon-Peretz, 2005; Sperber & Wilson, 1981).

There are several factors that make processing sarcasm distinct from metaphors and idioms. First is the consistency within the categories of language forms. Idioms are a closed set of items that have been established within a language or culture. Metaphors are a larger set, but typically take the form of a comparison. Thus, both of these forms have distinctive features that make them recognizable. Sarcastic remarks, on the other hand, can be created spontaneously for a specific communicative exchange and can take a variety of forms; thus, they are an open set and the form is unpredictable. Second, the nonliteral meaning of metaphors and some idioms can be derived from the words in the phrases. In contrast, with sarcasm the intended meaning is the opposite of the literal meaning. Comprehenders may have to recognize the inconsistency between the context and the literal meaning and then revise their interpretation. As mentioned above in relation to inferencing, revising interpretations can be affected by RHD. Finally, in verbal communication sarcasm is typically signaled by prosody. Individuals with receptive aprosodia (see Chapter 5) may have difficulty interpreting the prosodic cues. For written communication, the prosodic cues are not present, and thus the meaning must be derived from the other cues present in the context.

Nonliteral Language in the Intact RH

There is a large literature on comprehension and interpretation of nonliteral language in the healthy brain. The intact right hemisphere is activated during processing of metaphors and unfamiliar idioms more so than during comprehension of literal sentences (Burgess & Chiarello, 1998; Giora et al., 2000; Mashal, Faust, Hendler, & Jung-Beeman, 2007). However, this does not mean that the RH is dominant for nonliteral language processing. In fact, few

studies support this notion (e.g., Mashal et al., 2007). Most studies identify either a bilateral network (Coulson & van Petten, 2007; Diaz, Barrett, & Hogstrom, 2011; Lauro, Tettamanti, Cappa, & Papagno, 2007) or LH dominance (Eviatar & Just, 2006; Ferstl, Neumann, Bogler, & von Cramon, 2008; Lee & Dapretto, 2006; Mashal, Faust, Hendler, & Jung-Beeman, 2009).

Several reviews of the literature highlight a bilateral network used for figurative language comprehension (Bohrn, Altman, & Jacobs, 2012; Kasparian, 2013; Yang, 2014). This network spans frontal and temporal lobes in both hemispheres. The extent of lateralized activation patterns (either more RH or LH activation) differs based on the task. In their meta-analyses, Born and colleagues (2012) and Yang (2014) identified salience, context, and task processing demands as factors that influence hemispheric regions of activation.

Familiarity and Salience

In the Graded Salience Hypothesis (GSH), Giora and Fein (1999) proposed that familiarity or salience is a key factor in hemispheric language processing. Salient words/phrases are those that can be quickly retrieved. According to the GSH, salience is a more important determiner of LH/RH language processing than is literality. The LH is dominant for familiar or salient phrases, while the RH is more involved in processing unfamiliar or novel phrases. Thus, the LH processes familiar idioms and known metaphors and RH is important for comprehending novel metaphors or sarcasm. This hypothesis fits with many of the extant theories of hemispheric processing differences. The RH's coarse coding activates multiple, distantly related meanings (Beeman, 1986) and is important for integrating meaning within a local context (Bookheimer, 2002: Federmeier, 2007; Menenti et al., 2008). These processing characteristics make the RH more likely to generate meanings of unfamiliar or novel phrases (Cardillo, Watson, Schmidt, Kranjec, & Chatterjee, 2012; Diaz et al., 2011; Eviatar & Just, 2006; Lai, van Dam, Conant, Binder, & Desai, 2015; Lee & Dapretto, 2006; Mashal, Faust, Hendler, & Jung-Beeman, 2008). An RH advantage for sarcasm compared with idiom and metaphor processing also has been reported (Bohrn et al., 2012), which is consistent with the variety of forms of sarcasm described above.

Familiar idioms and known metaphors are processed primarily in the LH. There is extensive evidence that the figurative meanings of familiar idioms and metaphors are activated quickly and automatically (Giora et al., 2000; Glucksberg, 1998). Processing is akin to activation of multiple meanings of ambiguous words for which the different meanings are equally familiar (e.g., bat = animal and baseball equipment): both meanings are initially activated and then the contextually less appropriate meaning is suppressed in the left hemisphere but possibly remains active in the right hemisphere (Beeman, 1998).

Context and Task Demands

A variety of stimuli and tasks are employed in studies of nonliteral language processing. These include word pairs (e.g., STAR/sun versus STAR/actor) or triads (WARM/loving/kind), sentences or sentence pairs, story contexts, or video vignettes. Yang (2012) reported that greater RH activation occurs when more context is present. Thus, there is minimal RH activation when metaphoric processing is tested with word pairs, but greater RH activation when metaphors are embedded in sentences. This finding is consistent with the RH's role in contextual integration (e.g., Coulson et al., 2005; Xu et al., 2005).

Yang (2014) also found that the complexity or level of semantic processing required in the experimental task affected the amount of RH activation. Some researchers use valence judgments, asking participants to report whether or not the stimuli (word pairs, sentences, etc.) are generally positive, negative, or neutral. This requires fairly superficial semantic processing, and in some cases could be dependent on a single word (e.g., never, impossible). Other researchers use semantic relatedness judgment tasks, such as whether or not two words or sentences convey the same meaning. This task requires deeper semantic processing and may engage abstract or figurative language processing. This latter task is associated with greater RH activation.

The conclusions drawn from the extensive research on nonliteral language processing suggest that such processing requires a bilateral network. The relative contribution of the RH can be increased by using unfamiliar or novel stimuli, by providing sentence-level context, and by using a task that requires deeper semantic processing. The results are consistent with hypotheses suggesting that the intact RH is important for interpretation of novel linguistic constructions and contextual integration.

Nonliteral Language Interpretation After RHD

Difficulties interpreting or explaining nonliteral or figurative language such as idioms and metaphors have long been ascribed to RHD, often with the blanket conclusion that adults with RHD are overly literal or unable to comprehend figurative language (Brownell et al., 1986; Critchley, 1962, as cited in Critchley, 1991; Eisenson, 1962; Gardner & Denes, 1973; Myers & Linebaugh, 1981; Van Lancker & Kempler, 1987; Wapner et al., 1981; Winner & Gardner, 1977). However, like most of the deficits associated with RHD, the reality is much more complex and nuanced.

Evidence to support the notion that RHD impairs figurative language processing is not as strong as would be expected given the central role this deficit has in the RHD stereotype. When taken as a whole, the existing research suggests that the varieties of types and forms of nonliteral language, and the influences of familiarity and context, play a large role in how quickly and accurately figurative language is processed (Peleg, Giora, & Fein, 2001).

RHD and Indirect Requests

Weylman and Brownell (1989) reported that adults with RHD were less adept at interpreting the nonliteral or indirect meaning of such phrases compared with adults without brain injury. The phrases (e.g., "can you tell me the time?") were embedded into contexts that supported either a direct ("yes I can") versus an indirect ("yes I will") interpretation. The RHD group correctly selected the indirect meaning in about 75% of the contexts that sup-

ported it, while the non–brain damaged group was 90% accurate. The differences were significant, but the 75% accuracy clearly indicates that the process was not abolished. When performance was compared with a group of adults with aphasia, the results indicated that the RHD group did not have more literal interpretations than the LHD group.

The naturalness of the communication context has an effect on figurative language processing. One study reported that adults with RHD are able to process indirect speech acts with little or no difficulty in natural, or even pseudo-natural, communicative contexts, while showing difficulties in contrived situations (Vanhalle et al., 2000).

Interpretation of direct and indirect statements is part of the Montreal Evaluation of Communication (MEC; Joanette et al., 2004, 2015). In this subtest, participants hear a brief situation that ends with either a direct or an indirect statement. Their task is to explain what was meant by the statement. In their report of 112 adults with RHD from three countries (Argentina, Brazil, and Canada), Ferré and colleagues (2012) found that none of the averaged RHD scores fell below the cutoff for impaired performance on this subtest. Given that responses to both direct and indirect statements are combined in the total score, it is not possible (from this report) to determine whether or not interpretation of indirect statements is specifically impaired.

RHD and Metaphors

Processing of metaphoric meanings following RHD has been examined in a variety of studies with a variety of tasks and stimuli, including metaphor-picture matching, selection of related words based on literal versus metaphoric meaning, and verbal explanations of metaphoric phrases (Brownell, Simpson, Bihrle, Potter, & Gardner, 1990; Giora et al., 2000; Rinaldi, Marangolo, & Baldassarri, 2004; Winner & Gardner, 1977; Zaidel, Kasher, Soroker, & Batori, 2002). When taken as a whole, the results indicate that metaphoric processing can be impaired after RHD. Importantly, the ability to interpret metaphoric meanings is impaired but not absent. Whether or not the metaphoric meaning is correctly interpreted may be related to the complexity of the task, the familiarity of the metaphor (e.g., *The child is an angel* versus *The child is a hurricane*), or how similar or appropriate the comparisons are within the metaphor (e.g., *The bus is a snail* versus *The bus is a cheetah*).

According to Beeman's (1998) coarse coding hypothesis, the right hemisphere activates distantly related meanings. Given that figurative meanings generally are more distantly related than literal meanings (e.g., Coulson & Van Petten, 2002; Pynte, Besson, Robichon, & Poli, 1996), it could be concluded that RHD should impair the ability to activate figurative meanings of metaphors. In the contextual constraint treatment study for coarse coding, Blake and colleagues (2015) suggested that metaphoric meanings of words (e.g., "star") could be special cases of distantly related meanings, and thus adults with RHD who had a coarse coding deficit would have difficulty with metaphoric meanings not because they were nonliteral, but because they were distantly related. The results from their treatment study failed to support this assumption, as

increased speed of activation of distantly related words did not generalize to metaphoric meanings.

RHD and Idioms

Evidence for deficits in interpreting idioms after RHD is shaky at best. Several studies report deficits based on idiom-picture matching tasks (Kempler, Van Lancker, Marchman, & Bates, 1999; Myers & Linebaugh, 1981; Papagno et al., 2006; Van Lancker & Kempler, 1987). In the majority of these studies, however, the presence of visuospatial neglect and/or visuospatial processing deficits was not specifically assessed. Papagno and colleagues (2006) reported that scores on their idiom-picture matching task were meaningfully correlated with scores on visuospatial tasks, suggesting that the results may not reflect only idiom processing.

Defining idioms is another commonly used task to assess idiom interpretation. Again, results are contradictory. Tompkins, Boada, and McGarry (1992) reported that their RHD group was less accurate than a control group in defining familiar idioms. In Papagno et al.'s (2006) study of nonambiguous idioms representing a range of transparency, only 4/15 (27%) of participants exhibited a deficit. Myers and Mackisack (1986) assessed generation of definitions of both ambiguous and nonambiguous idioms and found no differences between their RHD and control groups, and no differences based on type of idiom. Interestingly, some participants in each group exhibited difficulties in generating explanations of idioms. In their attempts, many were able to demonstrate their understanding of the meaning, but struggled to create a definition. For example, some individuals may be able to provide another idiom with a similar meaning (e.g., "*to spill the beans* means *to let the cat out of the bag*") but still have problems generating a definition.

Online recognition of familiar idioms was examined by Tompkins et al. (1992). In this study, participants heard two-sentence "stories" in which the first sentence provided a context and the second contained either a contextually appropriate idiom (*she smelled a rat*) or a phrase that was not idiomatic but was worded very similarly to an idiom (she saw a rat). Participants had to respond as quickly as possible when they heard a target word, which was the final noun in the target phrase (rat). Results indicated that the RHD and control groups exhibited the same pattern of performance: they were both faster to respond to the target words in idioms than in literal sentences. This indicates that the RHD group had no idiom recognition deficit. The finding is consistent with the GSH (Giora & Fein, 1999), as the idioms were well known. Importantly, this intact idiom recognition was observed in the same group of participants described above that had difficulties generating definitions.

Together, the results of idiom studies are not convincing. While on the surface the results suggest that idiom processing may be affected for some adults with RHD, there are also visuospatial and metalinguistic demands that impact performance on the idiom-interpretation tasks.

RHD and Sarcasm/Irony

Only a few studies have been conducted to examine interpretation of sarcasm/irony, but the results are fairly consistent:

groups of adults with RHD have difficulty correctly interpreting the intended meaning of sarcastic comments embedded into short vignettes (Bihrle et al., 1986; Giora et al., 2000; Kaplan, Brownell, Jacobs, & Gardner, 1990; Shamay-Tsoory et al., 2005).

Giora and colleagues (2000) examined interpretation of sarcasm in adults with RHD or LHD and a control group with no brain damage. Participants heard a short scenario from the Right Hemisphere Communication Battery (Gardner & Brownell, 1986) and were asked whether a statement made by a character was sarcastic, a lie, a mistake, or a truthful response. The RHD group was less accurate, often selecting the "lie" interpretation instead of the "sarcasm" interpretation. It is important to note that while the RHD group misinterpreted sarcasm as lies, they did recognize that the statement was not truthful or simply a mistake; they recognized that it was a willful untrue statement, but were less accurate at determining the underlying intent (lie versus sarcasm). Adults with RHD may be less adept at using pragmatic contextual cues such as social relationships to aid in interpreting sarcastic intent (Cheang & Pell, 2006; Kaplan et al., 1990). Despite the consistency in the group results, individual variability exists (e.g., Cheang & Pell, 2006) and difficulties with interpretation of sarcasm should not be assumed of all individuals with RHD.

Assessment of Language Comprehension

Assessment of the types of semantic processing and language comprehension deficits associated with RHD is a tricky business. As described above, coarse coding and suppression deficits are characterized by slow or inefficient processes. Thus, traditional offline tasks (e.g., sentences or short paragraphs followed by comprehension questions) are not sensitive enough to detect the deficits. Tompkins and colleagues (2011; Blake et al., 2015) have devised an online, timed assessment to identify coarse coding and suppression deficits for research purposes, but it is not yet available for clinical use. While there are no specific measures to assess inferencing, nonliteral language, or use of context, many RHD batteries (see Table 2–5 in Chapter 2) include subtests for these areas.

Traditional discourse comprehension tasks also have a memory component that may affect performance and lead to inaccurate conclusions; a client may be diagnosed with a discourse comprehension deficit when he has an underlying memory impairment, and he was unable to keep the information in working memory long enough, or may not have been able to retrieve it at the right time to answer a question correctly. Another form of assessment task is to have clients provide a spoken or written interpretation; these commonly are used for assessing nonliteral language. This, too, conflates two processes: language comprehension and language production. A client who is unable to explain the main idea of a paragraph may have a comprehension deficit in which he is unable to derive the main idea from the contextual cues, but he also may have generated the main idea but then was unable to accurately or succinctly express it verbally.

Some RHD batteries have discourse comprehension subtests, but these are typically quite brief. The Discourse Comprehension Test (Brookshire & Nicholas, 1997) was designed for individuals with stroke or TBI and assesses comprehension of main ideas and details that are either explicitly stated or have to be inferred. Passages can be presented either auditorily or in writing to assess both auditory and reading comprehension. While the test does have good validity and reliability, one major drawback is the memory component. Additionally, it may not be sensitive enough to detect mild comprehension deficits.

Treatment of Language Deficits

There are few empirically tested treatments for language deficits in adults with RHD (Blake, Frymark, & Venedictov, 2013). As discussed in Chapter 2, in the absence of directly applicable evidence, clinicians have several options: select evidence-based treatments designed for other clinical populations with similar deficits that might be applicable; develop treatment tasks based on theories of the underlying deficits; and/or rely upon expert opinion (Blake, 2007).

Empirically Supported Treatment for Language Deficits

There are two treatments specifically for RHD language deficits that have been empirically studied. Tompkins and colleagues (Blake et al., 2015; Tompkins et al.,

2011, 2012) developed Contextual Constraint Treatment to remediate deficits in coarse coding and suppression processes. Lundgren and colleagues (2011) developed a metaphor training treatment. Each will be discussed in turn.

The Contextual Constraint Treatment (CCT) was designed to take advantage of the preserved ability to use strong contextual cues to implicitly facilitate inefficient coarse coding and suppression processes. The online, implicit nature of the treatment minimizes the metalinguistic and memory demands that are common in traditional language treatments. Both coarse coding and suppression deficits have been associated with general narrative comprehension. The goal of CCT, then, is to improve narrative comprehension by increasing the efficiency of the impaired processes.

In CCT, the participant/client listens to three-sentence "stories" (see example in Table 4–6). The first two sentences provide contextual cues that support the intended meaning of the final sentence. Participants make a response to a target that follows the final sentence—either a lexical decision (is it a real word?), or a relatedness judgment (is it related to the context?). For the treatment items, this target word is related to the intended meaning. Participants are encouraged to listen carefully to the whole story, but they do not make any explicit decisions about the story itself. The first two sentences are removed and/or added back in a hierarchical fashion, depending on how quickly and accurately the participant responds to the target word. If they respond quickly and accurately, the context is lessened; if they are slow or inaccurate, then the context is restored.

The key aspects of CCT are the following: strong contextual cues are used to bias towards the intended meaning, whether it be one meaning of an ambiguous word (suppression treatment) or a distantly related feature of a noun (coarse coding treatment). The repeated exposure to context and adding/subtracting contextual cues as needed to support fast, accurate responses is designed to increase the efficiency of coarse coding and suppression processes. The design of the treatment

Table 4–6. Example of Contextual Constraint Therapy Stimuli

Coarse Coding Stimulus	Suppression Stimulus	
The garment needed ironing. She smoothed the fabric. It was a shirt.	The surgery was difficult. The surgeon was skilled. He transplanted the organ.	1st sentence: strongly biasing 2nd sentence: moderately biasing 3rd sentence: ends with target noun
WRINKLED	MUSIC	Probe word: related to contextually biased feature/meaning

Note. Coarse coding: probe word reflects a distantly related meaning of the final word of the 3rd sentence. Suppression: probe word reflects one meaning of the ambiguous final word of the 3rd sentence.

reduces the demands on memory and does not create conflation of comprehension and production because no verbal explanations are required. Results from the coarse coding CCT indicate that participants did get faster and more accurate over time. More importantly, though, they showed an improvement in discourse comprehension that was maintained over time (Blake et al., 2015; Tompkins et al., 2011, 2012). Preliminary results from the suppression CCT show similar outcomes (Tompkins, Blake, Scharp, Meigh, & Wambaugh, 2013).

The CCT is not yet ready for clinical use; more work must be done to test the efficacy of the treatment and to create a delivery system that is feasible to use in clinical settings. However, there is important knowledge that arises from the studies that have been done. First, it is possible to increase the efficiency of coarse coding and suppression processes. Second, the increased efficiency improves general discourse comprehension. Third, changes in language processes were effected through the implicit training procedures. This last finding suggests that it is both feasible and beneficial to provide treatment that does not rely on traditional metalinguistic and memory-demanding tasks.

Lundgren and her colleagues (2011) developed a Metaphor Training Program to remediate deficits in metaphor comprehension. They began with a pool of novel comparator metaphors, such as *the child is a tornado*. To facilitate derivation of the meaning, they used a Bubble Map to list and link semantic features. First the participants would write down features of the word "child." Then they would be given the second noun, "tornado," and again

write down features of that word. Finally, the features of both words were examined, and any features common to both nouns (e.g., loud, messy) would be highlighted. These then would be used to derive the meaning: the child is a tornado means the child is loud, messy, and out of control.

Participants received approximately 10 hours of treatment. All five participants showed improvement in interpretation of novel metaphors. Only one showed improvement in nonliteral language comprehension more generally, and there was no measure of change in general discourse comprehension. While the treatment clearly improved the verbal interpretation of metaphors, it is unclear whether or how this change might affect daily communication.

Treatments Developed for Other Populations

Strategic Memory and Reasoning Training (SMART), also known as gist reasoning training (Anand et al., 2011; Chapman & Gamino, 2008; Chapman & Mudar, 2014), was designed to improve top-down reasoning skills using language-based comprehension and reasoning activities. The hierarchical stages include the following strategies: inhibiting, organizing/managing, inferencing, paraphrasing, synthesizing, integrating, and abstracting/generalizing. These strategies are used to facilitate the identification of main ideas and derive the meaning of a text using world knowledge. The treatment is based on the Fuzzy Trace theory (Rayna & Brainard, 1995), which suggests that gist meaning is stored and retrieved more easily than details.

An adapted version of gist reasoning was used with an adult with chronic cognitive-communication deficits caused by RHD with the goal to improve verbal reasoning and communication efficiency (Richardson & Blake, 2017). Following treatment, the client exhibited improvements in verbal reasoning that were maintained for six weeks posttreatment. Although gains were observed, the impression of the clinician, client, and spouse was that there were too many strategies for him to learn in a short amount of time and that focusing on one or two that could have the greatest impact may have been more beneficial. This restricted focus would also allow for repeated practice and development of the strategy as habitual practice, as is recommended for effective cognitive rehabilitation (Sohlberg & Turkstra, 2011; Ylvisaker & Feeney, 1998; Ylvisaker, Szekeres, & Feeney, 2008).

Metacognitive strategies, or strategies designed to break a task into steps and monitor progress towards a goal, are recommended for executive function deficits (refer to discussion in Chapter 8). Several of these strategies were designed to facilitate discourse or narrative comprehension. Two such strategies are provided in Table 4–7. The two strategies differ only in the acronym (PQRST versus SQ3R; Robinson, 1970; Spache & Berge, 1966). Both provide the same steps for breaking down a comprehension task. The client first should preview or survey the text to be read by reading the title and skimming over the text. The second step is to clarify the task: what is the purpose? Is it to read for details or to get the main idea or gist? How will I be tested on it? Are there restrictions on time? The third is to

Table 4–7. Two Metacognitive Strategies for Facilitating Comprehension of Narratives and Discourse

PQRST	SQ3R
Preview	Survey
Question	Question
Read	Read
Summarize	Recite
Test	Review

Sources: Robinson, 1970; Spache & Berge, 1966.

read the text, followed by summarizing or reciting the information. The final stage is to test or review the information. These strategies can be used to enhance reading and comprehension of any personally relevant material: newspaper articles for a discussion of current events, a label on a new medication to ensure understanding of the dosing schedule and any side effects that need to be monitored, a letter or e-mail written by a family member, etc. These specific strategies have not been assessed with adults with RHD, but relatively strong evidence supporting the use of metacognitive strategies for other cognitive deficits (see Chapters 6 and 8) suggest that they might be appropriate.

Treatments Based on Theory or Expert Opinion

In the absence of evidence of treatment efficacy, treatments can be constructed based on theoretical knowledge of the deficit and of relatively spared processes and abilities. Adults with RHD can use strong, consistent contextual bias to aid in interpretation. This can be exploited to facilitate comprehension of figurative language or generation of inferences. Importantly, the treatment suggestions described here have not been systematically evaluated to determine whether they are efficacious or effective.

Teaching interpretation of idioms has been addressed quite extensively in the second-language literature. Many idioms are specific to language or geography and cannot easily be translated. One method of addressing idiom interpretation is to treat them like vocabulary and teach the meanings directly or compare them to known idioms (e.g., "*to spit the toad*" means the same thing as "*to spill the beans*"; Steinel, Hulstijn, & Steinel, 2007). A second method involves teaching not only the meaning, but the derivation, to provide additional understanding of the origin of the idiom (Boers, Eyckmans, & Stengers, 2007; Noroozi & Salehi, 2013). The problem with these two methods is that learning occurs only for the idioms that are taught. There is no expectation of generalization, because learning one idiom will not aid in understanding another idiom. A third method is to teach a strategy of using the context to determine the meaning. Neither the efficacy nor the effectiveness of such a treatment has been assessed in adults with RHD, but given that strong, consistent contextual support facilitates other language processes, it may be a useful approach to treatment. One benefit of this method is that the strategy can generalize to untreated figurative language and to other language processes, such as inferencing. Table 4–8 provides an example using idioms that are relatively unfamiliar to Americans and are nondecomposable and nontransparent. It may be nearly impossible to guess the meaning if the idiom is presented in isolation; however, when embedded into a supportive context, the meaning is relatively easy to derive. A sample treatment procedure using a contextual strategy is provided in Table 4–9.

The contextualization procedure can be modified to use with novel metaphors, sarcasm/irony, inferences, or interpreting ambiguous words or phrases. The key aspect is to identify the information in the context that supports the correct interpretation (see example in Table 4–10).

Again, the contextualization procedure is based on our understanding of language

Table 4–8. Idioms in Context

Target Idiom	Sample Context	Interpretation
She has salt in her pumpkin	Ashley was the top student in her class. She was a quick learner and earned high grades on all of her exams. She had salt in her pumpkin.	She is smart
To spit the toad	Marisol had promised her mom that she wouldn't tell her cousin Alex that Santa Claus wasn't real, but he kept pestering her about it, and finally she got angry and spit the toad.	Tell a secret

Table 4–9. Contextualization Process for Interpretation of Novel Idioms

Step 1	Present idiom in isolation to check for familiarity. Do not ask for an interpretation, as this can lead to activation of an incorrect meaning that may then interfere with the correct interpretation.	"Have you ever heard the phrase, *she's got salt in her pumpkin*?"
Step 2	If the client is unfamiliar with the idiom, then present it embedded in a strongly biasing context.	"I've put that phrase into a short paragraph. See if that helps explain what the phrase means." [provide context, as shown in Table 4–8]
Step 3	Ask for interpretation.	"Now what do you think that phrase means?"
Step 4	Regardless of accuracy, ask for explanation for how meaning was derived. • If incorrect, guide client to the key words/phrases that lead to the correct interpretation (e.g., "top of the class," "quick learner," "high grades"); if any cues were omitted, point those out and discuss whether interpretation might change if only some of the cues were used. • If correct, reinforce the process of identifying cues that led to the correct interpretation.	"How did you figure that out? What information from the paragraph helped you figure out what the phrase means?" [can have them circle, underline, highlight key words as appropriate]

processing strengths and weaknesses but has not been evaluated to determine its efficacy or effectiveness.

Treatment Cautions

Suggested activities for nonliteral language deficits are commonly found in workbooks designed for adults with cognitive-communication disorders. These activities typically involve providing ambiguous words, metaphors, and idioms (often without supporting context) and asking clients to provide an interpretation. These types of tasks are problematic for several reasons.

▨ Underlying deficit: If a client has a suppression deficit, then asking her or him to generate multiple meanings will not target the deficit; the client can generate multiple meanings, but the problem is in suppression or inhibition of the meanings that are contextually inappropriate or irrelevant. If the client has a coarse coding deficit, this activity also may not target the

Table 4–10. Example of the Contextualization Process for Ambiguous Words or Phrases

Step 1	Present ambiguous word and ask for different meanings.*	"Tell me the different meanings of the word 'spring'" [season, stream of water, metal coil]
Step 2	Put the word into a sentence context and discuss the meanings that would be appropriate. Provide different contexts for different meanings; some contexts may still leave some ambiguity.	"If I said, 'When he took apart the clock he lost the spring,' what meanings would be appropriate? [coil] "What if I said, 'he went fishing in the spring'? [season/stream of water]. "What if I said, 'he liked to hunt in the winter but he went fishing in the spring'"? [season]
Step 3	Ask client to highlight/underline the cues that led to his/her choice of interpretation.	"When he took apart the <u>clock</u> he lost the spring." • A clock is a mechanical device with metal coils "He went <u>fishing</u> in the spring." • You fish in a body of water • You can fish in the spring season "He liked to hunt in the <u>winter</u> but he went fishing in the spring." • Contrast with winter leads to interpretation of "season" meaning
Step 4	Ask client to provide context that will support different meanings, highlighting the cues that support the intended meaning.	"The word is SPRING. Make up a sentence using the 'season' meaning of the word SPRING." "Now make up a new sentence using the 'stream of water' meaning of the word SPRING."

*While listing multiple meanings will not directly address either suppression or coarse coding deficits (see Treatment Cautions, above), in this case the client is asked to list the meanings so that they can then be embedded into different contexts. The focus of the treatment is using context to determine the appropriate meaning.

client's deficit; she or he may be able to list multiple closely related meanings or features of a word, because the deficit primarily affects distantly related meanings (e.g., Tompkins et al., 2012).

■ Familiarity of idioms: A person familiar with an idiom may be able explain it to some degree. It may not be possible to differentiate whether the problem is due to a comprehension/interpretation deficit or a production deficit (difficulty in putting an abstract idea or a well-known phrase into new words; Myers & Mackisack, 1986). If an idiom is not familiar, then success in describing the meaning will be highly dependent on the transparency and decomposability, and errors will tend to be literal interpretations because a decomposing strategy relies on literal meanings of the component words.

■ Absence of context: It is rare that in daily life we encounter ambiguous words or figurative language in isolation. We naturally use context to aid in comprehension and interpretation of language that is not immediately interpretable. Additionally, strong contextual support facilitates language processes, such as inferencing, in adults with RHD. Thus, emphasizing the use of context may facilitate comprehension by relying on a strength to overcome a weakness.

Conclusions

Language comprehension deficits associated with RHD tend to be processing inefficiencies that affect narrative comprehension. There are few assessments that can reliably and validly diagnose the language deficits exhibited by adults with RHD; the picture for clinically available, empirically based treatment is similarly bleak. On the positive side, there has been a dramatic increase in treatment-related research in the past 10 years. Additionally, the strong research evidence for specific language processing deficits provides a solid basis from which to develop theoretically based treatments. There are many good opportunities for empirical testing of such treatments and expansion of evidence-based practice in the near future.

5

Prosody

Prosody is a suprasegmental[1] feature of communication that conveys meaning through systematic variations in vocal pitch, loudness, and rhythm that are used to create intonation, stress, emotion, and tone. Prosody is commonly referred to as the "melody of speech." Throughout this chapter, the term "prosody" is used to refer to vocal manipulations that result in patterns of intonation, stress, emotion, and tone. It should be noted that while "intonation" refers to the manipulation of pitch within a sentence and is a component of prosody, some researchers use the terms "intonation" and "prosody" interchangeably.

Classification of Prosody Types

While there are a variety of ways to conceptualize prosody, it is broadly understood to be an integral part of language and should not be considered optional or peripheral (Crystal, 1976). Couper-Kuhlen (2015) describes several theoretical conceptualizations. One suggests that intonation can be considered a part of grammar and serves to link propositional content to the intents and beliefs of the speaker and listener. Another suggests that prosody is one form of contextualization cue (along with gestures, facial expression, and body language) that provide a structure or schema for linguistic forms.

Several classification schemes have been proposed to illustrate and differentiate types of prosody. The first was proposed by Monrad-Kohn (1947), who suggested four types of prosody: intrinsic, intellectual, emotional, and inarticulate. Intrinsic prosody is used to differentiate word forms (e.g., compound words from word phrases, such as hotdog versus hot dog) and sentence types (differentiating questions from statements such as: Sheri went to the movies? versus Sheri went to the movies.) but also underlies dialectal

---

[1]Prosody is considered suprasegmental because the variations typically extend over multiple phonemes (segments).

differences and individual or idiosyncratic characteristics of speech rate, fundamental frequency, pitch range, etc. Intellectual prosody is used to convey attitudes such as boredom, skepticism, enthusiasm, and doubt. Emotional prosody obviously is used to express emotions. Finally, he defined inarticulate prosody as nonlinguistic sounds such as sighs or groans that are used to enhance or embellish speech.

Another system of classification includes indexical, affective, grammatical, and pragmatic forms of prosody (compiled and reviewed by Peppe, 2009; Table 5–1). Indexical components are the idiosyncratic characteristics of Monrad-Kohn's intrinsic category. These are created by variations in fundamental frequency, frequency range, speech, rhythm, stress/intonation patterns, loudness, and dialect or accent patterns. Affective prosody includes both emotions and attitudes (see also Mitchell & Ross, 2013), which are conveyed through manipulation of rate, loudness, pitch height, and pitch span. Grammatical prosody, described as "spoken punctuation," is used to segment phrases, sections, and clauses to denote sentence types and to differentiate word forms. Grammatical prosody allows for the disambiguation of ambiguous syntactic structures and prevents comprehension problems with garden path sentences. Distinctions such as these are made by the manipulation of pauses, syllable and phoneme duration, pitch contours, and stress patterns. Finally, pragmatic prosody or "focus prosody" is used to focus a listener's attention on critical information. This includes emphatic stress to clarify or differentiate new from old information and the use of pauses and pitch changes

to signal either continuation or the end of a turn in a conversation.

Prosody and Communication

Prosody interacts closely with semantic and syntactic systems but is an independent component of language (Crystal, 1976; Honbolygó, Török, Bánréti, Hunyadi, & Csépe, 2016; Nakamura, Arai, & Mazuka, 2012; Pannekamp, Toepel, Alter, Hahne, & Friederici, 2005; Paulmann & Kotz, 2008). Prosodic distinctions can be quite fine. Hellbernd and Sammler (2016) indicate that manipulations of pitch within a single word can differentially convey criticism, doubt, warning, suggestion, naming, and wishes. Prosody also can be used to identify and signal correct referents such as large versus small items and fast versus slow items (Hupp & Jungers, 2013). Complex combinations of syntax, pitch, and pause duration are used to signal continuation versus the end of a turn in conversation (Wennerstrom & Siegel, 2003). All of these prosodic manipulations are rapidly processed and integrated by listeners to aid comprehension (Heeren, Bibyk, Gunlogson, & Tanenhaus, 2015; Kurumada, Brown, Bibyk, Pontillo, & Tanenhaus, 2014).

While many research studies isolate prosody, in normal communicative exchanges emotion is conveyed through not only prosody but also facial expression, body language, syntax, and semantics. These different modalities interact and influence each other. Emotional prosody influences the interpretation of semantics and facial expression (see brief review in Paulmann & Pell, 2010; also Pell, 2005;

Table 5–1. Classification of Types of Prosody

Type of Prosody	Description	Acoustic and Perceptual Components	Examples
Indexical	Individual or idiosyncratic characteristics of speech production	Fundamental frequency Frequency range Speed Rhythm Stress pattern Intonation pattern Loudness Dialect Accent	Deep, resonant voice of James Earl Jones Boston-accented speech of John F. Kennedy
Affective	Emotion and attitude	Rate Loudness Pitch height Pitch span	Fast rate, elevated loudness, and elevated pitch to convey excitement
Grammatical	Segment phrases, sections, clauses denote sentence types and differentiate word forms/types	Pauses Syllable and phoneme duration Pitch contours Stress patterns	The old men // and women sat on the bench versus The old men and women // sat on the bench Shannon got promoted? versus Shannon got promoted!
Pragmatic	Focus attention on specific syllables, words, or phrases. Clarify meaning. Differentiate old versus new information.	Loudness Duration Pauses Pitch changes	SHANNON got a promotion (not Julie). In my conversation with my boss YESTERDAY, I told her I would not lead the project (as opposed to another conversation today).

Source: Based on Peppe, 2009.

Pell, Jaywant, Monetta, & Kotz, 2011). The presence of congruent prosody and facial expression facilitates identification of emotion (Karow, Marquardt, & Levitt, 2013; Ethofer, Anders, Erb, et al., 2006). Semantics also influence the interpretation of emotional prosody such that an emotionally laden sentence can facilitate recognition of emotional prosody (Tompkins, 1991; Wambacq & Jerger, 2004). Schirmer and Kotz (2006) suggest that while emotional prosody does affect interpretation, its influence is more variable than semantics. Thus, results are more easily affected by task, context, and interindividual differences.

The integration of syntax and prosody may rely on interhemispheric connections via the posterior corpus callosum (Sammler, Kotz, Eckstein, Ott, & Friederici, 2010) and the anterior cingulate cortex is involved in interpretation of conflicting cues (e.g., when semantics and prosody do not match; Rota et al., 2008).

Gender differences have been reported in a few studies. There is some evidence that females are more sensitive to emotional prosody than males, particularly for unattended emotional cues (Schirmer & Kotz, 2006). In contrast, males may produce greater prosodic differences to mark semantic and syntactic meaning (Fitzsimons, Sheahan, & Staunton, 2001).

Emotional Prosody

Most of the work related to RHD has focused on emotional prosody, and that bias will be reflected in this chapter. Emotional prosody is a multifaceted construct and includes different valences (positive versus negative emotions), specific types of emotion (happy, sad, angry, fearful, etc.), intensity of emotional expression, and the influence of prosody on interpretation of semantics and facial expressions. In general, positive emotions tend to be recognized or identified faster and more accurately than negative emotions (Abbott, Wijeratne, Huges, Perre, & Lindell, 2014; Kucharska-Pietura, Phillips, Gernand, & David, 2003; Pell, 2005) regardless of the presence or location of brain damage, although there are some exceptions (e.g., Harciarek, Heilman, & Jodzio, 2006; Iredale, Rushby, McDonald, Dimoska-Di Marco, & Swift, 2013). Just as for facial expression, there is some evidence that different emotions are represented differently in the brain, and the ease of identifying emotions via prosody depends in part on the emotion conveyed. For example, Kotz, Kalberlah, Bahlmann, Friederici, and Haynes (2013) found that identification of surprise was the most accurate, followed by anger, sadness, and then happiness. Work from this same lab suggested that the judgment of emotional intensity appears to rely on a bilateral network, with a slight bias toward the LH (Kotz et al., 2003).

Prosody in the Intact RH

Just as with general emotional processing, there are a variety of hypotheses regarding the RH's role in prosody (see review in Baum & Pell, 1999). The right hemisphere hypothesis purports that the RH is dominant for all forms of prosody (Borod, 1993; Borod et al., 2000). The functional lateralization hypothesis suggests that the RH is dominant for affective and emotional prosody, while the LH controls linguistic prosody (Walker, Daigle, & Buzzard, 2002; Walker, Pelletier, & Reif, 2004).

Results from imaging research make both the right hemisphere and functional hypotheses untenable. Indeed, the use of accented syllables to draw focus or attention (pragmatic prosody) has been associated with an extensive bilateral network that includes the superior and inferior parietal lobes; superior and middle temporal lobes; and middle, inferior, and posterior frontal lobes (Figure 5–1). The network has extensive overlap with auditory attention networks (Kristensen, Wang, Petersson, & Hagoort, 2013). There also are bilateral networks for the recognition and production of emotional prosody (Adolphs et al., 2002; Ethofer et al., 2008, 2012; Frühholz, Gschwind, & Grandjean, 2015; Wildgruber et al., 2004, 2005). Regions within the network include the dorsolateral frontal, frontal operculum, orbitobasal frontal region, anterior insula, and superior temporal cortex (Wildgruber et al., 2004, 2005). In addition to the

hemispheric networks, the basal ganglia are involved in prosodic processing, and damage to these structures can affect explicit recognition of emotional prosody (Paulmann, Pell, & Kotz, 2008; Van Lancker Sidtis et al., 2006).

A slight RH advantage for emotional versus linguistic prosody has been reported (Wildgruber et al., 2004; see also a meta-analysis by Witteman, van Ijzendoorn, van de Velde, van Heuven, & Schiller, 2011). Kotz and colleagues (2013) also reported a right dominant fronto-operculo-temporal network for emotional prosody. They suggest that the temporal regions are important for processing suprasegmental acoustic features, while frontal regions are associated with emotional evaluation. Other proposed functions of the orbitofrontal regions include the differentiation of emotional prosody

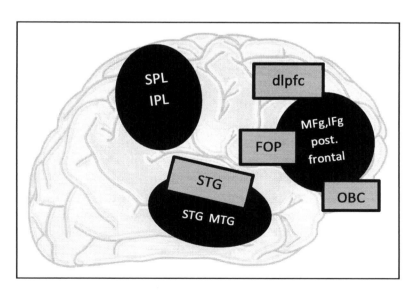

Figure 5–1. Regions involved in pragmatic (*black ovals*) and emotional (*gray rectangles*) prosody. *Notes.* dlPFC = dorsolateral prefrontal cortex; FOP = frontal operculum; IPL = inferior parietal lobe; MTG = middle temporal gyrus; OBC = orbitobasal cortex; SPL = superior parietal lobe; STG = superior temporal gyrus.

(Kotz et al., 2013; Paulmann, Siefert, & Kotz, 2010) and response to novel and behaviorally relevant prosodic emotional cues (Ethofer et al., 2012). Given the localization of the network within the fronto-temporal regions with a slight RH advantage, it is not surprising that decreased recognition and production of emotional prosody may be a marker of a behavioral variant of fronto-temporal dementia in which RH atrophy is prominent (Dará et al., 2012).

There also may be dual routes providing connections between the temporal and frontal regions (Frühholz et al., 2015). The dorsal pathway extends from the superior temporal cortex via the superior longitudinal and arcuate fasciculi to the inferior frontal gyrus. The ventral pathway extends through the inferior longitudinal fasciculus and extreme capsule and the inferior fronto-occipital fasciculus.

The acoustic or three-stage model suggests that individual acoustic cues may be differentially processed in the hemispheres. Rapid temporal variations may be processed more efficiently in the LH, while slower modulations of pitch are more easily decoded by the RH (Gandour et al., 2000; Guranski & Podemski, 2015; Iredale et al., 2013; Schirmer & Kotz, 2006; Van Lancker Sidtis, Pachana, Cummings, & Sidtis, 2006; Wildgruber, Ethofer, Grandjean, & Kreifelts, 2009; Zhang, Shu, Zhou, Wang, & Li, 2010). In the first stage, primary auditory processing occurs bilaterally in the temporal lobes. The second stage, localized in the superior temporal sulcus, involves integration of prosodic cues to create representations of meaningful suprasegmental patterns that allow for automatic emotion recognition. In the third stage the signals reach the frontal lobes (primarily the inferior frontal gyri), in which cognitive processing, including emotional judgment, occurs. The LH processes semantics and the RH makes evaluative judgments.

Prosody After RHD

Research related to RHD and prosody generally uses an oversimplified binary classification of "linguistic" versus "emotional." Linguistic prosody relates to both syntactic and semantic interpretations and includes the grammatical and pragmatic forms of prosody described above. Emotional prosody broadly matches Peppe's (2009) description, although most of the research focuses on emotion rather than attitude.

As described in Chapter 3 on pragmatics, RHD prosody research tends to explore comprehension or production of the six universal emotions (joy, sadness, fear, anger, disgust, and surprise). In some studies researchers evaluate only positive versus negative valence, while others evaluate specific emotions. Comprehension is assessed through a variety of tasks, including discrimination, identification, and recognition. Production is evaluated through repetition, cued production, and spontaneous production (Table 5–2). The type of sentence on which to overlay prosody varies, including emotionally biased (I thought I heard a burglar!), emotionally neutral (She's going to the movies), and nonsense (The flimmer was benked) sentences. Additionally in some studies researchers overlay prosody on a string of CV syllables ("ba-ba-ba-ba") or a sustained vowel to remove all semantic features.

Table 5–2. Examples of Tasks Used to Assess Prosody

	Instructions	*Task*
Comprehension		
Discrimination	You will hear two sentences. Tell me if the tone of voice was the same or different.	Same/different judgment
Identification	You will hear a sentence. Using the options (set of emotional labels), show which emotion was conveyed.	Identify what emotion was conveyed from a set of choices.
Recognition*	You will hear a sentence. Tell/show me what emotion was conveyed.	State what emotion was conveyed (no choices provided).
Production		
Repetition	Repeat the sentence, using the same tone of voice.	Repeat the sentence using the same prosody.
Cued production	Read/repeat this sentence in a [*sad/happy*] tone of voice.	Produce affective prosody with no example provided.
Spontaneous production	Tell me about a time in your life when you were very [*happy/sad*].	Spontaneous production of affective prosody.

Note. *In some studies this is referred to as identification with no choices provided.

The label "dysprosody" was first used by Monrad-Krohn (1947) to refer to difficulties in manipulating pitch, loudness, or timing during speech production. The label "aprosodia" was later coined by Ross (1981) to describe deficits in the production or recognition of affective prosody. Ross also proposed subtypes of aprosodia that mirrored the types of aphasia and that could be differentiated based on site of lesion (e.g., motor aprosodia related to anterior RHD, sensory aprosodia due to posterior RHD). The initial model was based on 10 patients, with a follow-up study with 14 additional patients (Gorelick & Ross, 1987). The diagnoses were based on nonstandardized assessments that relied on the examiners' ability to consistently and adequately both produce and judge affective prosody. These types of aprosodias and localization of lesions have not been consistently replicated by other researchers.

Aprosodia also has been broadly categorized by expressive and receptive modalities. Expressive aprosodia is characterized by decreased use or intensity of prosody during speech production. This can affect either linguistic or affective prosody in terms of pitch, timing, and/or loudness. Receptive aprosodia is a deficit in the ability to interpret others' prosody. Misinterpretation of questions, statements, or sarcastic remarks can occur, along with misinterpretation of another's emotional state. Expressive and receptive aprosodia are dissociable, meaning that they can occur separately (e.g., Ross, 1981; Ferré, Fonseca, Ska, & Joanette, 2012).

Estimates of the incidence of aprosodia following RHD vary widely. In a sample of patients in an inpatient rehabilitation unit, approximately 20% of patients were reported to have aprosodia (Blake, Duffy, Tompkins, & Myers, 2002), whereas nearly 80% of patients with acute stroke were diagnosed with receptive aprosodia (Dará, Bang, Gottesman, & Hillis, 2014). The extreme variability is likely due to a combination of different assessment approaches and spontaneous recovery.

Witteman and colleagues (2011) conducted a meta-analysis that included 38 studies representing over 500 participants each with RHD, LHD, and no brain damage. Results indicated a large effect of RHD on affective and linguistic prosody compared with LHD and no brain damage. LHD also consistently affected perception of linguistic and affective prosody. However, differences across RHD and LHD groups were significant only for affective prosody. There were no systematic differences between presence or type of aprosodia and localization of lesion, either frontal versus temporal lesions or cortical versus subcortical locations.

While linguistic prosody can be affected after RHD (see review by Witteman et al., 2011), the deficit is not found in all studies. Adults with RHD have been reported to use expressive linguistic prosody to convey intended syntactic meaning (Baum, Pell, Leonard, & Gordon, 2001) and differentiate meanings of ambiguous idioms

through alteration of the duration of syllables and pauses (Bélanger, Baum, & Titone, 2009). In a study of adults with RHD who speak Thai, results suggested that the participants correctly altered speech timing at the syllable, word, phrase, and sentence levels (Gandour, Ponglorpisit, Khunadorn, & Dechongkit, 2000).

There is little consistency in the results of studies that examine processing of different emotions. Some report that RHD differentially affects some emotions compared with others, but the affected emotions are not always the same (Charbonneau, Scherzer, Aspirot, & Cohen, 2003; Harciarek et al., 2006; Kucharska-Pietura et al., 2003). In other studies, the specific task (identification versus discrimination; comprehension versus production) affects performance on specific emotions (e.g., Charbonneau et al., 2003). Yet other reports suggest that different regions within the bilateral prosody network (frontal versus temporal versus basal ganglia) differentially affect recognition or production of specific emotions (Adolphs, Damasio, & Tranel, 2002; Guranski & Podemski, 2015; Rymarczyk & Grabowska, 2007). The intensity of emotional content also may play a role, with increased bilateral activation occurring with increased intensity (Ethofer, Anders, Wiethoff, et al., 2006).

As suggested above, another potential distinction in processing biases involves the acoustic cues. RHD can result in reduced manipulation of fundamental frequency (F_0) and intensity to express emotions (Guranski & Podemski, 2015; Schirmer, Alter, Kotz, & Friederici, 2001), while LHD primarily affects timing (Schirmer et al., 2001).

The vast majority of research studies focus on the recognition or identification of prosody but there are a few that examine broader implications of prosodic cues in relation to attitude or intent. Pell (2007) examined the use of prosodic cues to judge a speaker's level of confidence and degree of politeness. Adults with RHD were generally able to use both prosodic and semantic cues to judge confidence and politeness. When there were conflicts between the two types of cues, such as when a politely worded sentence was spoken in a harsh tone of voice, adults with RHD appeared to rely more on the semantics to make their judgment. The RHD group did show difficulties with determining the level of politeness. They tended to judge productions as either polite or impolite, whereas adults in the control group rated the productions along a continuum of politeness. In another study, Pell (2006) reported that as a group, adults with RHD were relatively insensitive to strength of emotional content. Thus, while they may be able to identify and use some emotional cues, some adults with RHD have difficulty with interpreting nuances of prosodic cues.

It is important to remember that, like all deficits associated with RHD, there is heterogeneity both within and across individuals. This is clearly shown in the study by Pell (2006) in which overall, the RHD group was poorer at identifying affective prosody compared with a control group. However, only four of the nine participants had clear deficits on one or more of the prosody tasks.

The presence of aprosodia in the acute phase of stroke may be a sensitive marker of RHD. Dará and colleagues (2014) reported that accuracy on an affective prosody recognition task accurately identified nearly 80% of patients with RH

stroke, compared with only about half (55%) who were identified using a test of unilateral neglect. This result suggests that the addition of a standardized assessment of prosody could facilitate the identification and/or diagnosis of RH strokes (see Chapter 1).

The functional, social, and vocational consequences of aprosodia are essentially unknown. Emotional recognition, through facial expression, prosody, or both, is not strongly related to outcomes for adults with traumatic brain injury (Milders, Fuchs, & Crawford, 2003; Milders, Ietswaart, Crawford, & Currie, 2008; Osborne-Crowley & McDonald, 2016; Saxton, Younan, & Lah, 2013; but see Spikman et al., 2013). The only data specific to aprosodia in adults with RHD are from a survey study conducted with spouses/caregivers and stroke survivors two years poststroke (Hillis & Tippett, 2014). Fourteen survivors of RHD and their caregivers were included and asked about the importance of various stroke-related impairments and disorders. Twenty-nine percent of the caregivers rated prosody in the top five impairments that caused them the most concern. This put prosody on par with their ratings of left motor function, the ability to walk, and spatial attention. None of the stroke survivors with RHD rated prosody in the top five. One could speculate that this could have been due in part to anosognosia for aprosodia.

Assessment

There are several standardized measures available for the assessment of aprosodia in adults (Table 5–3). In addition, many of

Table 5–3. Select Assessments of Prosody

Test	Authors	Areas Assessed	Reliability*	Validity*
Aprosodia Battery	Ross, 1981	Identification of affective prosody Production of affective prosody on command Identification and production via words (I'm going to the other movies), monosyllabic sentences (ba-ba-ba-ba) and asyllabic sentences (prolonged vowel)	None	None
Comprehensive Affect Testing System (CATS)	Froming et al., 2006	Facial expression, linguistic prosody, emotional prosody Includes conflicting semantic/prosodic	Weak	None
Florida Affect Battery	Bowers et al., 1991	Identification of facial expression Identification of emotional prosody Matching emotional prosody and facial expression	OK	OK (test-retest reliability available only up to age 55)
New York Emotion Battery (NYEB)	Borod et al., 1992	Identification, discrimination, and production of facial expression and prosody (linguistic and emotional) Includes conflicting semantic/prosodic	Weak	None
Perception of Emotion Test (POET)	Egan et al., 1990	Facial, prosodic, lexical emotion	None	None

Note. *Good = moderate–strong estimates of two or more types of reliability/validity; OK = moderate–strong estimates of one type of reliability/validity or mixture of weak and strong estimates; weak = weak estimates of one or more types of reliability/validity; none = no estimates reported. See Appendix for detailed information about reliability and validity.

the batteries designed for adults with RHD (see Chapter 1) include subtests for assessing receptive and/or expressive prosody. Unfortunately, the existing assessments tend to have substantial weaknesses in terms of reliability and validity. One major concern about these assessments is the subjective nature of evaluating or rating prosodic productions. Interrater reliability is not commonly reported but when it is it tends to be quite low (e.g., Joanette et al., 2015). Similarly, there is a concern regarding the adequacy of spontaneous production of prosodic patterns by examiners in tests for receptive aprosodia that do not include audio-recordings of the stimuli. Some examiners may be more adept at producing affective prosody than others, and there may be fluctuations in the adequacy or strength of the prosodic patterns over time, perhaps depending on the examiner's own mood or emotional state.

As another resource, Ben-David, Shaduf, & van Lieshout (2017) created a set of sentences that convey various emotions either prosodically or linguistically. These were validated for emotional intent with groups of young adults and could be used for either assessment or treatment activities. http://goo.gl/oNcfrI

Treatment

Empirically Based Treatment

Two systematic reviews, one on communication disorders associated with RHD (Blake, Frymark, & Venedictov, 2013) and one on treatments for disruptions of prosody (Hargrove, Anderson, & Jones, 2009), found only two aprosodia treatments that have systematically been evaluated (Leon et al., 2004; Rosenbek et al., 2004, 2006). The linguistic-cognitive treatment involves a six-step hierarchy to facilitate the production of affective prosody (Table 5–4). The theoretical basis for this treatment is the idea that the RH contains representations of affective prosody, comprising a lexicon of how different emotions are expressed through prosody. Damage to the system

results in a degradation or loss of this lexicon, such that individuals may not easily be able to access, for example, how anger should sound and how it is different from how happiness is conveyed. The treatment thus uses a combination of cues, including emotional labels, pictures of facial expressions, and written descriptions of emotional prosody characteristics.

The second treatment is an imitative treatment that also involves a hierarchy of fading cues (see Table 5–4). This treatment is based on the hypothesis that expressive aprosodia is similar to a motor speech disorder. The hierarchy thus involves production in unison, repetition, and cued production.

Results from a series of studies suggest that both treatments are effective for increasing the accuracy of production of emotional prosody (Leon et al., 2004; Rosenbek et al., 2004, 2006). While some patients responded better to one treatment than the other, both resulted in meaningful change that lasted for up to three months. In the studies, three emotions were trained: anger, happiness, and sadness. Results indicated that following treatment, production improved for the trained emotions not only on the trained sentences, but also on untrained sentences. However, gains did not generalize to untrained emotions. Thus, none of the participants showed a change in the ability to produce a fearful prosody because that emotion had not been addressed in treatment.

In a follow-up study (Jones, Shrivastav, Wu, Plowman-Prine, & Rosenbek, 2009) acoustic analyses were performed to determine what changes created the perceived improvement in emotional prosody. Analyses were conducted on productions by three of the participants who

Table 5–4. Treatment Hierarchy for Two Aprosodia Treatments

Imitative Therapy	Linguistic-Cognitive Therapy
1. Clinician models sentence using target emotional tone of voice; subject and clinician then produce sentence in unison.	1. Subject is given a written description of the characteristics of a given emotional tone of voice. Examples would be descriptors such as "loud," "harsh," or "fast rate." The subject reads the descriptors aloud and is asked to repeat the descriptors using her/his own words in order to ensure comprehension.
2. Clinician models same sentence using target tone of voice; subject imitates.	2. The subject is given cards listing names of emotions (happy, sad, etc.) and asked to pick which emotion matches the tone of voice she/he just described. The subject is then shown cards with black and white line drawings of faces demonstrating different emotions and is asked to pick the face that matches the tone of voice.
3. Clinician models same sentence using same target emotion with face covered; subject imitates.	3. Once the subject has the tone of voice descriptors, the name of the emotion, and the face representing the target emotion, the subject is given a sentence and asked to produce it using the descriptors.
4. Clinician produces same sentence using a neutral or flat tone of voice; subject continues to produce sentence with target emotional tone of voice.	4. Card with descriptors is taken away and subject is asked to remember descriptors and produce sentence.
5. Clinician asks subject a question ("Why are you angry, happy, sad . . . ") and subject responds with same sentence using target emotional tone of voice.	5. Card with emotion is also taken away and subject is reminded to remember the emotion name and the descriptors of the tone of voice and to produce the sentence.
6. Clinician asks subject to produce same sentence using same target emotional tone of voice while imagining that she/he is speaking to a family member.	6. Card with face representing the target emotion is now also taken away and subject is asked to produce the sentence as in previous steps.

Source: From Rosenbek et al. (2004). Novel treatments for expressive aprosodia: A phase I investigation of cognitive linguistic and imitative interventions. *Journal of the International Neuropsychological Society, 10,* 786–793. http://doi.org/10.1017/S135561770410502X. Used with permission from Cambridge University Press.

all first received the imitative treatment followed by the linguistic-cognitive treatment. The variability across participants was substantial, but the imitative treatment tended to result in changes to fundamental frequency (both mean F_0 and F_0 variability), while the linguistic-cognitive treatment affected intensity (both mean intensity and variability).

Treatment Based on Theory and Expert Opinion

Given the limited options for treatments with empirical support, clinicians often must rely on theoretically driven treatments and expert opinion. There are no published treatments for receptive aprosodia. Myers (1999) and Tompkins (1995) suggested pitch and prosody discrimination tasks (e.g., determine if two tones or two prosodic contours are the same or different). Another suggestion is to use a compensatory strategy of identifying cues other than prosody that convey emotion (Myers, 1999; Tompkins, 1995; Tompkins & Scott, 2013). In a naturalistic communication exchange, emotion is conveyed not only through prosody but through facial expression, body language, and lexical choice. These cues can be identified and discussed to aid in the determination of one's emotional state (Table 5–5). This form of treatment is based on evidence that prosody, linguistics, and facial expressions interact to convey emotional content (Karow et al., 2013; Paulmann & Pell, 2010;

Table 5–5. Sample Treatment Ideas for Emphasizing Affective Cues

Focus on . . .	Specifically Search for Affective Cues	Questions to Elicit Interpretations of the Cues
Facial expressions	Mouth: smile, frown.	What does a smile suggest?
	Eyes: open, squinting, looking away, looking down.	She's looking away, what could that mean?
	Eyebrows: elevated, scrunched together, creased forehead.	His forehead is creased, what could that mean?
Body language	Gestures: none, large, fast.	Why might he be using such big, fast gestures?
	Posture: stooped, erect, turned away from partner, facing partner.	Why might he be turning away?
Word choice	Neutral versus emotional.	What words is she using that help you figure out her emotions?
	Few versus many emotional words.	
	Highly emotional (furious) versus mildly emotional (mad).	

Note. These treatment ideas are theoretically based but have not been evaluated for efficacy or effectiveness.

Pell, 2005; Pell et al., 2011; Tompkins, 1991). Clients can view videos of monologs or communicative interactions while examining facial expressions, body language, or word choice to determine emotions and intended meaning. As noted above, this recommendation is based on theory but has not been systematically evaluated to determine the efficacy or effectiveness. Another approach (or adjunct approach) for clients with receptive aprosodia is to train family members and caregivers to explicitly state their emotion at the beginning of an exchange to lessen the possibility of misinterpretation.

One recommendation for treating expressive aprosodia is to use aspects of motor speech treatment (Myers, 1999; Tompkins & Scott, 2013). Similar to Rosenbek and colleagues' (2004, 2006) imitative treatment, this can involve repetition and cued production of affective prosody. For clients with expressive linguistic aprosodia, contrastive stress drills can be used to practice manipulation of pitch, duration, and intensity to alter intended meaning (Table 5–6). Compensatory strategies can be used either as an adjunct to impairment-level treatment or for clients with pervasive expressive aprosodia. Cli-

Table 5–6. Sample Contrastive Stress Drills for Targeting Expressive Linguistic Prosody

Word level	Differentiate verbs from nouns using stress on specific syllables.	Rebel versus **rebel** **Convert** versus **convert**
	Differentiate compound words from descriptors using stress on specific syllables/words.	Greenhouse versus the green house
Sentence level	Differentiate questions from statements using rising versus stable intonation.	Shannon got a promotion? versus Shannon got a promotion.
	Emphasize the critical information by using stress on specific words.	Michael scored 90% on his **MATH** test. versus Michael scored **90%** on his math test.
	Differentiate syntactic structures by using pauses to separate the clauses.	They evacuated the [old men] and women. (they evacuated elderly men and all of the women) They evacuated the [old men and women]. (they evacuated all elderly persons)

Note. These treatment ideas are based on suggested treatments for dysarthria or apraxia of speech but have not been evaluated for efficacy or effectiveness in the treatment of expressive linguistic aprosodia.

ents can explicitly state their emotional state or intent when they cannot express it through prosody. For example, starting a statement with "I'm really angry right now" will set the emotional tone of the conversation so that the speaker's affect is not misinterpreted.

Conclusions and Implications

Aprosodia appears to be a relatively common consequence of RHD in the acute phases, although the functional, social, and vocational consequences are essentially unknown. Research is needed to address these areas, as well as to improve the quality of the assessments and to further explore treatment options. Aprosodia is an area ripe for the use of practice-based research. Such work can add to the evidence of effectiveness of existing treatments and aid in the collection of data to support the effectiveness of some of the suggested treatments.

6

Attention

Attention is a broad concept that at first glance seems pretty straightforward. Everyone has experiences of being able to focus attention, even to the extent that unattended sights and sounds are not perceived, as well as times at which it seems nearly impossible to attend to any one thing in the midst of extraneous sights, sounds, or internal thoughts. While on one hand this makes it easy to discuss attentional deficits with clients and their families, on the other hand there is the risk of interpreting too many deficits as simply problems with attention and trivializing the complex attentional systems as an explanation for everything.

Attentional networks, forms of attention (e.g., sustained and divided attention), and characteristics of attentional processing such as limited capacity and top-down versus bottom-up processing will be covered in this chapter. Disorders related to both RHD and traumatic brain injury (TBI) will be addressed, because of the overlap in the presentation, assessment, and treatment. Unilateral neglect, which is considered a disorder of attention, will be addressed in the following chapter.

Attentional Processes and Networks

There are three distinct yet interconnected frontoparietal networks subserving attention (Table 6–1; Figures 6–1 and 6–2). One is a Default Mode Network (DMN) that is active when attention is directed inward and not focused on any specific external stimulus or task. Spreng and Grady (2010) describe it as "stimulus independent thought." The DMN has been proposed to underlie processes such as autobiographical memory, thinking about one's future, and considering the perspectives of others (a component of theory of mind). This network includes both the ventral medial and dorsolateral prefrontal cortices, the posterior cingulate gyrus, and the intraparietal sulcus (Buckner, Andrews-Hanna, & Schacter, 2008; Fox et al., 2005; Greicius, Krasnow, Reiss, & Menon, 2003).

The second network is the bilateral Dorsal Attentional Network (DAN; see Figure 6–1). This network is primarily responsible for sustaining attention and top-down attentional processes directed

Table 6–1. Fronto-Parietal Attentional Networks

Network	Function	Primary Regions
Default Mode Network	Broad-based activation in the absence of a specific task. Allows stimulus-free thoughts such as autobiographical memory, thinking about the future, or thinking about other people's perspectives.	Bilateral network. Ventromedial and dorsolateral prefrontal cortices. Posterior cingulate gyrus. Intraparietal sulcus.
Dorsal Attention Network	Sustained attention. Top-down attentional processes directed toward the contralateral visual field.	Bilateral network. Frontal eye fields. Dorsal parietal lobes (intraparietal sulcus and superior parietal lobule). Connected by axon tracts within the superior longitudinal fasciculus.
Ventral Attention Network	Attention to unexpected but relevant stimuli. Bottom-up attentional processes for salient, distinctive, or relevant stimuli.	Primarily right hemisphere. Middle and inferior frontal gyri. Anterior insula. Temporoparietal junction. Superior temporal gyrus and sulcus. Ventral supramarginal gyrus. Connected by axon tracts within the superior longitudinal fasciculus

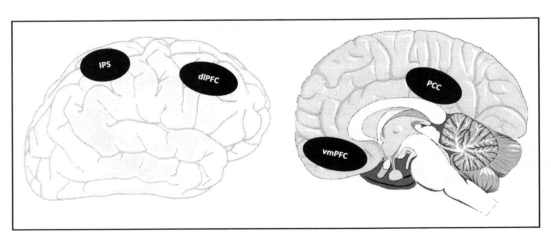

Figure 6–1. Components of the Default Mode Network. *Notes.* dlPFC = dorsolateral prefrontal cortex; IPS = intraparietal sulcus; PCC = posterior cingulate cortex; vmPFC = ventral medial prefrontal cortex. Regions are bilateral, although shown here only in the right hemisphere.

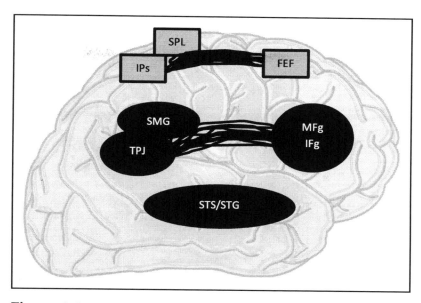

Figure 6–2. Components of the Dorsal (*gray squares*) and Ventral (*black circles*) Attention Networks. *Notes.* SPL = superior parietal lobe; IPS = intraparietal sulcus; FEF = frontal eye fields; MFG = medial frontal gyrus; IFG = inferior frontal gyrus; STS/STG = superior temporal sulcus and gyrus; TPJ = temporoparietal junction; SMG = ventral supramarginal gyrus. Lines represent sections of the superior longitudinal fasciculus. Regions are bilateral, although shown here only in the right hemisphere.

toward contralateral space (thus, the right hemisphere controls attention to the left side of space and vice versa) (Cabeza, Ciaramelli, Olson, & Moscovitch, 2008; Corbetta, Kincade, & Shulman, 2001). The core components include the frontal eye fields and dorsal regions of the parietal lobes, specifically the intraparietal sulcus and the superior parietal lobule (Bressler, Tang, Sylvester, Shulman, & Corbetta, 2008; Corbetta, Patel, & Shulman, 2008). The frontal and parietal regions are connected by a section of fibers within the superior longitudinal fasciculus (Thiebaut de Schotten et al., 2011). Top-down processes are cognitively driven, often

strategic processes that serve to increase the efficiency of the attentional system (see sidebar). One such process is expectation. Cues or strategies that aid in predicting when or where a target will appear or how frequently it will occur result in faster, more accurate responses (Gazzaley & Nobre, 2012).

The third network, the Ventral Attentional Network (VAN; see Figure 6–2), controls attention to unexpected but relevant stimuli or events. It is right-lateralized and includes the middle and inferior frontal gyri, anterior insula, temporoparietal junction, superior temporal sulcus/gyrus, and ventral supramarginal gyrus (Asanowicz,

Marzecová, Jaśkowski, & Wolski, 2012; Corbetta et al., 2008; Kucyi, Moayedi, Weissman-Fogel, Hodaie, & Davis, 2012). The frontal and parietal regions are connected by a section of fibers (distinct from the fibers of the DAN) within the superior longitudinal fasciculus (Thiebaut de Schotten et al., 2011). The VAN is associated with bottom-up attentional processes (see sidebar), in which attention is influenced by low-level features that are salient, distinctive, or relevant (Alho, Salmi, Koistinen, Salonen, & Rinne, 2015; Cabeza et al., 2008; Corbetta et al., 2001).

The functional connections are stronger within any one network than between networks (e.g., Greicius et al., 2003), but cross-network links facilitate attention modulation and switching. Connections between the DMN and the other two networks allow shifting of attention between internal and external stimuli (e.g., Uddin, Kelly, Biswal, Castellanos, & Milham, 2009). Connections between the Dorsal and Ventral Attentional Networks appear to occur in the right middle frontal gyrus (Corbetta et al., 2008) or the right superior temporal gyrus (Smith, Clithero, Rorden, & Karnath, 2013) and allow modulation of attention to external stimuli. During sustained attention, the DAN is most active, and suppresses activity in the VAN to maintain focus (Corbetta et al., 2008; Wen, Yao, Liu, & Ding, 2012). However, when a relevant but unexpected stimulus appears, the VAN can decrease activity in the DAN to allow a shift of attention (Corbetta et al., 2008; Weissman & Prado, 2012). Both the

---

SIDEBAR

Top-down processes: You're in the grocery store looking for spices. If you know that they are arranged alphabetically, you can use that knowledge as a strategy to narrow your search by estimating where the oregano might be and quickly skipping over the cinnamon and garlic in your search for spices that begin with "o."

Bottom-up processes: Looking at the text in this paragraph, the words printed in **bold** "pop out" because they are more intensely colored than the rest. *Italicized* words within a paragraph also may pop out if they are **distinctly** different from the surrounding font. In the grocery store, if there is only one kind of salsa that has a **yellow** label, that one will pop out from the others nearby on the shelf. If, however, there are multiple brands with similarly colored labels, then you must also consider the shape of the jar (*conjoined cues*—color and shape), which will slow down the search process. Similarly, in a letter cancellation task, a curvy letter (e.g., S) in the midst of angled letters (X, Y, T) may **pop out**, whereas searching for an angled letter (e.g., N) in the midst of other angled letters will require a slower, more methodical search.

DAN and the VAN are supramodal networks, meaning that they control attention to various modalities (e.g., visual, auditory, tactile) (Braga, Wilson, Sharp, Wise, & Leech, 2013).

The attentional networks subserve three functional components of attention: orienting, alerting, and executive control. Orienting refers to selecting and focusing on a stimulus. It has been linked to both the DAN and the VAN (Corbetta et al., 2008; Joseph, Fricker, & Keehn, 2015; Xuan et al., 2016). Alerting serves to increase the activation within the attentional system in preparation to locate or fixate on a target. Tonic alertness refers to the internally driven system that fluctuates relatively slowly, over minutes or hours. It is considered to be controlled by the DAN in conjunction with a broad-based noradrenergic system (networks of neurons that respond to the neurotransmitter norepinephrine) centered in the locus coeruleus (Asanowicz et al., 2012; Xuan et al., 2016). Maintenance of a high level of alertness has been compared to sustained attention (Degutis & VanVleet, 2010). In contrast, phasic alertness is a rapid and short-lived change usually driven by an external stimulus. It is controlled by the VAN (Asanowicz et al., 2010) in conjunction with left frontal and thalamic regions. Phasic alertness is important for orienting and selective attention (Alho et al., 2015; Degutis & VanVleet, 2010). Executive control has been linked to the dorsolateral prefrontal cortex, anterior cingulate gyrus, basal ganglia, thalamus, and cerebellum (Xuan et al., 2012). The frontal systems feed into modality-specific areas (e.g., temporal lobe for auditory stimuli, occipital lobe for visual) (Green, Doesburg, Ward, &

McDonald, 2011). Additionally, the posterior parietal lobes are important for conscious or controlled shifting of attention between items held in working memory (WM; Berryhill, Chein, & Olson, 2012). Just as with the networks, the three attentional components are separate yet interactional. For example, an alerting auditory stimulus can increase speed of orienting and responding to a subsequent visual target (Chica et al., 2012).

In this book, WM is discussed as a memory process (Chapter 10) as well as a component of executive function (Chapter 8), but it also has been conceived as part of attentional processes. There is extensive overlap in the functions of the WM and attentional systems. Both involve maintaining activation over time (as temporary storage and sustained attention) and have executive control components. Similar to the attentional control, the WM central executive has been described as the mechanism for selecting targets to be attended to and allocating or shifting attention between concurrent tasks or activities, particularly in reference to divided attention. In addition to the functional similarities, there is overlap between the anatomical networks for sustained attention and working memory (Awh & Jonides, 2001; Huang, Seidman, Rossi, & Ahveninen, 2013; Majerus et al., 2012; Soto, Rotshtein, & Kanai, 2014).

Limited Capacity of Attention

One critical feature of the human attentional system is that it has a limited capacity. The human brain cannot attend to the multitude of external sensory stimuli (e.g., somatosensory, auditory, visual, gustatory, olfactory) and internal thoughts that exist at any one point in time. Several neural mechanisms aid in solving this problem. One is habituation. A basic physiological process, habituation occurs in the presence of a constant stimulus. Fast-adapting sensory neurons respond when a stimulus begins, ends, or otherwise changes, but stop firing in the continuous presence of the stimulus. One might hear the air conditioning turn on, but then the auditory system habituates to the noise, and you are no longer consciously aware that it is on until the system turns off, and the change is noted. Habituation limits the sensory stimuli that reach the level of conscious processing. A second mechanism is a cognitive attentional filtering process. Although questions remain about specifically how and when the attentional filter works, the prevailing understanding is that all sensory stimuli are processed at a basic level and temporarily preserved in an attenuated state. Only the most important or salient are selected for further processing. Those that are filtered out are transiently available for higher-level processing if they become important (e.g., Treisman, 2009; see Wolfe & Robertson, 2012, for a collection of Treisman's extensive work on visual attention and perception).

Within the limited capacity, there may be separate "pools" of attentional resources for different tasks (e.g., language, motor, visuospatial). This helps explain why it is possible to divide attention between two different kinds of tasks but not between two tasks that require the same type of processing (e.g., language processing required for both talking on the phone and checking e-mail). One way this has been examined is through the use of divided attention methods in which participants are asked to complete two tasks at the same time. Performance is affected by several factors. First is the similarity of the tasks (see sidebar). Two tasks that require the same cognitive process (e.g., two language tasks) are more difficult to complete than different tasks (e.g., a language and a motor task) because they compete for the same "pool" of cognitive resources. Second is the similarity of the responses. Obviously, two tasks that require a similar response (e.g., must respond verbally to both) will be more difficult than when different responses are required (e.g., a verbal and a manual response) because similar responses must be temporally ordered. Finally is the level of automaticity of the tasks. A relatively automatic task that requires little conscious control and few attentional resources often can be conducted successfully even in the presence of a more demanding task that requires controlled cognitive processing. Experienced drivers generally have no difficulty carrying on a conversation while driving because the driving process has become automatic. If there are extreme weather conditions or if the driver gets lost, however, she may have to allocate more attention to the driving process and can no longer spare enough attention to continue the conversation. Two automatic tasks will be relatively easy to complete successfully; it is extremely difficult to conduct two cognitively demanding tasks concurrently.

An interesting phenomenon related to limited attention capacity is inattentional blindness (e.g., Simons & Chabris, 1999; Simons, 2000). This occurs when visual items that are not attended to are not reported as being seen. In Simon's classic experiment, when given a sustained atten-

---

SIDEBAR

Frequently, I can be found quilting during long meetings. The quilting I bring to meetings requires only motor control (moving the needle in and out of the fabric), allowing me to listen to the speaker (language processing) while keeping my hands busy (motor task). I rarely can crochet during a meeting, because most crochet patterns (at least for me) require counting stitches. I cannot count (language processing) and keep track of my stitches (WM) at the same time I am trying to listen (language processing involving WM).

---

tion task (count how many times a basketball is passed between several people), 50% of young adults failed to see a person in a gorilla suit walk through the scene. The work on inattentional blindness reveals that when attention is focused, even unexpected novel stimuli may fail to capture attention. Inattentional deafness has also been reported. For example, focused attention on a visuospatial task decreases the likelihood that an auditory stimulus will be detected (Dalton & Fraenkel, 2012; MacDonald & Lavie, 2011).

These concepts of limited capacity, attentional resources, top-down versus bottom-up processing, and automaticity of tasks are important for understanding the strengths and weaknesses of clients with RHD and how performance can vary under different conditions. These will be discussed in relation to treatment, particularly for unilateral neglect (see Chapter 7).

Clinical Classifications of Attention

Clinically, attention is often classified into several types: focused, selective, sus-

tained, alternating, and divided (Sohlberg & Mateer, 2001).

- Focused: attention to a specific stimulus in the absence of distractors. Controlled by the DAN.

- Selective: attention to one stimulus in the presence of distractors. Requires selection and orientation to the target and inhibition of distractors, which can be either internal (intruding thoughts) or external stimuli. Good selective attention has been called "freedom from distractibility." Controlled by the DAN, with suppression of the VAN to maintain focus.

- Sustained: either focused or selective attention over time. Time-on-task effects are measured to assess the consistency of attention over time. Typically, either speed or accuracy of responses decreases over time. Controlled primarily by the right frontal and parietal lobes, with input from regions of the brainstem and thalamus.

- Alternating: switching attention between two different stimuli.

Orienting, shifting, and reengaging are critical for alternating attention.

■ Divided: attending to two different stimuli/tasks at the same time. As described above, successful divided attention generally is possible only when the tasks use different kinds of processing (e.g., a language and a motor task) and/or when at least one of the tasks is relatively automatic.

Attention and the Intact RH

While attention is controlled by both sides of the brain, the right hemisphere has a greater role particularly in relation to the VAN and attention to stimulus-driven orienting (Chechlacz, Gillebert, Vangkilde, Petersen, & Humphreys, 2015; Corbetta et al., 2008; Smigasiewicz, Asanowicz, Westphal, & Verleger, 2014; Spotorno & Faure, 2011). Additionally, the RH attentional bias is greater for attention to near space than to more distant space (Longo, Trippier, Vagnoni, & Lourenco, 2015).

The RH dominance theory of attention purports that the LH controls directed attention (attention to a specific region or area) to the right side of space, whereas the RH can control attention to both the right and left regions (Dietz, Friston, Mattingley, Roepstorff, & Garrido, 2014; Duecker, Formisano, & Sack, 2013; Filley, 2002; Heilman & van den Abell, 1980). This theory is discussed in more detail in the following chapter. A recent study using functional MRI supported this theory of RH attentional bias, particularly for attentional control (Rosen, Stern, Michalka, Devaney, & Somers, 2015).

The orientation bias theory, in contrast, suggests that in the intact brain there is a balance between RH and LH attentional systems. Rapid shifts in hemispheric attention (shifting resources between hemispheres) have been found in normal attentional processes (Le, Stojanoski, Khan, & Keough, 2015). Disruption of the hemispheric balance, either by damage (e.g., Corbetta et al., 2008) or by magnetic stimulation (Plow et al., 2014), results in attentional deficits.

Attention After Stroke or Traumatic Brain Injury

Deficits in attention are not uncommon after stroke (Barker-Collo, Feigin, Lawes, Parag, & Senior, 2010; Duffin et al., 2012; Hochstenbach, Mulder, Limbeek, & Donders, 1998; Hyndman, Pickering, & Ashburn, 2007; Srikanth et al., 2003). Estimates of incidence range up to 75% of stroke survivors (Hochstenbach et al., 1998), with approximately equal rates for RH and LH stroke. Hyndman and colleagues (2007) examined different forms of attention in their participants with stroke. Approximately half of their patients had impairments in divided attention, and slightly over 35% had problems with sustained attention and selective attention in auditory and visual modalities. Murakami and colleagues (2014) reported that while visual attention deficits were more common after RHD, other forms of attentional deficits were more strongly related to LHD.

Following traumatic brain injury, the functional connectivity of the DMN can be altered. The extent of disruption between regions of the DMN is related to the presence and chronicity of attentional impairments (Bonnelle et al., 2011). Damage to the right parietal lobe can result in problems with attending to temporal events, specifically rapidly changing events (Tyler, Dasgupta, Agosta, Battelli, & Grossman, 2015). Brain injury can affect any of the types of attention (e.g., selective, sustained, alternating), although the more complex types (alternating and divided) are more likely to be affected than the "simpler" types.

Brain damage can affect either attentional capacity or the ability to allocate attention. If capacity is diminished, there are fewer attentional resources available. A phenomenon called "attentional blink" has been used as a measure of attentional capacity (Shapiro, Arnell, & Raymond, 1997). When two stimuli are presented close in time (e.g., less than 500 milliseconds apart), the second may not be reported if there is not enough attentional capacity "left over" to process it. The more complex the first stimulus (i.e., the more attentionally demanding), the more time is needed before a second stimulus can be processed. RHD can cause an increase in the attentional blink (Shulman et al., 2010), indicating a reduction in attentional capacity. The attentional blink also has been used to examine the size of space to which attention can be distributed. After RHD, attention may be limited to a smaller region of space, and focused attention to a central region can reduce the detection of targets presented laterally (Russell, Malhotra, Deidda, & Husain, 2013). Essentially, when adults with RHD focus on one region, they are more likely to miss stimuli outside of that specific region because they do not have enough capacity to spread attention beyond the focused area.

Alternatively, allocation of attention can be affected. Even if the overall attentional capacity was not decreased as a result of the stroke or brain injury, the client may not be able to effectively determine how much attention is needed for a given task, or be able to engage enough attentional resources to accurately complete a task. Compounding the problem, tasks that used to be automatic may require more attention following brain injury. The client has to then allocate more attention than he previously did in order to get the same result (see sidebar).

SIDEBAR

In her book *Over My Head: A Doctor's Own Story of Head Injury from the Inside Looking Out* (2002), Claudia Osborne describes her difficulty in efficiently getting dressed by explaining that it used to be automatic for her, as it is for most adults. Since her head injury she now has to think about every step of the process, and if she gets distracted and misses a step, the whole activity can get messed up (e.g., putting on shoes before pants). Success requires recognizing that more attention is needed for tasks that used to be automatic, allocating enough attention to complete each step of the process, and resisting distraction or checking for errors before beginning each subsequent step.

Clinically, attentional deficits can present as disinhibition, distractibility, impulsivity, slowed processing or response times, or perseverations (Sohlberg & Mateer, 2001). They can have substantial impact on recovery. Attentional deficits are related to poorer functional outcomes (see Chapter 1, Table 1–2), including poorer performance on activities of daily living (ADLs), general cognitive function, mobility and balance, as well as quality of life (Barker-Collo, Feigin, Lawes, & Senior Parag, 2010; Hyndman et al., 2007; Pearce, Stolwyk, New, & Anderson, 2016; van Zandvoort, Kessels, Nys, de Haan, & Kappelle, 2005).

Attention After RHD

Most of the research on attentional deficits following RHD has focused on unilateral neglect, and will be discussed in detail in Chapter 7. Studies specifically examining adults with RHD have reported deficits in sustained attention (Robertson, 2001; Robertson et al., 1997; Rueckert & Grafman, 1996; Saldert & Ahlsén, 2007) and attentional capacity, as measured by attentional blink (Russell et al., 2013). In contrast, Habekost and Rostrup (2007) reported no change in capacity of visual attention, but decreased processing speed during attentional tasks.

Attentional deficits associated with RHD have been suggested to affect pragmatics, language, and other communication abilities (Monetta, Ouellet-Plamondon, & Joanette, 2006; Saldert & Ahlsén, 2007) as well as unilateral neglect (Robertson, 2001; Robertson et al., 1997).

Assessment of Attention

A variety of tests have been designed to measure attention (Table 6–2). The tests vary in terms of what kind of attention is assessed and in which modalities. In addition to standardized tests, observations can provide a wealth of information about attentional abilities. Clinicians should observe clients in both quiet and noisy settings to get a sense of selective attention. Observing clients completing tasks that they find interesting versus those that are boring can provide information about their potential for focusing attention. Structured interviews of both clients and caregivers can provide additional information. Clients often will report being distracted, having difficulty concentrating, being unable to do two things at once, or being forgetful (as discussed in Chapter 10, attention is the first requirement for encoding memories).

Treatment of Attentional Disorders

Systematic reviews sponsored by government agencies and/or conducted by independent researchers suggest that in general, there are limited gains from treatment of attentional deficits related to TBI or stroke (Brasure et al., 2012; Cicerone et al., 2011; IOM, 2011; Park & Ingles, 2001; SIGN, 2013). These bleak conclusions are due in part to the limited number of randomized control trials (RCTs) from which to draw conclusions. Reviews that accept a broader group of studies, such as

Table 6–2. Select Assessments of Attention

Test	Authors	Domains Assessed	Reliability*	Validity*
Brief Test of Attention	Schretlen et al., 1996, 1997	Auditory divided attention	OK	Good
Moss Attention Rating Scale	Hart et al., 2009	Observation of behaviors indicative of attention deficits	None	Weak
Paced Auditory Serial Addition Test	Gronwall, 1977	Divided and sustained attention (also working memory, information processing speed)	Good	Good
Rating Scale of Attentional Behavior	Ponsford & Kinsella, 1991	Observational rating of behaviors indicative of attentional deficits	OK	OK
Ruff Selective Attention Test	Ruff, 1992	Sustained and selective visual attention	Good	Weak
Sustained Attention to Response Task	Robertson et al., 1997	Sustained attention	OK	Good
Symbol Digit Modalities Test	Smith 1973	Divided visual attention, processing speed	OK for alternate forms	Weak
Test of Everyday Attention	Robertson et al., 1994	Visual selective attention/ speed, attention switching, sustained attention, auditory-verbal working memory	Weak	Good

Note. *Good = moderate–strong estimates of two or more types of reliability/validity; OK = moderate–strong estimates of one type of reliability/validity or mixture of weak and strong estimates; weak = weak estimates of one or more types of reliability/validity; none = no estimates reported. See Appendix for detailed information about reliability and validity.

experimentally controlled group designs and controlled multiple baseline across subject studies (see Chapter 2 for discussion of systematic reviews and levels of evidence), provide a more positive outlook on attention treatment. Cicerone and colleagues (2011) generated treatment recommendations following an examination of existing evidence. Their three recommendation categories include: *practice standards* based on substantive evidence of effectiveness, *practice guidelines* based on evidence of probable effectiveness, and *practice options* based on evidence of possible effectiveness. Their recommendations, derived primarily from studies of adults with TBI, are provided in Table 6–3. Although etiology (stroke versus TBI) is not always considered an important factor, in one review (Virk, Williams, Brunsdon, Suh, & Morrow, 2015) differential results were found for groups of stroke survivors compared with individuals with TBI, suggesting that the etiology of the deficits may play a role in the response to treatment.

Broad-Based Treatment Approaches

Chen and Novakovic-Agopian and colleagues (Chen et al., 2011; Novakovic-Agopian et al., 2010) reported positive effects of an attentional control treatment that included aspects of metacognitive strategies, mindfulness meditation, and problem-solving approaches. Exercises in

the treatment program included reducing distractibility, using aspects of mindfulness training to redirect attention when needed, identification of relevant versus irrelevant information, and maintenance of relevant information in working memory. Following treatment, gains were observed not only on attention and executive control tasks, but also on memory and psychomotor speed.

In a systematic review and meta-analysis of attention treatments for adults with TBI or stroke, Virk and colleagues (2015) reported limited benefits. They focused on RCTs and found 12 studies that fit their criteria. Treatments for selective, sustained, alternating, and divided attention were assessed separately. The only significant treatment benefit was in divided attention for adults with stroke. This benefit was only seen, however, for immediate treatment gains and was not maintained over time.

Table 6–3. Recommendations for Treatment of Attention

Recommendation Level	Treatment for Attention
Practice standards	• Metacognitive strategy training to develop compensatory strategies and facilitate generalization to functional activities • Direct attention training in the post-acute period of recovery
Practice guidelines	None
Practice options	• Combining computerized treatment with behavioral treatment • Isolated computer treatments NOT recommended

Note. Practice standards are based on substantive evidence of effectiveness, practice guidelines are based on evidence of probable effectiveness, and practice options are based on evidence of possible effectiveness.

Source: Based on Cicerone et al., 2011.

Direct Treatment

The most efficacious and effective treatments for the majority of cognitive deficits are compensatory approaches. As described in other chapters, restorative (direct) treatments for memory (Chapter 10) and executive function (Chapter 8) are generally not very effective, while compensatory strategies can result in strong positive gains. The rehabilitation of attention is one of the few exceptions to this pattern. There is evidence that direct, restorative treatments can result in immediate, impairment-level improvements. Direct treatment has been recommended as a practice guideline for adults with attentional deficits related to acquired brain injury who are in the chronic phase of recovery (Cicerone et al., 2011; Sohlberg et al., 2003). However, there is limited generalization to functional tasks, and there is not enough evidence to suggest that it is effective in the acute phase of recovery from TBI.

The most commonly studied direct attention training program is Attention Process Training (APT; Sohlberg & Mateer, 2011). This program is based on the theories of attentional function and subtypes (e.g., focused, sustained, alternating, divided), uses a hierarchy of difficulty, and can be individualized to (a) begin treatment at the lowest level of difficulty for a given patient and (b) progress through levels based on mastery. Both visual and auditory attention tasks are included. Several studies of APT have demonstrated immediate gains on a variety of attention processes and executive function (Sohlberg, McLaughlin, Pavese, Heidrich, &

Posner, 2000; see also reviews by Cicerone et al., 2011; MacDonald & Wiseman-Hakes, 2010; Park & Ingles, 2001; Sohlberg et al., 2003). Clients most likely to benefit from direct attention treatment have good vigilance (sustained attention) and relatively mild attentional deficits (Sohlberg et al., 2003).

Reports of generalization to functional tasks are inconsistent (Zickefoose, Hux, Brown, & Wulf, 2013; see also reviews by Cicerone et al., 2011; MacDonald & Wiseman-Hakes, 2010; Sohlberg et al., 2003; SIGN, 2013). Sohlberg and colleagues (2003) recommended that metacognitive strategies focusing on feedback, self-monitoring, and development of compensatory strategies should be used in conjunction with APT in order to facilitate generalization to functional tasks and settings.

Sturm and colleagues (Sturm & Willmes, 1991; Sturm, Willmes, Orgass, & Hartje, 1997; Sturm et al., 2004) reported some gains from computerized attention training programs. Generally, the gains are specific to the type(s) of attention trained and do not generalize to untrained forms of attention. Adults with LHD tend to show greater gains than those with RHD (Sturm & Willmes, 1991). Physiological changes to the DAN were observed for adults with RHD who responded positively to the treatment (Sturm et al., 2004).

Metacognitive Strategies

Metacognitive strategies are systems for breaking problems into smaller steps to achieve a goal. They are described in greater detail in reference to executive functions in Chapter 8. There is some evidence that they can be effective components of treatment for attentional deficits (e.g., Cicerone et al., 2011; Sohlberg & Turkstra, 2011). Metacognitive strategies generally involve setting a goal, devising a plan to reach that goal, self-monitoring performance, and reviewing results. Self-instructional statements to facilitate sustained attention to task such as "focus on what is being said," "ignore intrusive thoughts," and "don't get distracted by irrelevant sounds" may be useful for certain clients.

Metacognitive strategies, as well as compensatory strategies discussed below, may affect impairment levels if they become automatic enough (e.g., Sohlberg & Turkstra, 2011). In essence they improve attentional functioning once the compensatory behavior becomes second nature. Additionally, strategies can be created to directly affect activity and participation levels. If a client has difficulty reading the morning newspaper due to deficits in sustained attention, a strategy for identifying specific articles, planning breaks as necessary depending on the length, and prioritizing the articles to create an order in which to read them may result in positive gains for this particular activity.

Compensatory Strategies

Compensatory strategies may be helpful in reducing the effects of attentional deficits on performance. Such strategies often are embedded in broader cognitive rehabilitation programs, so there is no evidence of efficacy for any one strategy. As with any strategy, to maximize the effectiveness, clinicians must match the strategy to the specific deficit(s) being targeted, engage the client in the development of the strategy to encourage ownership, make sure that the strategy is feasible given the client's cognitive and physical abilities, and measure its effectiveness.

Pacing can be used for clients with sustained attention deficits. This can include developing (a) realistic goals of productivity and time on task given how long attention can be sustained and/or (b) creating a structure for breaking tasks into steps with breaks scheduled in-between. For example, it may not be realistic to expect a client to focus attention for 10 to 15 minutes to complete an activity. The activity can be broken up into sets of steps that each can be completed within 3 to 5 minutes, with a short break planned in-between each step.

A key ideas log also can be effective in reducing the effects of distractibility and poor sustained attention in some clients (Sohlberg & Mateer, 2001). The purpose is to facilitate maintenance of attention on the task at hand by minimizing the effects of distractions. For some clients, ideas or questions may pop into their minds in the midst of a task. Relevant questions can be asked, but irrelevant or tangential questions will cause an interruption and shift focus away from the primary task. Some individuals may not be able to ignore the idea or question, and thus will not be able to maintain attention on the primary task. The log is simply a place in which the client can write down ideas or questions that come to mind. Once the idea is written down, the client can shift back to focusing on the primary task and can be

---

SIDEBAR

A client with moderate attentional, executive function and communication deficits related to RHD had significant difficulty staying on task. He would frequently get distracted by external stimuli (art on the wall, the color of the clinician's fingernail polish) or internal stimuli (an idea that he had been considering prior to the therapy session). Therapy activities were commonly interrupted by his comments about the external or internal distractors. The clinician began using a key ideas log. At the beginning of each session, she asked him to write down any ideas that were swimming in his head or things he wanted to comment on. Items that could be dealt with quickly, such as noticing a new color of nail polish, were addressed at that time. Other items that might lead to a broader discussion were kept until later. The clinician promised to save 5 to 10 minutes at the end of the therapy session to discuss the other items. The key ideas log was kept on the table throughout the session, and if other thoughts or ideas (unrelated to therapy) came to his mind, he would write them down. The client was then able to focus on the therapy activities because he knew that (a) he would not forget to mention the ideas he felt were important and (b) he would be given time to talk about them. The introduction of the key ideas log substantially reduced the negative effects of distractibility in the therapy setting. The client and his wife also began using a key ideas log during conversations at home to facilitate keeping the conversation on track.

---

sure that the idea will not be forgotten (see sidebar).

Education and Environmental Manipulation

Education of clients and families and changes to the environment can minimize the negative effects of attentional deficits. As noted at the beginning of the chapter, everyone has experiences with attention and challenges to attention, which in some ways makes educating families about attentional deficits easier than other kinds of deficits that are more abstract. Still, it is important for families to understand the extent to which attention can be affected and that there are different forms of attentional deficits. Clients and their families/caregivers should be educated about what kinds of attention are affected and explore what situations/environments/tasks will tend to be more difficult depending on the type and severity of attentional deficits. They can then use that information to avoid or modify settings that might cause problems (e.g., noisy restaurants, having a TV on in the background), or create realistic expectations for time on task or amount of work that can be done in one sitting. Identifying what times of day are "good" times, when the client is least likely to be fatigued and best able to concentrate, can help them to plan when to schedule important tasks or conversations.

Other environmental modifications can include using Do Not Disturb signs when the client is working on attentionally demanding tasks, removing auditory distractors (e.g., turning off the radio when working or conversing), and organizing personal spaces to remove physical or visual distractors.

Conclusions and Implications

Attentional deficits are common consequences of RHD and have substantial negative effects on prognosis and recovery. Attentional deficits are well understood and there is fairly good evidence for metacognitive and compensatory treatment strategies from the brain injury literature. Exploration of potential differences in attentional deficits and responses to treatment dependent upon etiology (RHD versus TBI) are needed to increase confidence in the use of treatments designed for adults with attentional deficits due to TBI.

7

Unilateral Neglect

Unilateral neglect (UN), also called hemispatial neglect, hemi-inattention, hemineglect, or simply neglect, is a reduction in the processing of and response to contralesional stimuli. It can affect the ability to perceive, attend to, orient to, explore, respond to, act on, or represent stimuli from the contralesional side. UN has been extensively studied and is the most researched disorder associated with right hemisphere brain damage (RHD). This chapter will cover the theories and characteristics of UN, the various types, and some related disorders that frequently co-occur with UN but should be treated as separate problems and not aspects of UN itself. Given the extensive research on UN, there are more assessment tools and evidence-based treatments than for other disorders associated with RHD.

Unilateral Neglect

The most widely accepted theory posits that UN is a disorder of directed attention; other theories of perceptual, representa-

tional, and sensorimotor transformational deficits have been proposed and provide explanations for some phenomena that do not fit with the attentional account (see Kerkhoff, 2001 for a review).

UN is not a unitary phenomenon, nor is it "all or nothing"; there are multiple forms of neglect which can vary in terms of severity across time and tasks (Baldassari et al., 2014; Harvey & Rossit, 2012; Rorden et al., 2012). Proposed core features of UN include an ipsilesional bias of attention and movement and a generalized deficit in attentional processes (e.g., focused or sustained attention; Baldassare et al., 2014; Rorden et al., 2012; Robertson, 2001). Lateralized deficits in representation (e.g., imagining a scene or location) also can occur.

Bartolomeo and colleagues (e.g., Bartolomeo & Chokron, 2002; Bartolomeo, Siéroff, Decaix, & Chokron, 2001) conclude that UN is characterized primarily by deficits in exogenous, or reflexive stimulus-driven orienting of attention, while endogenous, or voluntary strategy-driven orienting is relatively preserved. Thus, individuals with left UN may have a reflexive, magnetic attraction to stimuli in the right side of space but may be able to use strategies to reduce this reflexive orienting. Strategies do not always work, however, as endogenous orienting often is slowed after RHD, thus making it less likely that it can be useful in functional, daily activities (Bartolomeo & Chokron, 2002).

UN can affect a variety of modalities, including auditory, visual, tactile, and olfactory. Movement also can be affected, resulting in motor neglect. Focal damage to either hemisphere can cause UN. According to some estimates, right and left neglect (caused by left hemisphere brain damage [LHD] and RHD, respectively) occur at the same frequency (e.g., Bowen, McKenna, & Tallis, 1999), while a large disparity is reported in other studies (Azouvi et al., 2006; Becker & Karnath, 2007; Pederson, Jorgensen, Nakayama,

Raaschou, & Olsen, 1997; Stone et al., 1991) with right neglect occurring approximately half as often as left neglect. Azouvi and colleagues (2006), despite reporting a large discrepancy overall (44% of LHD cases and 85% of RHD), found that extra personal neglect occurred equally as often in LHD than in RHD (see summary in Table 7–1). Clinically, right neglect resulting from LHD is not often assessed or reported. This may be in part because right neglect tends to be less severe and often resolves quickly (Mesulam, 1981; Bowen et al., 1999), or because right neglect is masked by deficits such as aphasia (Bowen et al., 1999). Another reason may be that medical professionals do not expect UN to occur with LHD, and so do not often look for it.

Patients with UN are sometimes described as "ignoring" things on their affected side. This description is inaccurate and can be

Table 7–1. Incidence of Unilateral Neglect Following Right or Left Hemisphere Stroke

	RHD	LHD
Peripersonal or Unspecified Neglect		
Azouvi et al., 2006	19–85%	4–44%
Barker-Collo et al., 2010	24%	14%
Becker & Karnath, 2007	26.2%	2.4%
Bowen et al., 1999	13–82%	0–76%
Pederson et al., 1997	85%	39%
Stone et al., 1991	72%	62%
Personal Neglect		
Azouvi et al., 2006	16%	9%
Extrapersonal Neglect		
Azouvi et al., 2006	13%	13%

quite misleading to patients and families. In order to ignore something, one must be aware of it and consciously attempt to *not* attend to it. In the case of UN, patients are not fully aware of stimuli or movements on the contralateral side. It is important that families understand that the patient is not willfully ignoring things but rather is unable to easily attend to and process them.

UN has a substantial impact on recovery and eventual outcomes from stroke (see Chapter 1, Table 1–2). The presence of UN has been linked to reduced functional ability, overall greater impairment and disability, reduced independence, poorer prognosis for personal and instrumental activities of daily living, longer rehabilitation stays, reduced participation in rehabilitation, and slower progress in rehabilitation according to Functional Independence Measures of efficiency and effectiveness (e.g., Arene & Hillis, 2009; Azouvi et al., 1996; Di Monaco et al., 2011; Matano, Iosa, Guariglia, Pizzamiglio, & Paolucci, 2015; Punt & Riddoch, 2006).

Directed Attention and the Intact RH

Kinsbourne (1970) first proposed that the hemispheres directed attention to the opposite region of space and that damage to one hemisphere would result in an imbalance and attentional focus shifted to the ipsilesional side of space. In contrast, the RH dominance theory of attention suggests that the RH directs attention to both the right and left regions of space, while the LH directs attention only contralater-

ally to the right side of space (Dietz et al., 2014; Duecker et al., 2013; Filley, 2002; Heilman & van den Abell, 1980). This imbalance explains the clinical presentation of unilateral neglect and why left neglect is more common than right neglect. Damage to the LH can cause reduced attention to the right side of space, but this generally is not as severe and tends to resolve quickly because the RH attentional control serves as a "backup." In contrast, damage to the RH attentional systems can cause inattention to the left side of space that is more severe and less likely to resolve spontaneously because the LH cannot direct attention to the left side of space.

Several explanations of UN have been proposed based on hypothesized damage to the attentional networks (Baldassarre et al., 2014; He et al., 2007; Ptak & Schnider, 2011; Shulman et al., 2010; Smith et al., 2013). Difficulties ignoring distractors that are irrelevant to the task could be caused by interruption of the Dorsal Attentional Network (DAN; Ptak & Schnider, 2010). Alternatively, damage to the Ventral Attentional Network (VAN) could cause generalized attentional deficits and indirectly affect the functioning of the right hemispheric DAN, which results in left-sided UN (He et al., 2007; Shulman et al., 2010). Given that UN can be caused by interruptions to the attentional networks, it is not surprising that nonspatial attentional deficits often co-occur with UN (e.g., Butler, Lawrence, Eskes, & Klein, 2009).

Other explanations of UN are based on alterations of the interhemispheric connections. Corbetta et al. (2008) suggested that neglect results from an imbalance between the RH and LH attentional systems, which have some inhibitory control over each other. Damage to the right parietal lobe may result in hyperactivation of LH parietal areas (due to loss of RH inhibition), resulting in increased attention or "magnetic attraction" to the right side and neglect of the left side of space. Linking such ideas to physiology, Umarova and colleagues (2014) reported that decreased functional connectivity within the white matter of the unlesioned LH was associated with persistent neglect.

Finally, Karnath (2015) suggests that UN results in impairment of stimulus-driven attention and an alteration of body representation such that the body representation in space is shifted to one side.

Unilateral Neglect After RHD

UN has been linked to lesions in various areas of the RH, including the parietal lobe, temporoparietal junction, frontal lobe, thalamus, basal ganglia, and subcortical white matter (Arene & Hillis, 2007; Azouvi et al., 2002; Bartolomeo, de Schotten, & Doricchi, 2007; Buxbaum et al., 2004; Hillis et al., 2005; Karnath, Fruhmann Berger, Küker, & Rorden, 2004; Karnath & Rorden, 2012; Mesulam, 1981, 1985; Vallar, 1993; Vallar & Perani, 1986). The key factor is likely not damage to a specific structure, but rather disruption of the attentional networks (Bartolomeo et al., 2007; He et al., 2007; Shulman et al., 2010). The extent of leukoaraiosis, or white matter hyperintensities, has been associated with both the presence and the severity of unilateral neglect (Bahrainwala, Hillis, Dearborn, & Gottesman, 2014). Additionally, degenerating conditions that affect the right fron-

toparietal networks can result in unilateral neglect (Andrade et al., 2012).

The vast majority of research has been on left visuospatial neglect, which appears to be the most common form (compared with right neglect or neglect within other modalities). Thus, the examples provided throughout the rest of this chapter will nearly always reflect that. Unless otherwise specified, the left visual field can be assumed to be the contralesional visual space, and ipsilesional attentional bias refers to the right side of space.

Co-Occurring Disorders

There are several disorders that commonly co-occur with UN. In some cases, as with anosognosia (reduced awareness of deficits), the problems are conflated: some people consider reduced awareness a component of UN. There is good evidence, however, that the disorders described here (anosognosia, extinction, and hemianopsia) are not simply components of UN. Visual field cuts (hemianopsias) are included here to emphasize the differences between hemianopsia and UN both anatomically and in terms of clinical practice.

Anosognosia

Anosognosia, or reduced awareness of deficits (covered extensively in Chapter 9), frequently co-occurs with neglect. In a study of over 270 patients with first-time stroke, Appelros and colleagues (Appelros, Karlsson, & Hennerdal, 2007) reported that while 23% had UN, 17% had anosognosia and just under 10% had both. Anosognosia for neglect is more common with left neglect arising from RHD than for right neglect associated with LHD (Azouvi et al., 2006).

Extinction

Extinction occurs when a lateralized stimulus is perceived in isolation, but not when bilateral stimuli are presented simultaneously. Neurologists commonly use a finger wiggle test to assess visual extinction. The index finger of each hand is held within the patient's peripheral visual fields. The patient is asked to focus on the examiner's nose and report when he/she sees movement (wiggling) of one or both fingers. A patient with extinction will detect movement in both the right and left visual fields individually, but if both fingers move at once (called double simultaneous stimulation), the movement in the contralateral visual field will not be perceived. Extinction can occur within a modality (e.g., extinction of one of two visual or auditory stimuli), or across modalities: a right-sided tactile stimulus can cause extinction of a left-sided visual stimulus (Mattingley, Driver, Beschin, & Robertson, 1997). Similar to neglect, extinction is considered a deficit of attention (de Haan, Karnath, & Driver, 2012; de Haan, Stoll, & Karnath, 2015; Vuilleumier, Schwartz, Husain, Clarke, & Driver, 2001; Weinstein, 1994). It occurs at about the same frequency as visuospatial neglect and is more common after RHD than LHD (Becker & Karnath, 2007; Chechlacz, Rotshtein, Demeyere, Bickerton, & Humphreys, 2014).

Extinction is commonly associated with damage to the temporoparietal junction and/or the intraparietal sulcus (de Haan et al., 2012), and large cortical lesions have been associated with chronic extinction (Habekost & Rostrup, 2006). Compared with unilateral stimulation, bilateral stimulation requires increased activity of the RH VAN, plus bilateral parietal and visual association areas (Beume et al., 2015). However, both tactile and visual extinction have been found after strokes affecting the middle and posterior cerebral arteries (Chechlacz et al., 2014), suggesting that the ventral attentional network is not the sole location for such attentional processes.

Visual Field Cuts (Hemianopsia)

Hemianopsia, or a half-field visual field cut, can co-occur with visuospatial UN although it is not clear how often the co-occurrence is seen clinically. Visual field cuts are sensory impairments caused by damage to the neuronal pathways between the eye and the occipital lobe. The visual system is complicated, but the pathways can be described relatively simply. The right and left optic nerves extend posteriorly from the retinas into the cranium. At the optic chiasm, half of the nerve fibers from each eye cross over, while the remaining fibers stay ipsilateral. The result is that the images from the left visual field of each eye are carried to the right side of the brain, and the images from the right visual field (of each eye) end up in the left hemisphere. Lesions that occur posterior to the optic chiasm cause a homonymous visual field cut, meaning that the same part of the visual field (e.g., left or right region) is affected in each eye. A relatively small lesion can cause a homonymous quadrantanopsia, or loss of one quadrant of each visual field. A larger lesion can cause a homonymous hemianopsia, or loss of half of the visual field in each eye. Damage to the RH can result in loss of the left visual field of each eye (left homonymous hemianopsia). That means that if a patient closes his left eye, he can see only the right visual field from that eye. If he closes only his right eye, again he sees only the right visual field from that eye.

Given that UN and homonymous hemianopsia both can result from RHD and can co-occur, it is important to be able to differentiate them. A client with only homonymous hemianopsia will be aware of the visual impairment, be able to report it, and be able to compensate for it. In contrast, individuals with UN may not be aware of the deficit and/or may not spontaneously compensate for it. If neglect is present, it may be difficult to observe or diagnose the hemianopsia. Collaboration with neurologists and neuro-ophthalmologists is important for the diagnosis of visual field cuts.

Characteristics of Unilateral Neglect

Orientation Bias

A directional bias in gaze, visual search, and/or initiation of movement toward the ipsilateral space is considered by some to be a core component of UN (Rorden et al., 2012; Schindler, Clavagnier, Karnath, Derex, & Perenin, 2006). UN caused by RHD may reduce the ability to initiate a visual search or a movement into the left side of space (Harvey & Rossit, 2012; Husain, Mattingley, Rorden, Kennard, & Driver, 2000; Punt & Riddoch, 2006). Karnath and Dieterich (2006) suggest that the orienta-

tion bias associated with UN is caused by damage to a multimodal sensory processing region of the right parietal lobe. This region appears to be important for creation of body sense and the representation of one's body in space through integration of inputs from various sensory systems, including the visual and vestibular systems. At least one approach to treatment (see below) is based on this idea of a multimodal sensory region.

Magnetic Attraction

Some have described the attentional bias as a "magnetic attraction" to stimuli within the ipsilateral space (Bartolomeo & Chokron, 1999). In the case of left UN, attention is "stuck" on items or stimuli within the right visual field, and it is difficult to disengage attention in order to shift it to the opposite side (Posner, 1980; Posner, Walker, Friedrich, & Raphal, 1984). This was cleverly demonstrated by Mark, Kooistra, and Heilman (1988), who compared performance on a traditional cancellation task with a modified task in which the detected items were erased instead of cancelled. In the erasing task, the detected targets disappeared, leaving nothing to capture the attention on the right side, and allowing attention to be shifted leftward. Overall, the number of errors (undetected targets) decreased by two-thirds on the erasing compared with the cancellation task.

Unconscious Processing

Unlike a visual field cut in which items in the affected visual field are not processed even at a basic sensory level, items and features in the neglected region of space are unconsciously processed (e.g., Berti, Rizzolatti, & Umana, 1987; Driver & Mattingly, 1998; Kanne, 2002; Marshall & Halligan, 1988; Tamieto, Geminiani, Genero, & De Gelder, 2007; Vuilleumier et al., 2001; Vuilleumier, Schwartz, Clarke, Husain, & Driver, 2002). Results from priming studies suggest that features such as color and shape, word meanings, and even the identity of items can be processed in the absence of conscious recollection. Vuilleumier and colleagues (2002) conducted a study of repetition priming. Repetition priming occurs when individuals respond faster to an item that appeared previously (thus it is repeated) compared with an item that appeared only once. Adults with UN were shown a series of pictures presented in the left or right visual field. In some cases, two pictures were shown simultaneously, one in each visual field. Participants were asked to name the pictures seen. Participants with UN often did not report the pictures shown in the left visual field, particularly when they occurred along with pictures in the right visual field (extinction). In a second component of the study, the same participants were shown a series of fragmented pictures that they had to name/identify. Some of the pictures had been shown before, but others were new. Accuracy was better for pictures that had been presented in the first task, even if they had not been consciously processed (i.e., were not named when presented in the left visual field). The results indicated that the neglected items had been processed, even though the participants were not conscious of them. Semantic priming, or faster responses to words that follow a semantically related stimulus, also has been reported in adults with RHD (Driver & Mattingly, 1998; see illustration of semantic priming in Table 7–2).

Table 7–2. Illustrations of Semantic and Repetition Priming

Semantic Priming		
Stimuli	*Participants' Task*	*Result*
Pictures presented in either the right or left visual field followed by a centrally presented word	Push a button whenever you see a real word.	Button presses are faster in response to real words (tree) that follow a related picture (leaf) than those that follow an unrelated picture (house).
TREE		Responses to "tree" are faster after the leaf is presented, even when it appears in the neglected left space and the participants do not consciously recall seeing the leaf.

Stimulus Characteristics

Salient or relevant stimuli attract attention better than neutral stimuli. Emotionally laden pictures or words in the left visual field are more likely to be processed than neutral stimuli (e.g., Alpers, 2008; Grabowska et al., 2011). Lucas and Vuilleumier (2008) reported that adults with neglect were more accurate at identifying faces when there was an emotional facial expression than a neutral expression. Similarly, auditory extinction decreased when the stimulus coming from the left side was emotional prosody compared with neutral (Grandjean, Sander, Lucas, Scherer, & Vuilleumier, 2008).

Variability of Unilateral Neglect

Neglect is not an all-or-none phenomenon. As described above, the type of stimulus (e.g., emotional versus neutral) and the type of task (e.g., single item, double simultaneous stimulation, erasing versus cancellation) affect the ease of detecting and/or responding to items in the neglected visual field. Some individuals can direct or shift their attention to the neglected space when instructed to do so. Others exhibit excessive variability in how fast they respond to items in the neglected space (Anderson, Mennemeier, & Chatterjee, 2000), indicating that the ease of shifting attention is not necessarily consistent. Variability in severity of neglect also can change over time. This heterogeneity and the influence of task characteristics make assessment challenging, as will be discussed later in this chapter.

Scanning Characteristics

Individuals without UN tend to use a systematic, left-to-right pattern[1] of scanning during visuospatial tasks. In the presence of neglect, scanning is often disorganized or unsystematic, and includes more repetitions (e.g., re-cancelling items). These characteristics have been linked to various components of attention and UN, including a rightward attentional bias and reduced working memory (e.g., Butler et al., 2009).

Types of Unilateral Neglect

While visuospatial neglect is the most readily apparent clinically and has been studied the most extensively, UN also can affect auditory and tactile modalities. Additionally, patients with visuospatial neglect can exhibit motor neglect, or reduced use of the contralateral limbs. While in some cases only one modality is affected or dissociations between modalities are reported (e.g., Bisiach et al., 2004; Chokron et al., 2002; Kim et al., 2013; Laplane & Degos, 1983), in other studies UN affects multiple modalities, and relationships between types of UN are observed (e.g., Brozzoli, Demattè, Pavani, Frassinetti, & Farnè, 2006; Gainotti, 2010; Jacobs, Brozzoli, & Farnè, 2012; Pavani, Làdavas, & Driver, 2002; Schindler et al.,

---

[1]At least in languages with left-to-right reading patterns.

2006). Indeed, given the co-occurrence and interactions, some consider UN to be a multisensory disorder (e.g., Jacobs et al., 2012; Kerkhoff, 2001; Pavani et al., 2002).

Motor Neglect

Motor neglect is characterized by reduced use of contralateral limbs beyond what would be expected given any hemiparesis (Kim et al., 2013; Laplane & Degos, 1983). Estimates of incidence range from 8% to 75% (e.g., Sampanis & Riddoch, 2013). It is often assessed by observing how a person completes a bimanual task such as unscrewing the lid from a jar, lifting a large tray, propelling a wheelchair, or spontaneously gesturing. Motor neglect may be a result of damage to the motor intention system (Garbarini, Piedimonte, Dotta, Pia, & Berti, 2013). It is possible that the RH dominance for spatial attention and movement intention might explain why motor neglect is more common after RHD than LHD (Yan et al., 2012). Motor impersistence, or failure to maintain a position or movement, can be seen for leftward movements in patients with left motor neglect (Kim et al., 2013). As opposed to sensory forms of neglect, drawing a client's attention to the underutilization of the left side may result in improved movement (e.g., Laplane & Degos, 1983; Punt & Riddoch, 2006).

Tactile Neglect

Tactile neglect occurs when a person does not consciously process somatosensory stimulation on the contralesional side of the body, in the absence of a sensory defi-

cit that would prevent such processing. A variety of tasks have been used to assess tactile neglect, including estimation of rod lengths or marking the midline of a rod, grooved finger mazes, tactile search (e.g., find smooth versus rough patches on a board), and elevated shapes that can be identified with the fingertips (Beschin, Cazzani, Cubelli, Della Sala, & Spinazzola, 1996; Bisiach et al., 2004; Haeske-Dewick, Canavan, & Hömberg, 1996; Marsh & Hillis, 2008). Subtypes of tactile neglect have been identified, including allocentric (stimulus-centered) and egocentric (viewer-centered) forms (Marsh & Hillis, 2008).

There are varying estimates of the relative incidence of tactile neglect in relation to visuospatial neglect. Some suggest that tactile neglect is less common (Brozzoli et al., 2006; Fujii, Fukatsu, Kimura, Saso, & Kogure, 1991), while others report similar rates of occurrence (e.g., Bisiach et al., 2004; Marsh & Hillis, 2008). Gainotti (2010) reviewed 15 studies of visual and tactile neglect and found that while they tended to co-occur, visual UN was typically more severe than tactile (but see Vallar, Rusconi, Geminiani, & Berti, 1991).

Auditory Neglect

Auditory neglect is characterized by decreased response to, or processing of, auditory stimuli that arise from the contralesional region (Bisiach, Cornacchia, Sterzi, & Vallar, 1984; Pavani, Husain, Ladavas, & Driver, 2004). The deficits are more subtle than visuospatial neglect. First, poorer discrimination and identification typically occur only when there are bilateral stimuli. If sounds are presented only from the left side of space, identification and detection are often intact. However, if sounds are presented from both the right and left sides, auditory extinction may occur in which identification and detection will be less accurate for those sounds coming from the left (Pavani et al., 2004; Grandjean et al., 2008).

Auditory localization also can be affected. Adults with neglect can have difficulty localizing sounds, particularly those that arise from the left side of space but also when they differ along a vertical dimension (Guilbert et al., 2016; Pavani, 2002, 2004; Zimmer, Lewald, & Karnath, 2003). Auditory neglect has been shown to correlate with the severity of visuospatial neglect, suggesting that there is damage to a multimodal spatial attention system (Pavani et al., 2002).

Representational Neglect

Representational neglect, also called imaginal or imagery neglect, is a disorder of imagined spaces, locations, words, and/or objects. Salvato, Sedda, and Bottini (2014) provide a thorough review of the art and science of representational neglect since it was originally described by Bisiach and Luzzatti in 1978.

Representational neglect appears as difficulty describing locations (typically omitting landmarks or items on the contralesional side), drawing objects, or comparing imagined angles. It has been shown to be dissociated from visuospatial neglect, although the two forms commonly co-occur

(e.g., Vromen, Verbunt, Rasquin, & Wade, 2011). Clinically, representational neglect is not typically assessed, but estimates suggest it occurs in isolation in about 15% of adults with RHD and co-occurs with visuospatial neglect about 20% of the time.

Visuospatial Neglect

UN in the visual modality is the most researched form, and is the most common clinically. Estimates suggest that visuospatial neglect affects between 13 and 81% of patients with RHD (Barrett et al., 2006). The extremely large range is probably due to multiple factors. The most likely are timing and sensitivity of assessments. UN can spontaneously resolve within the first hours or days poststroke, and thus assessments beyond this point will underestimate the incidence. Individual assessment tasks, as will be discussed in more detail later in the chapter, vary widely in sensitivity to detect UN. Some individual tasks identify fewer than 25% of cases. Thus, if assessments occur several days after stroke and involve only one or two tasks, the likelihood of detecting UN will be substantially decreased.

There are several types of visuospatial neglect based on the region of space that is affected, and the frame of reference, or how "left" is defined (Table 7–3). In terms of region of space, there are three forms of neglect: personal, peripersonal, and extrapersonal (Appelros, Nydevik, Karlsson, Throwalls, & Seiger, 2004; Buxbaum et al., 2004).[2] Personal space refers to one's own

---

[2]Some researchers combine peripersonal and extrapersonal into one category called extrapersonal neglect. In some cases a distinction between near versus far extrapersonal space is made, which appears to be synonymous with what others refer to as peripersonal and extrapersonal space.

Table 7–3. Types of Unilateral Visuospatial Neglect

Types Based on Region of Space		
Type of Neglect	*Area Affected*	*Sample Problem*
Personal	One's own body	Failure to comb left side of hair, shave or apply makeup to the left side of the face. Failure to dress the left side of the body.
Peripersonal	Space within an arm's reach	In cancellation tasks, miss items on the left side. In reading tasks, words on the left side may be omitted or read incorrectly. Writing begins at the midline.
Extrapersonal	Space beyond an arm's reach	Difficulty finding items within a room (e.g., TV, window, people) that are on the left side.
Types Based on Frame of Reference		
Viewer-centered (egocentric)	Left defined by viewer's visual fields	Reduced attention to all stimuli/items to the left of the person's midline
Stimulus-centered (allocentric)	Left defined for each stimulus/object in the visual field	Reduced attention to the left side of each stimulus/item, regardless of the position within the visual field

body. Personal neglect results in such problems as only dressing or grooming the right side of the body. Peripersonal neglect affects the region of space within an arm's reach. Reading, writing, copying, and cancellation tasks are used to assess peripersonal neglect. Extrapersonal neglect affects space beyond an arm's reach. Difficulties with navigation (bumping into the left side of doorways) or problems finding items within a room may be indicative of extrapersonal neglect. The three forms can be dissociated and can co-occur in various patterns (Azouvi et al., 2002; Butler, Eskes, & Vandorpe, 2004; Hillis, 2006). Peripersonal neglect appears to be the most common form. In a group

of 37 patients with neglect, all but one evidenced peripersonal neglect, 62% had personal neglect, and just under 40% had extrapersonal neglect (Appleros et al., 2004). It is important to note that the vast majority of neglect tasks assess peripersonal neglect; thus the prevalence in comparison to the other types may be overestimated because personal and extrapersonal neglect are underdiagnosed.

While there is no direct relationship between localization of lesion and type of neglect, personal neglect has been linked to posterior lesions of the right hemisphere (Azouvi et al., 2002), particularly the supramarginal gyrus (Bartolomeo et al., 2007), whereas more anterior lesions in the superior temporal gyrus and inferior frontal gyrus have been found to cause peri- and extrapersonal neglect (Bartolomeo et al., 2007).

Appleros and colleagues (2004) reported differing patterns of recovery for these three forms of UN. While the most recovery occurred within the first six months poststroke for all forms, only 13% of those with peripersonal neglect had fully recovered after one year. In contrast, over 50% of those with personal neglect had recovered by six months, and approximately 65% of those with extrapersonal neglect recovered by one year poststroke.

Two additional types of neglect are based on the frame of reference, namely, how "left" is defined (Chatterjee, 1994; Tipper & Behrmann, 1996). In viewer-centered neglect, also known as egocentric neglect, the frame of reference is the patient's visual field. In this form, items to the left of the person's midline are likely to be neglected. Because the frame of reference is based on the viewer, when the patient turns his head, the midline of the visual field shifts. In contrast, in stimulus-centered, or allocentric, neglect, left and right are defined for each stimulus/object. The placement within the broader visual field does not matter, because each item has an intrinsic right and left side. For example, on a keyboard the Q, W, S, and D keys are on the left regardless of whether the keyboard is at a person's midline or within the right visual field.

There is disagreement about whether these two types of neglect are separate disorders or represent different forms of the same underlying disorder. Hillis and colleagues (Hillis, 2006; Khurshid et al., 2012; Marsh & Hillis, 2008) suggest that the two forms are dissociable and that co-occurrence is rare. Karnath and colleagues (Karnath & Rorden, 2012; Rorden et al., 2012), on the other hand, argue that they are two forms of the same disorder that is characterized by a bias in gaze and visual search to the contralateral visual space along with reduced awareness of the symptoms (Karnath & Rorden, 2012). They suggest that the apparent dissociation in diagnoses is due to the practice of identifying the types of neglect as simply present or absent. This binary distinction prevents the consideration of severity and results in classification into either viewer-centered or stimulus-centered neglect while missing the overlap between the two forms. Additionally, there is some evidence that the severity of stimulus-centered neglect is related to the position of items within the visual field; if stimuli are in the left visual field, the extent of stimulus-centered neglect is greater than if they are placed in the right visual field (Karnath, Mandler, & Clavagnier, 2011).

Viewer-centered and stimulus-centered neglect appear to be associated with lesions in different regions of the right hemisphere. More ventral and posterior regions (e.g., temporo-occipital) have been linked to stimulus-centered neglect and its recovery, while frontoparietal regions are associated with the presence and recovery of viewer-centered neglect (Grimsen, Hildebrandt, & Fahle, 2008; Karnath & Rorden, 2012; Khurshid et al., 2012). Viewer-centered neglect is by far the more common, occurring in approximately 17 to 28% of large groups of adults with RH stroke, whereas stimulus-centered is apparent in only 5% (Hillis, 2006; Marsh & Hillis, 2008).

Additional features of visuospatial UN, such as distortions of spatial representation that affect not only the horizontal, but also the vertical plane, have been reported (e.g., Funk, Finke, Müller, Preger, & Kerkhoff, 2010; Kerkhoff, 2001).

Neglect Dyslexia

Neglect dyslexia is characterized by errors in reading that are restricted to the left sides of words or lines of text. It is considered a peripheral form of dyslexia, as it affects the perception and initial processing of the letter forms rather than the central phonological and graphemic reading processes. Neglect dyslexia is typically considered to be a component of UN but can occur in the absence of visuospatial neglect (Behrmann, Black, McKeeff, & Barton, 2002; Vallar, Burani, & Arduino, 2010). The presence of neglect dyslexia has been related to severity of visual UN (Lee et al., 2009), the occurrence of perseverative behaviors on cancellation tasks (i.e., repeatedly cancelling the same targets; Ronchi et al., 2016), and abnormal eye movement patterns that suggest a disruption of the fine-motor exploratory eye movements required for reading (Primativo, Arduino, De Luca, Daini, & Martelli, 2013). Neglect dyslexia has been estimated to occur in 40 to 70% of individuals with UN (Lee et al., 2009; Siéroff, 2015).

Reading errors in neglect dyslexia most often are letter omissions (THREAD becomes READ) or substitutions (LINK becomes SINK). Additions (OAT becomes COAT) are relatively rare (Ptak, Di Pietro, & Schnider, 2012). A variety of word-level effects have been found in neglect dys-

lexia, providing interesting insights into reading processes. According to reviews by Vallar and colleagues (2010) and Siéroff (2015), individuals with the disorder read real words better than nonwords (lexicality effect), short better than long words (word length effect), high-frequency better than low-frequency words (word frequency effect), nouns better than verbs (grammatical class effect), concrete better than abstract (concreteness effect), and regularly better than irregularly spelled words (word regularity effect). Several studies have also reported semantic, syntactic, and morphophonological effects in which errors are less common for standardized phrases (e.g., hit and run) or idiomatic constructions (*kick the bucket*) (Acara et al., 2012; Friedmann & Gvion, 2014).

There are several models of reading designed to explain neglect dyslexia. The dual mechanism model (Daini et al., 2013; Martelli, Arduino, & Daini, 2011) includes visuospatial exploration and perceptual integration mechanisms. A deficit in exploration results in omission errors, while a deficit in integration causes substitutions. The perceptual integration component is modeled after a phenomenon reported in healthy adults, in which target letter identification is more difficult (a) when the target is surrounded by other letters and (b) when it appears within the periphery of the visual field. This effect, referred to as letter crowding, can be lessened by increasing spacing between the letters. With neglect dyslexia related to perceptual integration problems, increasing the spacing does reduce the substitution errors but also increases the omission errors, presumably because it increases the demands on the visual exploration mechanism.

An older model suggests three levels of reading processes, again with predictable patterns of errors related to each (Caramazza & Hillis, 1990). In the first stage, a retino-centric map is created in which spatial location is coded. Deficits in this stage cause modality-specific (visual reading, not spelling) errors based on the physical location within the visual fields (e.g., increasing errors the further leftward the stimulus appears). Omission of the entire word can occur (Ptak et al., 2012; Reinhart, Schaadt, Adams, Leonhardt, & Kerkhoff, 2013; Vallar et al., 2010). In the second stage, a stimulus- or object-centered letter shape map is created in which the shapes and features of letters and spacing between letters are coded. A problem in this stage will result in omission or substitution errors on the neglected side of the word string regardless of its placement in the left or right visual fields. The third stage results in a word-centered grapheme description in which the specific letters (but not their font, size, or case) are coded in sequence. Damage affecting this third stage of processing results in a rare form of neglect dyslexia in which omissions or substitutions will occur based on the canonical form of the word (i.e., how it typically appears) regardless of spatial orientation. This has been termed word-centered neglect dyslexia (Savazzi, 2013). Assuming the left is the neglected side, the word HIKING may be read as KING when it appears in typical horizontal alignment, but also when it is written vertically or backward (Caramazza & Hillis, 1990).

Neglect dyslexia has been associated with lesions in the intraparietal sulcus as well as the middle temporal gyrus and angular gyrus (Ptak et al., 2012). Lee and colleagues (2009) reported that their participants with neglect dyslexia had lesions in the fusiform and lingual gyri along with lesions in the temporoparietal region.

Neglect Dysgraphia

Neglect dysgraphia is a writing disorder characterized by letter or stroke repetitions (e.g., crossing the letter "t" multiple times or adding extra "humps" to the letter *m*) and omissions, sloping lines of text, a tendency to write on the right side of a page, and splitting errors in which there are larger-than-normal gaps between letters within a word (Figure 7–1). As with neglect dyslexia, neglect dysgraphia is considered a peripheral dysgraphia in that it affects the visuo-spatio-motor processes of writing as opposed to central, linguistic processes more commonly associated with agraphia or aphasia (Ellis, 1988; Ellis, Young, & Flude, 1987).

Two forms of peripheral dysgraphia associated with RHD have been proposed (Cubelli, Guiducci, & Consolmagno, 2000). Afferent dysgraphia is caused by an impairment of a control mechanism that uses sensory (afferent) feedback (primarily visual) to monitor and control writing movements. Errors include letter or stroke repetitions and omissions. In contrast, spatial dysgraphia is a component of a broader visuospatial deficit and results in sloping or wavy lines, splitting errors, and a tendency to write on the right side of a page. Despite the clear distinction in the descriptions, the labels are not consistently used in the literature (e.g., Ellis,

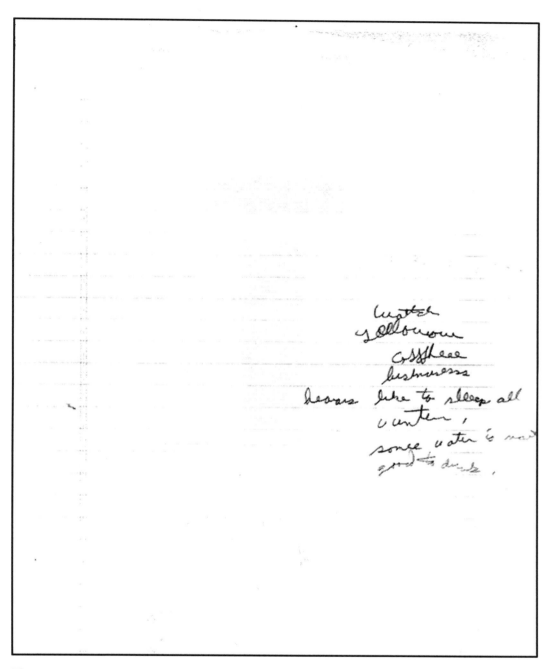

Figure 7–1. Example of neglect dysgraphia. A patient with RHD was asked to write the following words and sentences to dictation: watch, yellow, coffee, business, bears like to sleep all winter, some water is not good to drink. Note that the writing began on the right side of the page. Letter repetitions can be seen in most words (e.g., wattch, yelllowow).

Young, & Flude, 1988), and in many cases the label "neglect dysgraphia" is used to encompass both of these types. Little is known about the prevalence of neglect dysgraphia or how commonly it co-occurs with neglect. While spatial dysgraphia appears to share some characteristics with UN, such as the right-sided focus, the letter and line perseverations have been associated with UN.

Assessment of Unilateral Neglect

The rate of assessment of UN in acute care hospitals has been estimated to be relatively low. As noted in Chapter 1, the most commonly used stroke scales (National Institutes of Health Stroke Scale, Brott et al., 1989; and the Scandinavian Stroke Scale, 1985) have few if any items dedicated to UN. In an examination of 10 hospitals in Canada, Menon-Nair, Korner-Bitensky, Wood-Dauphinee, and Robertson (2006) reported that only 38% of patients admitted for stroke who were medically able to participate were assessed for UN within 48 hours. While the authors did not examine differences based on side of lesion (LHD versus RHD), assessments of neglect occurred more often when there was an orientation deficit or upper extremity weakness.

Assessment of Visuospatial Neglect

Visuospatial neglect is the focus of the majority of UN research, and this focus

extends into assessment and treatment. Traditional assessment of visuospatial UN relies on paper/pencil tasks such as cancellation, line bisection, picture description, and figure copying/drawing (Table 7–4). Some assessments also include observation of personal care activities such as mimicking shaving or combing hair to assess personal neglect. Standard paper/pencil assessments can underestimate the presence of neglect for a variety of reasons. First, no one task has been shown to be sensitive enough to identify neglect in more than half of patients. Individual tasks range in sensitivity from 13% to 50% (Azouvi et al., 2002, 2006). Lindell et al. (2007) suggested that a minimum of 10 different tasks are needed to detect neglect, establish severity, and explore dissociations of performance. Second, even groups of tasks administered in traditional settings may not be sensitive enough. One reason is that for most testing situations, distractors are removed and the client is given the opportunity to focus exclusively on the task (Appelros, Nydevik, Karlsson, Thorwalls, & Seiger, 2003). Third, there is a strong bias toward assessment of peripersonal, viewer-centered, visuospatial neglect given the tradition of using paper/pencil and picture description tasks.

The clock drawing task (i.e., draw a clock, including all of the numbers, and set a time) is commonly used in assessment of UN, but there is disagreement about what exactly the task assesses. In many cases it is interpreted as a measure of visuospatial UN. However, it requires object representation, and thus may measure representational or imagery neglect (Salvato et al., 2014). It also requires visuoconstruction skills. Thus, impaired construction of the

Table 7–4. Select Assessments of Unilateral Neglect

Scale	Authors	Domains Assessed	Reliability*	Validity*
Apples Test (part of BCoS)	Bickerton et al., 2011	Peripersonal viewer- and stimulus-centered visuospatial neglect	OK	Good
Balloons Test	Edgeworth et al., 1998	Extrapersonal, viewer-centered, visuospatial neglect	OK	Good
Behavioural Inattention Test	Wilson et al., 1987	Peripersonal viewer-centered visuospatial neglect	Good	Good
Catherine Bergego Scale	Azouvi et al., 1996, 2003	Personal, peripersonal, and extrapersonal neglect	Weak	Good
Comb & Razor Test	Beschin & Robertson 1997	Personal neglect	OK	OK
Line Bisection Test	Schenkenberg et al., 1980	Peripersonal, viewer-centered, visuospatial neglect	OK for severe neglect	OK
Ota/gap detection task	Ota et al., 2001 Marsh & Hillis, 2008	Peripersonal viewer- and stimulus-centered visuospatial neglect	OK	OK
Vest Test	Glocker et al., 2006	Personal neglect	Good	Good
Wheelchair Collision Test	Qiang et al., 2005	Extrapersonal visuospatial neglect	OK	OK

Note. *Good = moderate–strong estimates of two or more types of reliability/validity; OK = moderate–strong estimates of one type of reliability/validity or mixture of weak and strong estimates; weak = weak estimates of one or more types of reliability/validity; none = no estimates reported. See Appendix for detailed information about reliability and validity.

clock face and the placement of the numbers may reflect visuoconstruction deficits (particularly due to lesions in parietal, supramarginal regions, also frontal and temporal sites). Finally, problems with time setting have been associated with LHD, primarily inferior frontal lesions (Tranel, Rudrauf, Vianna, & Damasio, 2008).

Assessment of Neglect Dyslexia

In regard to neglect dyslexia, Reinhart and colleagues (2016) reported that compound words or words in which a shorter real word exists when the leftmost letter(s) are omitted (e.g., cowboy = boy; paragraph

= graph; understand = stand/and) are more sensitive than words that cannot be broken into separate words (e.g., pencil, mountain). They also found that their specialized list of words that could not be subdivided was more sensitive than a paragraph reading task for detecting stimulus-centered (in this case word-centered) errors.

Galletta and colleagues (Galletta, Campanelli, Maul, & Barrett, 2014) reported that reading words or sentences within columns (e.g., like a menu or newspaper article) was more sensitive for detecting neglect dyslexia than single word reading. The types of errors were not defined, and thus the errors seen in the menu and article reading tasks may have been viewer-centered errors as opposed to stimulus-centered errors.

Specific UN Tests and Batteries

One commonly used assessment for visuospatial UN is the Behavioural Inattention Test (BIT; Wilson, Cockburn, & Halligan, 1987). The six conventional subtests include line, shape, and letter cancellation; copying; drawing; and line bisection tasks. The functional tasks include reading maps, menus, texts, and clocks, as well as identifying coins. The BIT has good reliability and validity, primarily for the conventional subtests.

The Catherine Bergego Scale (CBS; Azouvi et al., 1996) assesses a variety of forms of UN, including personal, peripersonal, and extrapersonal, perceptual, representational, and motor neglect. The test has strong validity (see review in Chen, Hreha, Fortis, Goedert, & Barrett,

2012), although there are few studies of reliability. Azouvi and colleagues (2002, 2006) later added the Bisiach scale for anosognosia (see Chapter 9) and a measure of extinction. They then compared the expanded CBS with a set of paper/pencil tasks (cancellation, line bisection, figure copying and drawing, reading and writing). Results indicated that of the paper/pencil tasks, the starting point for the cancellation task was the most sensitive measure. The behavioral assessment of functional tasks was more sensitive than any other single task but remained less sensitive than the battery as a whole.

The CBS has been shown to have two primary factors: spatial perceptual attention and motor exploration (Goedert et al., 2012). Detailed instructions for administration of the CBS and observation of behaviors were developed as part of the Kessler Foundation Neglect Assessment Process (KF-NAP) to enhance the reliability and the amount of information that can be obtained from the CBS (Chen et al., 2012). Despite the positive aspects of the CBS, it may not adequately predict safety and independence or the fluctuations in UN that occur in daily life when common distractors or unpredictable stimuli cannot be controlled (Klinke, Hjaltason, Hafsteinsdóttir, & Jónsdóttir, 2016).

The Apples Test, a subtest from the Birmingham Cognition Screen (BCoS; Humphreys, Bickerton, Samson, & Riddoch, 2012), is a paper/pencil cancellation task designed to assess both stimulus-centered and viewer-centered UN (Bickerton, Samson, Williamson, & Humphreys, 2011). The test paper contains an array of line drawings of apples. There are small and larger apples, and some of the apples have a gap, or a "bite" in either the right or left side. The task is to cancel all of the complete apples. Viewer-centered neglect is assessed by determining the asymmetry between the numbers of apples cancelled on the right versus the left side of the page. Stimulus-centered neglect is scored by determining the difference between the numbers of incorrectly cancelled apples with gaps on the right versus the left side. The task has reasonable reliability and good validity.

Rorden and Karnath (2010) developed the computerized Center of Cancellation (CoC) score as a measure of severity of visuospatial neglect. Clinicians can administer cancellation tasks and then input a patient's performance (i.e., which items were cancelled versus not cancelled). The program then generates a CoC score to indicate the extent of lateralized targets that were neglected. A similar measure for object-centered neglect (Rorden et al., 2012) is also available on the researchers' website (http://www.mccauslandcenter. sc.edu/crnl/tools/cancel).

Virtual Reality Assessment of UN

Virtual reality (VR) has been suggested as a potentially more valid and sensitive measure of UN than traditional paper/pencil tasks (e.g., Baheux, Yoshizawa, Seki, & Handa, 2006; Baheux, Yoshizawa, Tanaka, Seki, & Handa, 2005). This technology has the potential to facilitate dynamic assessment through the detection of changes in eye movement, reaching behaviors, and reaction time in response to changes in visual scenes, complexity of scenes, or the addition of auditory or visual cues (Broeren, Stibrant-Sunnerhagen, Blomstrand, & Rydmark, 2007; D. Kim et al., 2010; K. Kim et al., 2004; Navarro et al., 2009; Navarro Lloréns, Noé, Ferri, & Alcañiz, 2013; Tsirlin, Dupierrix, Chokron, Coquillart, & Ohlmann, 2009).

D. Kim and colleagues (D. Kim et al., 2010) created a street-crossing task in which the patient's avatar is attempting to cross a street and cars approach from either the left or the right side. The patient's task is to indicate when he/she (as a pedestrian) detects a car. Visual (headlights turn on) and auditory (honking) cues are added as a car gets closer to the crosswalk without being detected. Results indicate that adults with RHD and UN have slower response times and need more cues to detect a car than those without UN. In the most recent study, participants were included if they showed UN on any one of many functional tasks, including ADLs, wheelchair navigation, response to auditory cues, and detecting objects in both near and far space, thus resulting in a pool of participants with heterogeneous deficits. This and other VR tasks tend to assess viewer-centered, extrapersonal visuospatial neglect. Few researchers examine individual performance on the VR task in relation to the type or severity of neglect exhibited by the participants. Thus, it is not clear how the assessment of extrapersonal neglect might inform clinical practice in terms of diagnosis or treatment of the various forms of UN. Indeed, there were few meaningful relationships between performance on the extrapersonal VR task and peripersonal paper/pencil tasks (line bisection and letter cancellation).

Treatment for Unilateral Neglect

There are many systematic reviews of treatments for visuospatial unilateral neglect (Bowen, Hazelton, Pollock, & Lincoln, 2013; Cappa et al., 2005; Cicerone et al., 2011; Luauté, Halligan, Rode, Rossetti, & Boisson, 2006; Pernet, Jughters, & Kerckhofs, 2013; Pierce & Buxbaum, 2002; Yang, Zhou, Chung, Li-Tsang, & Fong, 2013). As noted in Chapter 2, conclusions from individual systematic reviews can differ based on the criteria for inclusion of studies. For example, Yang and colleagues (2013) included only randomized control trials (RCTs) that used the Behavioural Inattention Test (BIT; Wilson, Cockburn, & Halligan, 1987) as the primary outcome measure. Their results indicated large effects for immediate treatment gains, but nonsignificant long-term gains. In contrast, Luauté and colleagues (2006) reviewed studies that reported functional outcomes. Of the 18 types of treatment they examined, evidence of long-term functional

gains was reported for 6 of them. There was not enough consistent evidence at the time to make recommendations for 10 other treatments. Recommendations from Cicerone et al. (2011) are provided in Table 7–5.

Integrating results from the various systematic reviews and meta-analyses, the following conclusions can be drawn: there is reasonably strong evidence that visual scanning treatments and prism adaptation are effective for treatment of visuospatial UN. Evidence supporting other treatments is weaker, although positive results have been reported for visuo-spatio-motor approaches and the use of visual and verbal feedback.

As with the research on UN assessment, the vast majority of treatment studies focus on visuospatial neglect, and most address viewer-centered, peripersonal neglect. Additionally, the diagnosis of UN is typically quite general and does not include careful assessment of different forms of UN; thus, it is difficult to determine which treatment(s) might be most effective when more than one form

Table 7–5. Recommendations for Treatment of Visuospatial Unilateral Neglect

Recommendation Level	Treatment for Unilateral Visuospatial Neglect
Practice standards	• Visual scanning treatments • Metacognitive strategy training
Practice guidelines	• Isolated computer treatments have NOT been shown to be effective and are NOT recommended
Practice options	• Limb activation treatment • Computer training in conjunction with behavioral treatment

Note. Practice standards are based on substantive evidence of effectiveness, practice guidelines are based on evidence of probable effectiveness, and practice options are based on evidence of possible effectiveness.

Source: Based on Cicerone et al., 2011.

of neglect is present. Finally, most studies examine impairment-level outcomes, although some also include activity-level measures.

Treatments for UN generally can be divided into top-down and bottom-up approaches. Top-down treatments focus on awareness and use of strategies to reduce the UN or lessen the effects of UN on function. In contrast, bottom-up approaches are designed to affect the impairment and do not rely on awareness of the deficit. Saevarsson, Halsband, and Kristjansson (2011) suggest that a more comprehensive classification scheme should include not only top-down versus bottom-up distinctions, but also active versus passive and compensatory versus restorative. For purposes of this discussion, treatments will be divided simply in terms of top-down versus bottom-up. Within each of these categories, the treatments with the strongest evidence for efficacy and/or effectiveness are discussed first.

Top-Down Treatments

Visual Scanning Treatment

There is solid evidence from a variety of well-controlled experimental studies that visual scanning treatment (VST) is effective for the reduction of neglect (primarily peripersonal viewer-centered neglect). Gains are noted on impairment-level measures as well as functional measures and are maintained for several weeks or months (see reviews in Cicerone et al., 2011; Luauté et al., 2006, Yang et al., 2013). Cicerone and colleagues (2011) recommend that VST should be considered a practice standard.

VST can take different forms, but at its core it revolves around repeated practice with scanning across the visual field. The treatment may involve cancellation tasks, picture description, finding and picking up objects, or reading text. It often involves practicing the process of scanning, beginning in the upper left quadrant, moving across left to right, and then returning to the left margin to begin again. In some cases external physical cues such as a red line or Velcro strip is placed along the left side of the page to draw attention back to the left margin. Verbal cues such as "look to the left" or "begin at the red line" often are part of the treatment.

Immediate gains commonly are found, particularly for outcome measures similar to the tasks used in treatment. Generalization to other kinds of tasks does occur, but not as consistently. Thus, if reading is a goal for a client, then reading tasks should be used in treatment to facilitate achieving the goal. Several early studies suggested that extensive treatment (40 hours) led to greater long-term gains (Antonucci et al., 1995; Pizzamiglio et al., 1992).

Visuo-Spatio-Motor Treatments

Visuo-spatio-motor treatments rely on combinations of visual, visuospatial, and motor components. Limb activation treatment involves the purposeful movement of the affected (left) limb. The rationale behind the treatment is based on the theory of UN as an attentional imbalance (Kinsbourne, 1970). As described earlier in this chapter, the attentional imbalance theory suggests that the two hemispheres mutually inhibit each other. Damage to the RH thus results in excessive inhibition of the RH by the LH due to imbalance of the interhemispheric connections. Given this imbalance, movement of the unaffected right limb is associated with activation within the intact left hemisphere, which may further exacerbate the inhibitory imbalance. Conversely, movement of the left limb requires activation within the RH, which may help to reduce the imbalance (Bailey, Riddoch, & Crome, 2002).

Limb activation treatments generally involve movement of the left limb (cued by a buzzer or the clinician) during an unrelated task (e.g., card sorting) (Bailey et al., 2002; Brunila, Lincoln, Lindell, Tenovou, & Hämäläinen, 2002; Robertson, McMillan, MacLeod, Edgeworth, & Brock, 2002). Results differ, with gains reported in UN, motor control, and/or scanning and reading. In several studies comparing limb activation to VST, results indicate that both treatments result in reduction of neglect immediately following treatment. There is no clear benefit of one treatment over the other (Bailey et al., 2002; Luukkainen-Markkula, Tarkka, Pitkänen, Sivenius, & Hämäläinen, 2009; Priftis, Passarini, Pilosio, Meneghello, & Pitteri, 2013). In fact, Luukkainen-Markkula and colleagues (2009) compared 30 to 40 hours of arm activation with 10 hours of VST combined with traditional cognitive rehabilitation and found that while gains related to UN were equivalent at six months posttreatment, the participants who had the less intensive VST + cognitive rehab also evidenced gains in other cognitive and motor areas.

Another form of visuo-spatio-motor treatment is the Lighthouse Strategy (Niemeier, Cifu, & Kishore, 2001). It combines visual, spatial, motor, and imagery components. Clients are instructed to think about a lighthouse with its light moving

from left to right across the sky, and to move their head and eyes in a similar pattern during scanning tasks. This imagery and movement is then paired with a scanning or reading task. Outcomes include reduction of severity of UN (Bailey et al., 2002) and improved navigation (Niemeier et al., 2001).

Virtual Reality

Just as for assessment, a variety of VR tasks have been created for treatment of UN (see review by Pedroli, Serino, Cipresso, Pallavicini, & Riva, 2015). These include street-crossing tasks, navigation within a house, and detection of targets against a landscape background. Several of the VR environments are functional and appear to target activity- and participation-level outcomes (e.g., safely moving around a house or city). In these early stages of development there is a disconnect between the treatment and the outcomes: the treatments address viewer-centered extrapersonal neglect at the activity level, while the outcome measures are traditional viewer-centered peripersonal tasks that assess impairment-level changes.

Katz and colleagues (2005) examined the activity-level benefits of a street-crossing VR training compared with computerized visual scanning tasks. Few group differences were noted on paper/pencil tasks following treatment, but only the group that received VR training showed gains on the VR measures. An additional, real-life outcome was included. Aided by a clinician, participants in this study completed an actual street-crossing task. Performance was judged based on the number of times they looked to the left and their judgment of when it was safe to cross. Neither group showed improvement on the real-life task following treatment.

While results appear promising, weaknesses in the literature include small sample sizes and lack of control groups or comparison treatments. Barriers to adoption of VR technologies in assessment and treatment include the costs of the systems, the need for technical support, adaptation of VR mechanisms for adults who are in wheelchairs and adaptation of controls for one-handed use (Pedroli et al., 2015).

Computerized Training

Cicerone and colleagues (2011) recommended that computerized scanning training should not be used in isolation to treat UN. In one study, there was no benefit of general (non-individualized) computer training on UN, either in isolation or paired with hemifield glasses (Aparicio-López et al., 2015).

External Cues

As described above, external cues such as a red line or other marker along the left side of a page or verbal exhortations to "look to the left" have been described as components of VST. They are also exceedingly common in clinical practice. However, there are no empirical studies on the cues themselves to determine their efficacy or effectiveness. In the literature on cognitive rehabilitation after TBI, there is

---

SIDEBAR

This example illustrates some of the limitations of external cues. One gentleman, approximately 4 years poststroke, had mild visuospatial UN and good awareness of his UN. He had been through rehabilitation that included treatment for UN. When given a letter cancellation task, he said, "Aha! I need to make my line" and proceeded to make a line with his pen along the left margin. He then began the task, missing most of the targets that were on the far left side of the array. Once he was done, he went back to check his work and eventually found all of the targets on the left side, but this was through slowly shifting attention from the right over to the left along a line of letters. Although he drew the line in the left margin at the beginning, he never used it during the task itself to aid in shifting his attention over to that side or to pace his scanning from the end of the right side back to the leftmost side of the next line in the array.

He completed two other cancellation tasks as part of the assessment, but did not draw a line for either of them. Perhaps it was the orderly array of lines of letters compared with the more random appearing stimuli in the other two cancellation tasks; whatever the reason, the strategy of drawing a line in the margin was not used consistently, and not effective when it was used.

good evidence that external cues are not as effective as internal cues. One primary reason is that they are external, and thus if there is no one available to provide the cue (e.g., someone to mark a red line on the left), then the cue does not exist for the client. It is possible that "look to the left" or some other such cue could be trained through spaced retrieval training (see Chapter 10) or as part of a metacognitive strategy. However, extensive practice is necessary to create the transition from verbal knowledge ("I know I need to look to the left") to use of the strategy in daily activities when needed (e.g., transition from intellectual to emergent or anticipatory awareness, as described in Chapter 8).

Bottom-Up Treatments

Prism Adaptation

Prism adaptation (PA) is a phenomenon resulting from recalibration and realignment of the visual and motor systems in response to prism-shaped glasses (see tutorial and review in Newport & Schenk, 2012). The prisms are created such that the left visual field is shifted into the right visual space. During PA treatment, the client wears the prism glasses/goggles and repeatedly reaches for items placed within arm's length in the left region of space. The initial reaches will be off target, as the objects appear to be in the right visual field due to the prism distortion, but actually are in the left. The person rapidly adapts such that she is able to accurately grasp the objects. These direct effects of treatment (adaptation while the glasses

are on) are a combination of strategic recalibration or conscious error fixing and an unconscious realignment of visual and proprioceptive maps. In a typical session, clients complete about 30 reaches with the glasses on. Once the glasses are removed, the reaching task is conducted again, and aftereffects are observed in which clients reach too far to the left, because they are used to a mismatch between what they see and the actual physical location. The aftereffects last longer in clients with UN than healthy adults and result in repeated reaches into the previously neglected space.

Prism adaptation has been reported to reduce tactile as well as visuospatial neglect (Maravita et al., 2003). Transient effects of PA on representational neglect also have been reported, although the benefits disappear within 24 hours after treatment (Rode, Rossetti, Boisson, Bernard, & Cedex, 2001). Limited benefits for neglect dyslexia (Rusconi & Carelli, 2012) and neglect dysgraphia (Rode et al., 2006) have been reported.

In a comparison of treatments, Priftis and colleagues (2013) reported that gains from PA were equivalent to those of either VST or limb activation treatment. The required or optimal intensity of treatment of PA has yet to be determined, although Goedert, Zhang, and Barrett (2015) provide preliminary evidence that relatively long-lasting effects might be possible with four to six sessions of treatment.

PA must be conducted in collaboration with a neuro-ophthalmologist, neurologist, or other professional to aid in preparing glasses/goggles with the appropriate prisms and to monitor the effects of the treatment on the visual system.

Sensory Stimulation

Karnath and Dieterich (2006) suggested that UN is a result of damage to a multimodal sensory processing region of the right parietal lobe. This region integrates information from auditory, vestibular, somatosensory, and visual modalities to generate and update one's body representation. In the case of UN, when there is an imbalance and a resulting rightward bias, stimulation of any other sensory modality might aid in realigning the representation. Treatments involving neck muscle vibration, vestibular stimulation, and optokinetic stimulation (OKS) all fit with the multimodality theory. Such treatments must be conducted in collaboration with the appropriate professionals, namely, physicians, neurologists, and/or neuro-ophthalmologists to ensure safe and optimal use while minimizing potential side effects of sensory stimulation.

Caloric vestibular stimulation involves inducing nystagmus (repetitive "beating" movement of eyes with a slow phase of lateral movement and rapid return to midline). In the case of left neglect, cold water introduced into the contralesional (e.g., left) ear canal or warm water to the ipsilesional canal will stimulate the lateral semicircular canal, resulting in nystagmus with the slow phase toward the left. Reported outcomes include transient improvements of visuospatial, tactile, and representational neglect as well as reorienting of gaze and reduction of anosognosia (see Kerkhoff & Schenk, 2012 for a review). Ronchi and colleagues (2013) replicated the transient effects of caloric vestibular stimulation on UN, but also reported longer-lasting effects on anosognosia for UN.

Longer-lasting effects have been reported with OKS, which involves a visual display with vertical bars in apparent motion from the right to the left side of the screen. In large displays, this motion causes the illusion of movement to the left, with compensatory rightward reorienting. Smaller displays create instead a nystagmus as described above. Reductions of both visual and auditory UN with maintenance for up to two weeks have been reported following OKS (Thimm et al., 2009; also see review in Kerkhoff & Schenk, 2012), although other studies have not found benefits beyond those from "usual care" (Machner, Konemund, Sprenger, von der Gablentz, & Helmchen, 2014).

The benefits of OKS for neglect dyslexia are mixed. Reinhart, Schindler, and Kerkhoff (2011) reported a reduction of viewer-centered errors on a reading task (i.e., the number of whole words omitted from the left side of a paragraph) but no effect on the stimulus-centered errors (i.e., omission or substitution of the left-sided letters of words, regardless of position within a paragraph). Daini and colleagues (2014), in support of their dual-mechanism model of neglect dyslexia, reported that OKS improved performance in a participant with primarily visual scanning errors (e.g., omissions). In contrast, a participant with substitution errors linked to a faulty perceptual integration mechanism demonstrated no improvement following OKS.

Neck muscle vibration is another form of sensory stimulation. Vibratory stimulation of the muscles on the left side of the neck create the illusion of leftward head and trunk rotation and the increased orienting to the left in adults with UN (e.g., Kerkhoff & Schenk, 2012).

While each of the sensory stimulation techniques have shown some promise, it appears that pairing such stimulation with another treatment (e.g., neck muscle vibration plus VST or PA) results in greater and longer-lasting effects (e.g., Kerkhoff & Schenk, 2012; Pitteri, Arcara, Passarini, Meneghello, & Priftis, 2013; Saevarsson et al., 2011).

Alertness and Attention Training

Based on the theory that UN is a component of a broader attentional deficit (e.g., Robertson Tegnér, Tham, Lo, & Nimmo-Smith, 1995), training alertness or sustained attention has been suggested to be a logical approach to treatment of UN. However, the evidence for efficacy is not strong (Degutis & Van Vleet, 2010; Robertson et al., 1995; Sturm, Thimm, Kust, Karbe, & Fink, 2006). The Tonic and Phasic Alertness Training (TAPAT) program (Degutis & Van Vleet, 2010) involves sustained attention and a go/no-go task (respond to target stimuli and withhold responses to distractors). As with the other alertness and sustained attention training programs, immediate improvements in both spatial (neglect) and non-spatial attention were observed but the gains were not maintained.

Mirror Therapy

Mirror therapy has been used to address both UN and limb movement and has shown promise in reducing UN (Pernet et al., 2013). The essence of this treatment is to view movement of the unaffected (e.g., right) limb through a mirror so that it appears as if the affected (left) limb is moving. The rationale is that visualization of movement that appears to be of the affected limb causes activation in the RH motor and attentional systems (Pandian et al., 2014). Pandian and colleagues (2014) reported that mirror treatment in addition to limb activation, compared with limb activation alone, resulted in significantly greater gains on UN tasks such as star cancellation and line bisection that were maintained for six months.

Neuromodulation

Transcranial direct cortical stimulation (tDCS) and repetitive transcortical magnetic stimulation (rTMS; see brief review in Chapter 2) have been used in several studies to treat unilateral neglect. The theoretical rationale for application of neuromodulation is based on the idea of interhemispheric inhibition and the imbalance caused by a lesion to the RH. Such a lesion can reduce the RH inhibitory control over the LH and change the balance of the interhemispheric inhibition. This can cause either increased inhibition of the RH from the LH, or a reduction of inhibition of the LH from the RH. Either might result in increased attention to, and difficulty shifting attention from, the right side of space. Excitatory (anodal) stimulation to the posterior parietal lobe in the RH and inhibitory (cathodal) stimulation to the LH have both been explored (Agosta, Herpich, Miceli, Ferraro, & Battelli, 2014; see reviews in Cazzoli, Müri, Hess, & Nyffeler, 2010; Convento, Russo, Zigiotto,

& Bolognini, 2016; Hesse, Sparing, & Fink, 2011; and Oliveri, 2011). Results from both types of stimulation indicate that a short-term reduction in peripersonal, visuospatial neglect or left-sided extinction occurs on some but usually not all outcome measures.

Bottom-Up Treatments Without Empirical Evidence

Several suggestions for treatment tasks involve manipulation of stimulus characteristics to increase attention to items in the neglected region of space. These are based on theories of attention, such as salience or emotional characteristics of stimuli, but have not been empirically tested to assess the efficacy or effectiveness. Examples are provided in Table 7–6.

Stimulus Characteristics

As described earlier, salient stimuli are more likely to capture attention, even when items appear in the neglected visual field. Thus, the use of emotional, personally relevant, or vividly colored stimuli

Table 7–6. Sample Stimulus Choices to Increase or Decrease Likelihood of Leftward Attentional Shifts

	Facilitates Leftward Attentional Shifts	*Decreases Likelihood of Leftward Attentional Shifts*
Emotionally laden stimuli	Crying/laughing baby, snake, spider, beautiful sunrise	Neutral facial expression, toothbrush, spoon, desert scene
Salient stimuli	Client's name on the left side of the page	Neutral word on the left side of the page
Overlapping versus separate stimuli		
Connectors between stimuli		
Boundaries around stimuli		
Asymmetrical versus symmetrical pictures		
Noncompound versus compound words	mountain oblivious pencil	paragraph (graph) thinking (king) staircase (case)

may aid in drawing attention to the left. For scanning or cancellation tasks, targets that are clearly different from the distractors (e.g., curved letter targets [S] in an array of angled letter distractors [X, T]) will be easier to identify than if the targets and distractors are more similar. Note that these stimulus characteristics will aid in attention capture, but not necessarily attentional control. Such manipulations could be used to demonstrate to clients that they *can* shift their attention to the left. Working on controlling the attention and developing voluntary shifts to the left may require other approaches, such as VST.

Connectors between stimuli or a border around a group of stimuli might increase the likelihood of identifying stimuli in the left side of space. Similarly, the leftmost item in a set of overlapping stimuli may be identified more often than if the stimuli are touching but not overlapping, and those may again be identified more easily than if the stimuli are not touching.

Another suggested manipulation is to use pictures for which the critical information is on the left side. For example, shown a picture of a hammer lying horizontally with the head on the left side, it would be impossible to know what kind of tool it was without processing (at some level), the disambiguating information on the left side. Pictures of items that are symmetrical can be identified with information only from one side, and thus are unlikely to facilitate a shift in attention to the neglected side.

Another way to draw attention over to the left region of space is to present words that cannot be subdivided into shorter words if the leftmost letters are omitted

(e.g., PENCIL, MOUNTAIN). Such words may aid in the shifting of attention leftward in order to determine what word it is. In contrast, words that can be subdivided, such as COWBOY or THINKING, are less likely to draw attention to the left, because real words (BOY and KING) can be read without the initial letters.

Stimuli that capitalize on lexical, semantic, and syntactic components of meaning also may aid in drawing attention to the left. As described above in reference to neglect dyslexia, idiomatic phrases (e.g., *kick the bucket*) or common irreversible binomials (e.g., *sugar and spice, hit and run*) are read more accurately than reversed binomials (e.g., *spice and sugar*).

Combined Treatments

Saevarsson and colleagues (2011) reviewed the UN treatment literature and suggested that combinations of treatments might be more effective than any one treatment in isolation. They identified nine studies in which treatment combinations were used and reported that the gains typically were greater than gains reported from individual treatments (e.g., VST in combination with neck vibration was more effective than VST alone).

More work is necessary to determine the best combinations of treatments and whether simultaneous or sequential application of treatments is most effective. Additionally, exploration of what forms of treatment should be combined (e.g., compensatory and restorative; restorative active and restorative passive) is needed. Saevarsson and colleagues (2011) caution that combinations of two active, top-down treatments may cause fatigue and thus would not be recommended.

Treatment for Stimulus-Centered Neglect

Only two treatments have been proposed specifically for stimulus-centered neglect (Hillis, 2006). These have not been empirically studied; they each appear only once or twice in the literature as part of case studies. Thus, their efficacy and effectiveness are unknown.

One stimulus-centered treatment is based on the idea of an "attentional window" in which attention is focused. If the window can be increased in size, then the features within that window, even on the left side, might be fully processed. In one task, participants are shown a page with randomly placed circles. Some of the circles have gaps on either the right or the left side (Figure 7–2). The task is to cancel each incomplete circle. Individuals with stimulus-centered neglect will perceive the circles with a left-sided gap as complete, as the left portion is not fully processed. In treatment based on an attentional window, the idea is that if the window is approximately the size of the individual circles, then the left-gap circles will not be identified. However, if the page contains both small and larger circles, then the attentional window may expand to the size of the larger circles. The left-sided gaps in the small circles then will be detected because the leftward extent of the attentional window extends beyond the small circle stimulus.

Another suggested approach to treatment involves adding irrelevant information to the left side of a stimulus (Hillis, 2006). For example, given the word "HIKING," an individual with stimulus-centered neglect may read it as "KING,"

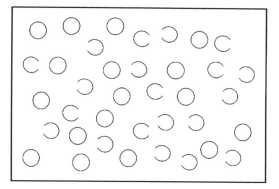 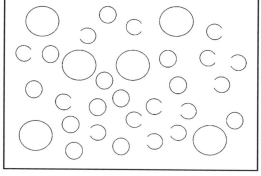

A   **B**

Figure 7–2. A. Gap-detection task: cross out each incomplete circle. Individuals with stimulus-centered neglect will miss circles with a gap on the left side. **B.** Attentional window treatment task: large circles are interspersed with small circles. The task is to cross out each incomplete circle. The presence of the large circles expands the attentional window to a larger region of space. Thus, the left-sided gaps in the small circles will be detected because even though they are on the left side, they are well within the region of attended space (based on Hillis, 2006).

even if it appears within the right visual field. Adding irrelevant stimuli to the left side, such as "xxHIKING" will increase the size of the stimulus itself, and thus if the leftmost portion ("xx") is neglected, the entirety of the target word may be processed.

Conclusions and Implications

The presence of UN can have a substantial effect on outcomes from RHD, and thus presents an important clinical challenge. Thinking about UN as an attentional deficit aids in the understanding of the variability of the deficit and the influence of stimulus and task factors that impact performance. The extensive research provides a solid base from which assessments and treatments have been developed. There is good evidence for both top-down and bottom-up treatment approaches. Work is still needed in relation to the assessment and treatment of stimulus-centered UN and the clinical consideration of the various forms of UN that may coexist in a single patient/client. Additionally, the effectiveness of treatment for neglect dyslexia and dysgraphia is relatively unknown.

Executive Functions

"Executive functions" (EFs) is an umbrella term that encompasses a variety of high-level cognitive functions that are required to manage, monitor, and regulate goal-directed behaviors (Cicerone et al., 2011). They are necessary to complete tasks that are not automatic, routine, overlearned, or overly familiar[1] and are controlled primarily by the frontal lobes. There is no single agreed-upon definition of EFs; over 30 different definitions are listed in a recent edition of the Handbook of Executive Functioning (Goldstein, Naglieri, Princiotta, & Otero, 2014). Some authors make a clear distinction between specific executive functions (e.g., inhibition, task persistence, self-regulation) and other high-level cognitive functions (e.g., reasoning, judgment, problem solving), while others tend to group all of them together. In this chapter, the label "executive function" will be used to encompass all functions related to nonautomatic goal-directed behaviors. However, in discussions of existing research, the terminology used by the authors will be preserved.

The goal-directed behaviors requiring executive functions can be differentiated from overlearned, routine, or automatic tasks. The latter are activities that can be completed with little demand on working memory or executive control. These are generally preserved after RH stroke or traumatic brain injury, and can be used to facilitate performance on more complex tasks or with new learning. This will be discussed in relation to treatment later in this chapter.

Executive Functions and the Frontal Lobes

Executive functions are controlled primarily by the frontal lobes (both right and left), although there are extensive connections with both subcortical structures of

---

[1]Automatic, routine activities can be goal directed but generally are so overlearned that they use few working memory or executive function resources. Making a pot of coffee achieves a goal but for many people is such a habit that they can complete the task with little conscious or controlled thought.

the basal ganglia and thalami as well as the rest of the cerebrum; thus, lesions that disrupt any of the connections or circuits can result in EF deficits. The frontal lobes also receive inputs from the limbic system, allowing emotion and motivation to impact cognitive function.

Over the years, several models have been proposed to explain the core functions of the frontal lobes (Table 8–1). Shared components of the models include working memory, attentional control, goal-directed behaviors, problem solving, decision making, planning, inhibition, integration, and the bidirectional influence of emotion (e.g., Damasio, Tranel, & Damasio, 1991; Hasher, 2007; Hasher & Zacks, 1988; Kimburg & Farah, 1993; Mesulam, 2002).

Working memory (WM) is the function that allows both temporary storage and manipulation of information. Its function as part of memory systems will be discussed in Chapter 10. WM also has been conceived as a component of frontal lobe or executive function. Kimberg and Farah (1993) proposed that weakened WM associations were the key factor in their Unified Theory of frontal lobe function. According to this model, after damage to the dorsolateral prefrontal cortex, representations of goals and world knowledge as well as the perception of stimuli are all generally intact, but the WM associations between these components is weak, thus causing the core "frontal deficits" such as perseverations, disinhibition, and poor planning.

Mesulam (2002) provides a broader view of frontal lobe function in his Default Mode model. According to this model, the default mode of behavior is one of routinized stimulus-response behaviors that lack novelty and creativity and do not change depending on context or experience. The function of the frontal lobes is to override the default mode. This is done through five systems delineated in Table 8–1. When the frontal lobes are functioning properly, individuals can attend and respond to select stimuli without being distracted by extraneous stimuli; they can make choices and seek out novelty; emotional stimuli can affect their cognitive processing, and executive control can be used to modulate emotional responses; and all of these abilities can be altered based on the specific contexts in which they occur. Damage to the frontal lobes can affect any or all of these in various ways.

Clinical Models of Executive Functions

Focusing on clinical contexts, there again are multiple definitions, conceptualizations, and models of executive functioning, each with somewhat different use of terminology (see summary by Constantinidou, Wertheimer, Tsanadis, Evans, & Paul, 2012). However, there are general consistencies across the models. Sohlberg and Mateer's (2001) clinical model of executive function includes most of the components proposed in other models. They describe six components:

- ▪ **Initiation and drive.** The motivation to start a task and the ability to initiate it are related to the limbic system inputs to the frontal lobes. Deficits appear as apathy or poor initiation.

Table 8–1. Models of Frontal Lobe Function

Model and Authors	Description
Somatic Marker Hypothesis (Damasio, 1991, 1996)	Frontal lobes attach somatic markers to potential responses and consequences, creating a "gut feeling" or general positive/negative sense for any given consequence.
	Damage decreases the activation of somatic markers (although aspects of the situation, potential responses, and potential consequences are all intact).
	Damage results in difficulty selecting responses and making decisions.
Unified Theory (Kimberg & Farah, 1993)	Frontal lobes use working memory to create and maintain associations between representations of goals, stimuli, and stored/world knowledge.
	Damage affects the associations (although representations of the individual components remain intact).
	Damage results in perseveration, disinhibition, motor sequencing, and memory for context.
Inhibition Theory (Hasher & Zacks, 1988)	Frontal lobes inhibit vast amounts of information that is automatically activated.
	Damage results in decreased inhibition.
	Damage results in perseveration and memory deficits (activation of irrelevant information impacts efficiency of both encoding and retrieval)
Default Mode Hypothesis (Mesulam, 2002)	"Default mode" of function involves patterned stimulus-response behaviors that are resistant to context or to experience
	Frontal lobes function to override default mode through five components:
	• Working memory and attention
	• Inhibition
	• Pursuit of choice and novelty
	• Emotional significance
	• Encoding context, perspective and mental relativism
	Damage causes return to aspects of default mode, generally in two patterns: Abulic (reduced creativity, initiative, concentration and affect, along with apathy) and Disinhibition (distractibility, perseveration, decreased judgment, insight and difficulty learning from experience or feedback).

▣ **Response inhibition.** The ability to inhibit a response (e.g., not picking up and flipping through a magazine on a table, not verbalizing the thoughts and ideas that pop into your head) is critical for goal achievement. Deficits appear as impulsivity or stimulus-bound behavior, in which a client will initiate a behavior when a familiar stimulus or object is present. For example, upon seeing a therapy workbook on a table, a client may open it and begin to look through it prior to any instruction, unable to inhibit the automatic response stimulated by the presence of the object.

▣ **Task persistence.** The ability to stay on task over time or as difficulty increases is called task persistence. It requires good WM (to remember what the task and goal are) as well as good response inhibition necessary for maintaining focus on a task and not being distracted by internal or external stimuli. Behaviorally, clients with poor task persistence will appear distractible and have difficulty completing tasks. Their performance may decrease over time on lengthy tasks.

▣ **Organization.** Organization encompasses the ability to find or create patterns and to sequence stimuli, thoughts, and actions.

▣ **Generative thinking.** Creativity, fluency of thought, brainstorming, understanding others' perspectives, and cognitive flexibility are all part of the generative thinking concept. It allows one to generate multiple ideas and possible solutions. Deficits of generative thinking appear as rigid or narrow thought processes and difficulties in thinking of new ways to do something or generating multiple strategies for solving problems. Clients may have a limited point of view, being unable to see things from others' perspectives.

▣ **Self-regulation.** Sometimes described as "awareness" (e.g., Sohlberg & Mateer, 2001), self-regulation involves monitoring one's performance, detecting errors, and changing behavior based on error detection or external feedback. This self-regulation and self-monitoring require awareness of performance but are not synonymous with anosognosia (reduced awareness of deficits), which is discussed in depth in the following chapter.

The following processes, as mentioned above, are variously described as part of executive functions or as higher-level cognitive skills.

▣ **Integration.** Integration requires synthesizing pieces of information into a whole. Integration can involve combining new and old information (e.g., from short-term memory and from long-term memory/world knowledge) or combining information or cues across modalities or from various sources. Key elements and relationships must be identified and differentiated from extraneous or irrelevant information. As described in the chapter on pragmatics (Chapter 3), correct interpretation of a speaker's intent might require integration of linguistic, prosodic, and facial expression cues along with knowledge of the speaker's personality and the environment in which a conversation is taking place.

▪ **Reasoning.** "Reasoning is thinking with a conscious intent to reach a conclusion" (Lezak, Howieson, & Loring, 2004, p. 593). It involves use of logically justified steps to determine relationships and to make judgments. Formal reasoning includes deductive reasoning and syllogisms (e.g., if Peter is taller than Patrick, and Patrick is taller than John, then Peter is taller than John). Verbal reasoning involves deriving a meaning or conclusion based on linguistic material, such as determining the meaning of a nonword embedded in a sentence context. Providing explanations of proverbs is considered by some to be a verbal reasoning task.

▪ **Problem solving.** Problem solving allows the achievement of purposeful and novel goals. It is a complex process that depends on multiple other executive functions. For example, for an individual in an in-patient rehabilitation center, figuring out how to alert the

nurse when the call button cannot be found (perhaps it is on the nightstand on the left, neglected, side of the bed) might involve the following: initiation to begin a response; generative thinking to generate multiple options, such as calling out, or trying to find it through searching around the room; analysis to identify the relevant information (one's roommate is sleeping); reasoning to infer what might have happened and where it might be (on the floor, on a bedside table); integration; and task persistence (staying on task until the goal has been met).

Reports of localization of specific executive functions within the frontal lobes are quite variable. The variability may be due in part to the use of different tasks to assess EFs and different methods for identifying localization, including lesion studies versus functional imaging techniques. Initiation, response inhibition, and task switching have all been linked to both dorsolateral and inferior medial regions. Maintenance is often associated with inferior medial regions (Aron, Robbins, & Poldrack, 2004; Sohlberg & Mateer, 2001; Stuss et al., 2002).

Executive Function After RHD

The presence of EF deficits following stroke in general has been fairly well studied. Results consistently suggest that stroke affects EF and other cognitive processes

(Adamit et al., 2015; Levine et al., 2015; Middleton et al., 2014; Oksala et al., 2009; Park et al., 2015; Pedersen, Jorgensen, Nakayama, Raaschou, & Olsen, 1996; Zinn, Bosworth, Hoenig, & Swartzwelder, 2007). Slowed information processing (Hochstenbach, Mulder, Limbeek, & Donders, 1998; Visser-Keizer, Meyboom-deJong, Deelman, Berg, & Gerritsen, 2002) and psychomotor speed are commonly seen after stroke, as are other executive dysfunctions (Middleton et al., 2014). Unfortunately, few researchers separately evaluate RH and LH stroke groups. It is thus impossible to determine the incidence of such deficits related to laterality of lesion. Additionally, in most studies participants with moderate to severe aphasia are excluded because of their inability to complete the language-based cognitive tests. This creates several problems with the participant pool: those with perisylvian LH lesions are often excluded, while all those with comparable lesions in the RH would be included; similarly for size of lesion, those with larger LH lesions may have more severe aphasia and be excluded, while participants with all sizes of RH lesions would be included. The result is a potential overrepresentation of RHD in the participant samples. Without direct comparison between LHD and RHD participants, however, these assumptions cannot be confirmed and the interpretations of the results remain limited.

There is general consensus that RHD impacts executive functions. However, few studies have directly assessed this question. Several studies conducted in the 1980s and 1990s reported deficits in organization and planning as well as generative thinking. Regarding the latter, adults with RHD tend to generate fewer novel ideas and produce more perseverative responses than adults without brain injury (see review in Lezak et al., 2004).

Other EF deficits have been assessed in the context of language tasks. RHD-related impairments in generative thinking, strategy use, and organization have been identified through verbal fluency tasks. Verbal problem solving has been reported to be deficient, including difficulties identifying missing information, self-monitoring, and judging the adequacy or completeness of one's own response. As discussed in Chapters 3 and 4, planning and organizing deficits have been reported in other language tasks, such as picture arrangement, and integration deficits have been reported in inferencing, joke completion, picture description, and pragmatic tasks (Bihrle, Brownell, & Powelson, 1986; Brownell, Michel, Powelson, & Gardner, 1983; Cheang & Pell, 2006; Marini, Carlomagno, Caltagirone, & Nocentini, 2005).

McDonald (2000) and Martin and McDonald (2003, 2006) explored the idea that RHD pragmatic deficits might be caused by executive function deficits. Reports of difficulty with abstract reasoning, using themes as organizers (Delis, Wapner, Gardener, & Moses, 1983; Schneiderman, Murasugi, & Saddy, 1992), and rigid thinking (Brownell & Martino, 1998; Brownell, Potter, & Bihrle, 1986; McDonald & Wales, 1986; Siegal, Carrington, & Radel, 1996) suggest that EFs might underlie the other problems evident after RHD. McDonald (2000) examined correlations between pragmatic performance and measures of EF (word association and similarities tasks), and found no meaningful or significant correlations. Martin and McDonald (2006) again explored the potential correlations. In this study they used interpretation of causal inferences as a measure of general EF, confounding language and EF processing. Once again, no clear relationships between EF and pragmatics were observed, suggesting that pragmatic and EF deficits (measured by causal inferencing) are not closely intertwined.

Impact of Executive Function Deficits

Clinically, EF impairments have important influences on long-term stroke outcomes (see Chapter 1, Table 1–2). The presence of cognitive deficits acutely predicts chronic cognitive deficits (Nys et al., 2005). Cognitive and EF deficits are related to performance of instrumental activities of daily life (IADLs; Middleton et al., 2014), functional recovery (Park et al., 2015), participation-level outcomes, and quality of life (Adamit et al., 2015). Oksala and colleagues (2009) reported lower survival rates for adults with poststroke EF deficits compared with patients without cognitive deficits (5.8 versus 10 years survival). Stroke survivors with EF deficits are four times less likely to participate in moderate physical activity one year poststroke than those without EF deficits (Påhlman, Sävborg, & Tarkowski, 2012). Given the positive relationship between exercise and cognitive function, this reduction in participation can have important consequences for recovery and well-being (Austin, Ploughman, Glynn, & Corbett, 2014; Kluding, Tseng, & Billinger, 2012; Liu-Ambrose & Eng, 2014).

A few studies have focused on the long-term impact of specific executive function deficits. Viscogliosi, Belleville, Desrosiers, Caron, and Ska (2011) examined the effects of EF deficits on patterns of change over time in regard to participation-level outcomes. Results indicated that patients with deficits in inhibition tended to show a greater rate of change over time in participation compared with patients with deficits of memory, attention, visuoperception, or language. Purposive behavior and self-regulation have been reported as primary predictors of return to work following stroke (Ownsworth et al., 2007). Planning, self-monitoring, and self-regulation are related to productivity, such that stroke survivors with deficits in these areas tended to have alterations to their work responsibilities that reduced their productivity compared with colleagues (Ownsworth & Shum, 2008).

Assessment of Executive Functions

Thorough assessment of EFs requires a combination of both standardized and nonstandardized tools as well as observation of the patient in a variety of settings. Impairment, activity, and participation-level EF abilities also should be assessed. Contextual factors that could impact premorbid EF abilities and treatment planning, such as education level and social and vocational expectations, should also be considered. Ideally, assessment should occur in collaboration with a neuropsychologist and other clinical/rehabilitation professionals to identify the client's strengths and weaknesses. The basic goals of cognitive assessment, as laid out by Constantinidou and colleagues (2012), include:

- Evaluation and identification of a client's strengths and weaknesses in relation to their return to daily activities

- Development and implementation of treatment goals

- Development of compensatory strategies

- Identification of the information necessary for personalized education of the client and family about the challenges they will face during the recovery process

- Establishment of a baseline against which to measure change.

Standardized assessments provide objective measures that allow for comparison against norms or criteria. Such assessments are valuable in identifying impairments and quantifying the severity of those impairments. However, they often have limited ecological or predictive validity (Alvarez & Emory, 2006; Burgess et al., 2006; Constantinidou et al., 2012; Turkstra et al., 2005). Thus, performance on standardized tests may not help in determining how well a patient will do in an everyday situation, or predict prognosis.

Nonstandardized measures are useful for assessing behaviors and successes in real-world activities or settings, determining what kinds of strategies are used and how effective they are, exploring the effectiveness of communication partners using different kinds of supports, and identifying the kinds of demands on cognition and communication that arise in daily activities (Coelho, Ylvisaker, & Turkstra, 2005; Ylvisaker, Szekerez, & Feeney, 2008). Nonstandardized assessments provide greater insight into what kinds of strategies might be effective and what situations/environments facilitate or impede performance. On the other hand, these measures are more subjective and performance may be difficult to quantify.

Standardized Assessment

There are a variety of cognitive and executive function assessments that are appropriate for adults with RHD (Table 8–2). Conti and colleagues (Conti, Sterr, Brucki, & Conforto, 2015) reviewed the assessments most commonly used for examining EF deficits due to stroke[2]. Of the 35 studies published between 1999 and 2015 on this topic, the most commonly used assessments were the Stroop test (Stroop, 1935), digit span, and the Trail Making Test (Rietan, 1958). Others included the Wisconsin Card Sorting Test (WCST; Grant & Berg, 1981), verbal fluency, and the Behavioral Assessment of Dysexecutive Syndrome (BADS; Wilson, Emslie, Evans, Alderman, & Burgess, 1996). Success on these measures is dependent upon

---

[2]The studies reviewed all were designed to assess executive function in adults post-stroke. However, they all were basic or applied research studies, not clinical studies, and thus the results likely do not reflect the assessments used most often in clinical practice.

Table 8–2. Select Measures of Executive Function

Scale	Authors	Domains Assessed	Reliability*	Validity*
Behavioral Assessment of the Dysexecutive Syndrome (BADS)	Wilson et al., 1996	Organization, planning, problem solving, self-monitoring	Weak	Good
Behavior Rating Inventory of Executive Function (BRIEF) –Adult Version	Roth et al., 2005	Self-regulation in natural environment	Good	OK
Brixton-Spatial Anticipation Test	Burgess & Shallice, 1997	Rule derivation and shifting, fluid ability	Good	OK
Delis-Kaplan Executive Function System	Delis et al., 2001	Nine separate tests of executive function: Word Context test, Sorting Test, Twenty Questions test, Tower test, Color-Word Interference test, Verbal Fluency test, Design Fluency test, Trail Making test, Proverb test	OK (varied by subtest)	Weak
Dysexecutive Questionnaire (DEX)	Burgess et al., 1998; Wilson et al., 1996	Intentionality, inhibition, executive memory, affect	None	OK
Functional Assessment of Verbal Reasoning and Executive Strategies (FAVRES)	McDonald, 2005	Verbal reasoning, executive function	OK	OK
Frontal Systems Behavior Scale	Grace & Malloy, 2001	Intentionality and disinhibition	OK	Good
Hayling Sentence Completion Test	Burgess & Shallice, 1997	Response inhibition, fluid ability	Good	OK
Iowa Gambling Task (IGT)	Bechara et al., 1994	Executive function, decision making, & emotional signals	None	OK

continues

Table 8–2. *continued*

Scale	Authors	Domains Assessed	Reliability*	Validity*
MicroCog: Assessment of Cognitive Functioning, 2004 Edition	Powell et al., 2004	Computerized assessment of attention, memory, EF, reaction time, speed of processing, general cognitive functioning	OK	OK
Multiple Errands Test	Shallice & Burgess, 1991	Strategy allocation, planning	Good	Good
Naturalistic Action Test	Schwarz et al., 2002	Planning, sequencing, and strategy allocation	Good	Good
Revised Strategy Application Test	Levine et al., 2000	Executive function and strategy allocation	None	OK
Ruff Figural Fluency Test (RFFT)	Ruff, 1996	"Cognitive fluency"— shift, cognitive set, planning strategies, executive ability	OK	Good
Tower of Hanoi	Newell & Simon, 1972	Planning	Good	Weak
Tower of London	Shallice, 1982	Planning	Good	Good
Trail Making Test	Reitan, 1958	Attention, planning, working memory	None	OK
Wisconsin Card Sorting Test (WCST)	Heaton et al., 1993	Switching/perseveration	Good	Weak

Note. *Good = moderate–strong estimates of two or more types of reliability/validity; OK = moderate–strong estimates of one type of reliability/validity or mixture of weak and strong estimates; weak = weak estimates of 1 or more types of reliability/validity; none = no estimates reported. See Appendix for detailed information about reliability and validity.

a variety of executive functions, and clinicians cannot determine merely from an overall score the reason for the deficient performance (Constantinidou et al., 2012). The relationship between performance on standardized assessments and functional abilities is questionable. The most widely used measures were not initially developed for clinical purposes, but were adopted for such uses without much evidence to suggest that they would be appropriate for making clinical decisions or predictions (Burgess et al., 2006). Functionally based assessments, such as the Multiple Errands Test (Shallice & Burgess, 1991) and the Zoo-Map Test (Alderman, Evans, Emslie, Wilson, & Burgess 1996; also included as a component of the BADS), have been shown to be more ecologically valid, in that they more closely predict functional abilities. Burgess and colleagues (2006) indicated that the development of valid, reliable measures of functional cognitive abilities is long past due.

In 2005, a systematic review of standardized assessments available for use by speech-language pathologists (SLPs) was published by the traumatic brain injury (TBI) writing group of the Academy of Neurologic Communication Disorders and Sciences (ANCDS; Turkstra et al., 2005). The authors identified 78 tests that met their criteria and reviewed 31 of them that were designed or conceptualized with TBI in mind. They also described the assessment recommendations provided by experts in the field. They provided four practice options for approaching assessment.

1. Caution must be taken in using and interpreting standardized tests for cognitive-communication deficits. This is based on limitations of the reliability and validity of specific tests and the focus of the tests. The vast majority of standardized assessments focus on the impairment level, whereas cognitive-communication deficits are most apparent at activity and participation levels. Additionally, standardized tests typically involve strict administration procedures and a quiet room free of distractors, and provide patients with the materials needed. These environmental characteristics make the testing situation very different from everyday situations, and the impairment scores may not accurately reflect the potential for success in familiar daily activities.

Standardized test scores may either over- or underestimate a client's functional abilities. Underestimation can be related to the novel, decontextualized tasks that are often part of EF assessments, test anxiety that decreases performance, and a focus on impairments as opposed to activities or participation. In a familiar setting with familiar supports, a patient may do better than would be expected by impairment-level scores. Some patients are able to use areas of strength to compensate for areas of weakness in familiar environments. In semi-independent living, daily functioning is structured primarily by established routines.

The opposite may also occur, such that standardized scores overestimate a client's ability to function in daily life because of the structured environment, absence of distractors, and specific instructions. Additionally, novel situations that occur in daily life may be accompanied by emotional responses that impact a person's ability to respond appropriately. Imagine a client is making toast, a routine task, and there is an electrical short that causes the toast to catch on fire. The fire may elicit anxiety and fear that will impact the person's ability to think through the possible solutions. Such emotional responses are not addressed in standardized tests. Asking someone to describe what she would do if the toaster caught on fire might yield a reasonable response in a testing situation, but the ability to verbally respond may not (and often does not) generalize to how the person will respond in the actual situation.

2. Standardized testing must be interpreted in the broader context of each client's life, including social and caregiving networks, pre-injury characteristics, and personal needs and wants including the demands of daily social and vocational activities. Due to the limitations of standardized tests in terms of predicting current or future performance in "real-life" settings, nonstandardized, dynamic assessments must also be used to identify strengths and weaknesses at the activity and participation levels.

3. Collaboration with colleagues in related fields is important for developing a more valid understanding of a client's cognitive and behavioral status and potential. Neuropsychologists have extensive training in administration and interpretation of cognitive assessments; SLPs provide critical expertise for understanding the impact of cognitive deficits on communication; occupational therapists have expertise in how cognition affects activities of daily living. Input from all of the rehabilitation team members will provide a broader, more realistic view of a client's impairments and the impact they have on daily functioning.

Nonstandardized Assessment

The ANCDS writing committee also made recommendations regarding nonstandardized assessments to complement the use of standardized assessments (Coelho et al., 2005). Most of these are relevant for communication efficiency and effectiveness, and were discussed in Chapters 3 and 4. Specifically for cognition and executive function, collaborative, contextualized hypothesis testing is valuable in determining what kinds of cognitive and behavioral supports are most effective for a particular patient.

Ylvisaker and colleagues (Ylvisaker et al., 2008) provide an in-depth discussion of dynamic assessment. They describe assessment as a form of "contextualized hypothesis testing," in which clinicians seek to identify both strengths and weaknesses and explore what kinds of structure, support, and strategies are beneficial and which are not. Through this process, clinicians can obtain a wealth of information that can be used to tailor therapy. They can identify how much support is necessary to create success through enhancing and fading cues; what specific contexts or environments facilitate performance and to what extent; and what level of complexity (in various areas—memory, EF, attention, language) is appropriate versus too easy or too difficult.

The process should involve:

■ Observing a client in different settings and interacting with different people with an eye toward identifying settings, environments, and people that either facilitate or hinder success

■ Observing how a client reacts to a situation or problem, including emotional and behavioral responses

■ Identifying whether a client spontaneously uses any strategies, when they are used, and whether they are beneficial or not.

Environmental assessment is an important part of the process. As described in Chapter 2, knowledge of the structures and people in a client's environment and the level of support they provide will assist in determining the impact of EF deficits on daily functioning.

Treatment for EF Deficits

There are no studies of treatment for EF/cognitive deficits specifically for adults with RHD. However, the TBI literature provides important recommendations that should be applicable to the RHD population. Most of the research focuses on adults with chronic brain injury, with a greater focus on moderate-to-severe injury compared with mild TBI. Additionally, most of the research describes general "cognitive rehabilitation," which likely includes not only aspects of EF but also other cognitive abilities such as attention and memory.

There are many reviews of the efficacy and effectiveness of cognitive rehabilitation following stroke or TBI (AHRQ, Brasure et al., 2012; Cicerone et al., 2011; IOM, 2011; Langhorne, Bernhardt, & Kwakkel, 2011; Poulin, Korner-Bitensky, Dawson, & Bherer, 2012). In general, the results are not very positive. There are not enough well-controlled, carefully documented, experimental studies of rehabilitation from which to generate conclusions about the effectiveness of rehabilitation or to make recommendations about specific treatment methods.

Three reviews will be briefly discussed to provide a sense of the current state of knowledge. The conclusions differ somewhat depending on the criteria for including studies in the review (e.g., some included only randomized control trials, while others also included well-controlled single subject designs; see discussion in Chapter 2) and the outcomes assessed (e.g., short- versus long-term gains; gains in impairment, activity, or participation levels). Despite the differences in the recommendations, all conclude that more work is needed to develop and assess treatments that will make a meaningful difference in the lives of adults with cognitive disorders.

A review by the Institute of Medicine (2011) included 90 studies of treatments specifically for adults with TBI that reported either impairment-level outcomes or maintenance of gains on patient-centered goals. The authors reported the level of evidence (e.g., modest, limited, or not informative) for a variety of cognitive and language domains. Results indicated that for treatments specifically for executive function deficits, there was not enough evidence to determine the effects of treatment on (1) patient-centered outcomes such as quality of life or functional status; (2) generalization outside of treatment for patients with moderate–severe TBI in the chronic phase of recovery; or (3) maintenance of gains.

Examination of the evidence for multimodal cognitive rehabilitation similarly was not strong enough to support recommendations regarding the impact on patient-centered outcomes, maintenance of treatment gains, or domain-specific impairment-level outcomes when treatment was provided in the subacute phase of recovery. When treatments specifically for adults with mild TBI were examined, there was evidence, albeit limited, supporting impairment-level and patient-centered outcomes from comprehensive or multimodal treatments with maintenance of gains up to three months (IOM, 2011).

Despite the seemingly gloomy results, the IOM committee emphasizes that "the limitations of the evidence do not rule out meaningful benefit" (p. 14–1). While there are not enough well-designed studies to provide strong support for the use of one treatment over another, the committee encourages the use of cognitive rehabilitation for individuals with cognitive deficits as well as additional research to add to the evidence base.

The Agency for Healthcare Research and Quality (AHRQ; Brasure et al., 2012) evaluated 16 studies of multidisciplinary postacute cognitive rehabilitation programs for adults with moderate–severe TBI that reported participation-level outcomes. The committee concluded that there was insufficient evidence to determine the effectiveness of multimodal cognitive rehabilitation, either in individual or in group treatments. They reported that many of the programs were poorly described and few were theoretically based. Other factors that limit the conclusions are the heterogeneity of the TBI population, the variety of treatments and methods used in the programs, and individual responses to specific treatment programs that cannot be captured by group results.

Cicerone and colleagues (2011) reviewed 112 studies of language and cognitive disorders resulting from acquired brain injury (both TBI and stroke). Based on their review, they recommended practice standards (substantive evidence of effectiveness), practice guidelines (evidence of probable effectiveness), and practice options (evidence of possible effectiveness). For executive function and problem solving, Cicerone and colleagues (2011) provide several standards and guidelines, as well as one practice option. A summary of their recommendations is provided in Table 8–3.

Based on these reviews, three treatment approaches with some supportive evidence will be described: metacognitive strategies, problem-solving strategies, and comprehensive-holistic rehabilitation.

Metacognitive Strategies

Metacognition is thinking about one's own thinking. Metacognitive strategies are systems for breaking problems into smaller steps to achieve a goal. The strategies typically include some "self-talk" to pace oneself through a task, and include the following components: generating goals, self-monitoring performance, self-recording performance, and adjusting a plan of action based on feedback (internal or external). In some cases, clients will be asked to predict how well they will do, and then compare their prediction with the actual results. The strategies typically are designed to be fairly general, so that

Table 8–3. Recommendations for Treatment of Executive Function and Problem-Solving Deficits

Recommendation Level	*Treatment*
Practice standards	• Metacognitive strategy training • Comprehensive-holistic rehabilitation
Practice guidelines	• Formal problem-solving strategies with application to everyday situations and functional activities • Individualized and interpersonal therapies in a comprehensive program
Practice options	• Group treatments

Note. Practice standards are based on substantive evidence of effectiveness; practice guidelines are based on evidence of probable effectiveness; and practice options are based on evidence of possible effectiveness.

Source: Based on Cicerone et al., 2011.

they can be implemented with a variety of tasks or activities (Table 8–4). In order to achieve success, extensive practice is needed with different tasks and in a variety of contexts. Metacognitive strategies have been shown to be effective in treatment for a variety of cognitive domains, including attention, memory, awareness, social skills, and higher-level cognition (Cicerone et al., 2011). Publications by Ylvisaker (Ylvisaker & Feeney, 1998; Ylvisaker et al., 2008) and Sohlberg and Turkstra (2011) provide in-depth explanations of developing and implementing metacognitive strategies based on the authors' extensive work with clients post-TBI to supplement the basics provided here.

There is compelling evidence that metacognitive strategies are effective in improving problem solving in adults with cognitive deficits related to TBI and that they have a beneficial effect on activity- and participation-level outcomes (Cicerone et al., 2011; Sohlberg & Turkstra,

2011). Importantly, clients with mild-to-moderate TBI can learn to implement the strategies, even though they are cognitively demanding by nature. This suggests that while many adults with RHD tend to have more difficulty with cognitive and language tasks that have metacognitive demands compared with those that are implicit (Blake, 2007; Tompkins & Scott, 2013; see also Chapter 4), this should not prevent them from being able to learn and implement metacognitive strategies.

The majority of the treatment research has been conducted with patients in the chronic phase of recovery from TBI. While the results are promising, there is little information about whether strategy training might be effective earlier in recovery or with stroke survivors. Skidmore et al. (2015) examined the effects of metacognitive strategy training on executive functions when provided within a month following stroke. Participants were stroke survivors (2/3 of whom had an RH

Table 8–4. General Metacognitive Strategies

WSTC Lawson & Rice, 1989	What should I be doing? Select a strategy Try the strategy Check the strategy
Ylvisaker et al., 2008	Goal Plan (predict) Do Review
Goal Management Training (GMT) Levine et al., 2011	STOP ("what am I doing?") DEFINE the main task LIST the steps LEARN the steps (if not already known) DO IT (execute the task) CHECK ("am I doing what I planned to do?")
IDEAL Byrnes, 1996	Identify problem Define problem Explore alternative approaches Act on the plan Look at the effects

stroke) with at least one cognitive impairment who were in an inpatient rehabilitation facility. Outcome measures included Functional Independence Measure scores and measures of inhibition and cognitive flexibility. Participants were randomly assigned to either strategy training or reflective listening. Results indicated significantly greater increases on the outcome measures for the strategy group compared with the listening group. The improvements were observed at the end of treatment as well as at 3 and 6 months following treatment. The results suggest that strategy training may be effective for patients with cognitive deficits related to stroke and that such treatment in the subacute phase of recovery can have long-lasting positive effects.

There are three important components of metacognitive strategy training prior to beginning the extensive practice. First, selection or development of strategies must be done in consideration of the client's goals and with input from the client (Sohlberg & Turkstra, 2011). The strategy must be one that he/she is comfortable with and would be likely to use outside of the therapy setting. Education about the strategy is critical. The education should include knowledge about the strategy and the procedure for implementing it; when and where the strategy should be used; and how the strategy will help the client.

If it is a strategy for organizing thoughts to tell a story, then it might be used only in certain conversational settings. If it is a strategy for identifying and repairing communication breakdowns, then it might be used in any conversational setting.

Second, the clinician must assess the client's feelings toward the strategy and motivation to use it. A client who does not like the strategy or who does not feel it "fits" him or her is unlikely to use it independently. If the client believes it will help and is comfortable using it, he/she will be more motivated to learn and practice the strategy. The inclusion of the client in the selection/development of the strategy, as described above, will be beneficial in increasing the motivation.

Third, the clinician must make sure that the client's cognitive abilities are adequate for determining when and how to use the strategy. For clients with more severe cognitive impairments, task-specific strategies might be used. These strategies would be designed for a specific activity or situation. The client needs to learn to identify a specific situation or task and employ the strategy every time that situation presents itself. In contrast, clients with better executive functions may be able to learn and use a more general strategy that is designed to address a general problem that could occur in many different activities or settings. In this case, clients need to recognize a variety of situations in which the problem may surface and employ the strategy in each one.

The essential components of metacognitive strategies are as follows:

a. **Task preparation.** This involves getting ready for the task. The goal should be set along with a series of steps to achieve the goal. The preparation can include self-instructional phrases such as "get ready to focus," "clear my thoughts," or something similar that is relevant to the client. All of the necessary tools or supplies should be collected during the preparation stage to minimize interruptions during the task itself. A prediction of how successful he/she will be can also be added at the end of the preparation stage.

b. **Task execution.** The client should pace him/herself through the steps planned out earlier, monitoring performance along the way to ensure that progress is being made. Self- instructional phrases to "keep going" or "do one step at a time" also can be used.

c. **Posttask.** Once the task is completed, the client should review the process, check his/her success by checking answers or solutions, and summarize the process. If the goal was not met, the source of failure should be explored. If the client made a prediction, the result should be compared with the prediction.

Any treatment involving strategy training must include extensive practice in order for the strategy to become habitual (Ylvisaker et al., 2008). There are several reasons. First, adults with brain injuries often have difficulty learning new information and learning from experience. Thus, they need repeated practice to learn the strategy and to recognize the link between successes occurring with the use of a strategy and failure (or less than optimal performance) without it. Second, there is a well-known dissociation between knowing and doing that can occur in adults with acquired brain injury.

A client may know what to do, and be able to verbally describe a deficit or provide a logical, feasible plan for solving a problem but may not be able to enact that plan when in a relevant situation. Finally, there is a hierarchy regarding when clients realize they need to use a strategy. At the lowest level is awareness once failure has occurred; the second level is awareness during a task, when a client realizes that he is not going to succeed; the highest level is anticipatory awareness, in which a client can anticipate that a problem will occur unless a strategy is employed (Crosson et al., 1989; see discussion in Chapter 9). Repeated practice with strategies in a variety of settings (see discussion of treatment generalization and maintenance, below) will improve a client's ability to develop anticipatory awareness.

Rath, Simon, Langenbahn, Sherr, and Diller (2003) found that the addition of an orientation phase prior to treatment increased the positive outcomes of their problem-solving treatment. The orientation included examining the clients' initial reaction to a problem situation in terms of affect, attitude, and motivation, and discussing these with the client. Next, they identified and removed potential blocks to effective problem solving. These included eliminating negative self-talk and maladaptive responses, identifying contexts or situations that decreased success, and stopping or preventing impulsive responses. Finally, they increased motivation to use problem-solving strategies by providing positive self-talk to replace the negative, and encouraged self-efficacious feelings —feelings that the client could succeed.

All cognitive treatments should include phases for acquisition, mastery, and generalization (Sohlberg & Turkstra, 2011). Different treatment techniques and practice schedules can enhance the success of each phase. During the acquisition phase, Sohlberg and Turkstra recommend the following steps, conducted using errorless learning and massed practice:

- The client describes the strategy, the purpose for the strategy, how and when it should be used (e.g., to achieve what goals) and lists the steps.

- The client uses the strategy, with cues and supports from the clinician. Cues may be external, such as a checklist or cue cards, or internal, such as talking through the steps.

Following acquisition, treatment moves into the mastery and generalization phases.

- External cues should be faded and replaced with internal cues; checklists may be memorized due to repeated use; talking through steps out loud may be converted to "inner speech."

- Extensive practice should involve different stimuli and environments.
  - ☐ The client should begin identifying cues or triggers that suggest the strategy should be used.
    - The clinician should vary the environmental triggers so that the client learns to identify them.
    - Different people should provide the cues/triggers, so that they are not associated only with one person.

◾ The cues/triggers should be provided in different environments and settings so that the client learns to recognize them in all relevant settings.
☐ Strategies are practiced in everyday contexts.
☐ Home programs are developed and practiced with the client and his/her family or caregivers so that they can be practiced at home.
☐ The clinician provides everyday reminders to increase the likelihood of use and practice of the strategy.

◾ Throughout the process, motivation must be maintained. This can include having the client take data on his/her own successes versus failures to assess and visualize the usefulness of the strategy.

Throughout the training process, clinicians must continually evaluate the effectiveness of the strategy. This includes the efficiency (time and effort), effectiveness (number of errors, rate of successes versus failures), and ease of task completion when the strategy is implemented. The effectiveness of the strategy in different contexts also should be monitored. It is possible that a conversation-organizing strategy works well when used in a social gathering or when meeting new people but is ineffective in a home setting, where conversational patterns may be more informal and are less amenable to change. The impact of a strategy in daily life should also be evaluated. If there are generalized, large increases in effective problem solving, the strategy may clearly be making an impact. If the changes are more restricted to certain environments, yet there are distinct improvements for those settings, then it still may be useful to maintain the strategy but limit its use to those settings. If a strategy is only minimally effective, then small changes, major alterations, or elimination of the strategy altogether may be necessary.

Task-Specific Problem-Solving Strategies

Task-specific (or task-oriented) strategies, as the name indicates, are those that are designed to promote success for a specific task, with no expectation of generalization (e.g., Myers, 1999; Sohlberg & Turkstra, 2011).These should be highly individualized, created to solve a specific problem for a specific client. For example, if a client has difficulty grocery shopping, takes an inordinate amount of time, and returns home with some items that he/she does not need but without some items that were needed, a strategy for shopping might be needed. The strategy might include creating a standard list with commonly needed items arranged in the order they would be found in the store. Prior to going to the store, the client should review the list and check whether each item is needed. Those that he needs to buy should be highlighted. Any special items not on the list should be added at the bottom. At the store, the client would use the strategy of going through the store in the same direction, aisle by aisle, each time. This would increase the efficiency and effectiveness of trips to the grocery store. The strategy likely would not generalize to shopping at a hardware store, and thus would be task specific.

Holistic Cognitive Programs

Comprehensive rehabilitation programs are typically designed and implemented through collaborations across rehabilitation professionals, including physical therapists, SLPs, occupational therapists, neuropsychologists, social workers, and others. Details of the programs and primary areas of focus are often site specific. For example, in the milieu approach pioneered by Ben-Yishay (1996; Ben-Yishay & Diller, 2011; Prigatano, 1999) the relationship between clinicians and clients is paramount. Cicerone and colleagues (2011) recommend individualization within the larger program to enhance outcomes.

There is emerging evidence that participation in exercise programs can improve EF in adults with cognitive deficits related to stroke (Austin et al., 2014; Kluding et al., 2012; Liu-Ambrose & Eng, 2014). Providing exercise as part of a holistic program may aid in achieving gains in EF and other cognitive functions.

Environmental Manipulation

Environmental manipulation can be used at any stage of recovery to increase participation and potentially quality of life. The goal of environmental manipulation is to minimize the effects of deficits. It is not a treatment strategy *per se*, because there is no expectation that the client will "get better" or that the impairments will decrease. Instead, providing organization, structure, and cues in the client's environment can increase independence and participation. Examples of manipulations that might be effective for clients with EF deficits include putting labels on cupboards and organizing spaces and making sure necessary materials or tools are available. If a client wants to talk about a TV show with his daughter during their weekly phone conversation, then placing a pad of paper and pencil where he can reach it while watching TV will act as a cue to make notes about the show to discuss later. A white board in a visible place in the kitchen or near the front door can be used for reminders. A system of organizing medications and alarms to take the medications may be needed to increase the adherence to medication schedules.

Clinically, environmental manipulation often appears to create meaningful benefits but there is little research evidence to support the efficacy or effectiveness of such manipulations for clients with TBI or stroke. There is some evidence that participation and quality of life can be improved for clients with dementia by altering the environment, specifically the behaviors of communication partners (e.g., Bourgeois & Hickey, 2009; Hopper, 2007; Zientz et al., 2007).

Conclusions and Implications

EF deficits are common after stroke and can have substantial impacts on long-term outcomes. These are especially important for younger stroke survivors whose goals include returning to the workforce. Although more work is necessary to explore patterns of impairments and their effects on activity and participation levels in adults with RHD, the work with adults with TBI provides a solid foundation on which to plan and implement treatments.

9

Awareness

Awareness of one's own abilities, deficits, strengths, and weaknesses can impact performance in daily life, vocational success, and participation in rehabilitation. Awareness can be impaired following brain injury, particularly when the RH is damaged. This chapter will cover definitions, types, and models of awareness, how the RH is involved, and how to assess and treat deficits of awareness.

Anosognosia

The word "anosognosia" comes from Greek and means "without knowledge of disease." In clinical practice it is used to refer to the reduced awareness of either acquired deficits or the consequences of those deficits. The term was initially coined in 1914 by Babinski in reference to reduced awareness of hemiplegia (Babinski, 1914; translated by Langer & Levine, 2014). However, descriptions of reduced awareness first appeared over 30 years earlier when von Monakow described such a

deficit in relation to symptoms of Korsakoff's syndrome. Anton and Pick (known today as namesakes of types of cortical blindness and frontotemporal dementia) also described aspects of reduced awareness in the late 1800s (Prigatano, 2010a).

As with many disorders, there are inconsistencies in terminology (Table 9–1). "Anosognosia" is commonly used for reduced awareness of specific impairments, most often hemiparesis and unilateral neglect. Anosognosia is the label used in research with stroke survivors, while "Impaired Self-Awareness" (ISA) is preferred in the literature on TBI. ISA is defined more broadly; in addition to referring to reduced awareness of a specific deficit, it encompasses the functional implications of that deficit, the patient's expectations for recovery, differential awareness for different domains, and adherence to treatment (Orfei, Caltagirone, & Spalletta, 2009). Some even use ISA synonymously with metacognition (Schmidt, Lannin, Fleming, & Ownsworth, 2011), as both refer to one's understanding of one's own strengths and limitations and

Table 9–1. Terminology Related to Anosognosia

Terms	Description
Anosognosia	Reduced awareness of acquired deficits; typically used in relation to reduced awareness of specific impairments
Denial of deficit	Connotes that there is some awareness that allows for psychological refusal to acknowledge the deficit (conscious or unconscious)
Impaired self-awareness	Commonly used in TBI literature to refer to reduced awareness; can be used for specific impairments or general awareness; often includes insights about consequences and motivation to participate in therapy
Lack of insight	Connotes higher-level cognitive deficit implicating higher-level reasoning; reduced understanding/awareness of the consequences of an impairment
Types of Unawareness	
Explicit awareness	Ability to verbally report the presence of a deficit
Implicit awareness	Changes in behavior related to the presence of a deficit (e.g., to avoid failure related to a deficit)
Related Disorders	
Alexithymia	Reduced use of emotion-related words
Anosodiaphoria	Reduced emotional reaction to, or concern for, deficits
Asomatognosia	A form of disturbed sense of ownership in which a patient believes his impaired limb is missing or does not belong to him
Misoplegia	Hatred of one's limbs or body part(s)
Personification	Refer to and treat a limb as if it were its own being (e.g., naming one's arm)
Somatoparaphrenia	A form of disturbed sense of ownership in which a patient feels her impaired limb belongs to someone else

how those will impact performance on daily activities. Prigatano and Morrone-Strupinsky (2010) use the label "anosognosia" to refer to a complete unawareness of a specific impairment, and use "ISA" to refer to partial unawareness that may be a stage of recovery from anosognosia.

"Lack of insight" can be described as a component of ISA. It connotes a cognitive deficit implicating higher-level reasoning. This may occur in some patients who have a reduced awareness of the *consequences* of a deficit, even if they do have awareness of the deficit itself. A patient who can describe his hemiparesis, but in the next sentence talk about how he plans to resume his weekend bike rides with his son once he is discharged from the hospital could be described as having reduced insight.

The phrase "denial of deficit" often is used synonymously with anosognosia in clinical practice (Prigatano & Klonoff, 1998). However, denial is very different from reduced awareness. In order to deny that something exists, you must be aware of it and consciously reject it. Using the phrase "denial of deficit" may cause families to erroneously believe that the patient is being difficult or refusing to admit a problem, when in reality the patient is not aware of the existence of the deficit at a conscious level.

Another commonly used but not quite accurate label is "unawareness." While some researchers and clinicians use "unawareness" synonymously with anosognosia, the former suggests a complete loss of awareness and does not convey the nuances of the disorder, in which a patient may be aware of hemiparesis but not of cognitive deficits; have different levels of awareness of upper and lower extremity weakness (Berti, Ladavas, & Della Corte, 1996); demonstrate awareness that appears to increase or decrease depending on the questions asked; or may not verbally report hemiparesis but never try to stand up unassisted (Mograbi & Morris, 2013; Nurmi & Jehkonen, 2014; Orfei et al., 2007). For these and other reasons, Prigatano (2013) cautions that anosognosia should not be considered a unitary disorder.

Nurmi and Jehkonen (2014) highlight some of the difficulties and inconsisten-

cies in research on anosognosia. First, as described above, there are inconsistencies in definitions and terminology. Second is the distinction between explicit and implicit awareness (Fotopoulou, Pernigo, Maeda, Rudd, & Kopelman, 2010; Mograbi & Morris, 2013; Moro, Pernigo, Zapparoli, Cordioli, & Aglioti, 2011). Explicit unawareness is measured by verbal responses to questions (e.g., is there anything wrong with your arm?). Implicit unawareness, in contrast, is observed in patients' behaviors. A patient who does not verbally acknowledge her hemiplegia but who never attempts to get out of bed without assistance might have implicit but not explicit awareness of her deficit. Another example of implicit awareness comes from studies that employ bimanual tasks (e.g., Cocchini, Beschin, Fotopoulou, & Della Sala, 2010; Moro et al., 2011). Some individuals with explicit anosognosia will use strategies to complete bimanual tasks that suggest implicit awareness of upper limb paralysis. For example, when asked to lift a two-handled tray, they will lift with one hand in the middle of the tray instead of attempting to lift from the two ends. In studies of Alzheimer's disease, some patients may have emotional reactions to failure despite not being able to explicitly acknowledge the poor performance (Mograbi & Morris, 2013). Not all individuals with anosognosia have preserved implicit awareness. Evidence from priming studies (Fotopoulou et al., 2010; Nardone, Ward, Fotopoulou, & Turnbull, 2007) suggests that some patients with anosognosia show reduced activation of relevant disability-related words (e.g., weakness, walk) compared with individuals with hemiparesis but intact awareness, indicating that explicit and implicit awareness can be affected differentially.

Vocat and Vuilleumier (2010) suggest that the dissociation between implicit and explicit awareness could be due to two separate monitoring systems. One is a subcortical system that provides implicit, automatic monitoring of "affective relevance of a mismatch between a goal and the outcome" (p. 267). The other is a cortical system residing in frontal and parietal lobes which provides "conscious error detection based on the quality of feedback and on access to attentional and executive networks" (p. 267). Damage to the former would cause a deficit of implicit awareness, and the latter would result in problems with explicit awareness.

Models of Anosognosia

There have been a variety of theories of anosognosia over the years. Some of the earliest were motivational or psychodynamic theories in which anosognosia was described as a form of psychological denial that was used as a defense mechanism (Weinstein & Kahn, 1955). While the terminology "denial of deficit" lingers, strong versions of these theories have been discarded in light of disconfirming evidence. Anosognosia has been identified in acute stages of stroke recovery, before patients have had a chance to experience their deficits (e.g., attempting to walk to the bathroom with a hemiparetic leg) or the broader consequences of them (e.g., not being able to drive with hemiparesis). Without the experience of the loss, there is no need for a psychological defense against it. Other evidence against this theory is the fact that some patients

can be aware of some deficits (e.g., hemiparesis) but not others (e.g., unilateral neglect) (Berti et al., 1996; Bisiach, Vallar, Perani, Papagno, & Berti, 1986). Turnbull, Fotopoulou, and Solms (2014) argue that such evidence does not spell the death knell for the idea that anosognosia may have an emotional component related to a defense mechanism. They argue that emotional deficits associated with RHD result in the person viewing the world as he would like it to be, as opposed to the reality. Thus, for some clients, emotion and motivation may play a strong role in anosognosia.

Geschwind (1965) suggested a disconnection model, in which verbal reports of awareness were disrupted by a disconnection between the RH sensory and proprioceptive processing areas and the LH language areas. If this were true, then there should be dissociations between verbal and nonverbal assessments of awareness. These dissociations have not consistently been found.

More recent theories use anatomical models and include different levels of awareness. Higher-level, conscious awareness is thought to be controlled primarily by the prefrontal regions. Low-level, modality-specific awareness is localized posteriorly, in the temporal and parietal lobes. Damage to either region could result in reduced awareness.

McGlynn and Schacter's (1989) Conscious Awareness System (CAS) resides primarily in the prefrontal regions and works in concert with judgment, insight, and self-reflection processes. Damage to the CAS may result in a global unawareness of self. The input from modality-specific systems (visual, somatosensory) is intact, but the signals are not processed correctly by the damaged CAS, thus resulting in incorrect interpretation and self-monitoring of the sensory input. In this model, cognitive and affective states may be part of the presentation of anosognosia.

In contrast to the CAS model are the modality- or domain-specific accounts of anosognosia (Bisiach, 1990). Damage to the temporal and parietal sensory processing areas may result in disruptions to connections or signals sent to the frontal lobes for processing by the CAS. For example, an RH parietal lesion may result in unilateral visual neglect. If information about the incomplete visual representation is not sent to the frontal lobes, or if erroneous information is sent (e.g., the visual representation is complete), then the central processor will not detect a problem, resulting in reduced awareness of the unattended visual field.

The theories with the most empirical support purport that anosognosia for hemiparesis is caused by a disruption in the motor control system. The motor system is thought to control intention to move, the movement itself, and a comparison between the intended movement and the actual movement based on sensory feedback. Disruption to either the intention or the comparator system has been implicated. According to the feed-forward model (Heilman, 1991; Wolpert, 1995), there is a loss of intention to move. In the intact system, the intended movement would be compared with the actual movement, and discrepancies would be noted. However, if there is a loss of intention, then there would be no discrepancy with an absence of actual movement. In the feedback model (Berti & Pia, 2006; Spinazzola, Pia, Folegatti, Marchetti, & Berti, 2008; Wolpert, 1995), the disruption occurs

in the comparison process. The intended (desired) and predicted results match, but the "comparator" does not correctly identify a mismatch between these two states and the actual movement. If no mismatch is identified, then there is no awareness that the movement was incorrect or did not occur as planned. This model can explain the phenomenon of illusory movement, in which patients report that they felt a movement occur, even in the face of contradictory visual and sensory feedback (Feinberg, Roane, & Ali, 2000; Fotopoulou et al., 2010). Jenkinson, Edelstyn, Drakeford, and Ellis (2009) reported that adults with anosognosia for hemiparesis are impaired in determining whether they had seen or imagined pictures or had performed, observed, or imagined actions. They tend to recall having seen pictures or performed actions that had only been imagined, indicating a deficit in reality monitoring.

Related Disorders

There are several disorders that are related to, or commonly co-occur with, anosognosia (see Table 9–1). In some cases, the disorders are erroneously considered to be parts of the same problem. First is unilateral neglect. Some researchers appear to equate unilateral neglect and anosognosia: "right hemispheric stroke is usually associated with neglect, which reduces awareness of neurological deficits" (Foersch et al., 2005, p. 392). While patients with unilateral neglect often have anosognosia for neglect, the deficits are distinct disorders that can be dissociated (Appelros, Karlsson, & Hennerdal, 2007; Berti et al., 1996; Bisiach et al., 1986; Vocat et al., 2010).

Additionally, some individuals with anosognosia for unilateral neglect can be aware of other deficits, such as hemiplegia.

Second is anosodiaphoria, which is a reduced concern for deficits, or reduced emotional expression related to those deficits (Babinski, 1914/Langer & Levine, 2014). This too has been dissociated from anosognosia. Some patients may be aware of their deficits and be able to identify and describe their hemiparesis but show no apparent concern over the loss of motor control. It is not clear whether there is reduction in emotional experience or if the problem is in the expression of emotion. Related to the latter is alexithymia, a reduced use of emotional words (Heilman & Harciarek, 2010; Jorge, 2010). Again, these two deficits may co-occur, but just because a person is not using many emotional words does not mean that he or she is not experiencing emotional responses.

Third, some individuals with anosognosia develop delusional beliefs about their hemiparetic limbs (Bottini et al., 2010; Giacino & Cicerone, 1998). Several of these fall under the category "disturbed sense of ownership" in which patients do not feel that a paretic limb really belongs to them (Karnath & Baier, 2010). One form of this is asomatognosia, in which they believe their limb is missing. In another form, somatoparaphrenia, patients attribute the impaired limb to someone else.

Other phenomena include misoplegia, in which patients develop a hatred for the impaired limb, and personification, in which patients develop a name and personality for the impaired limb. For example, a patient who names her hemiplegic arm "Connie" and gives reports about how Connie is doing on a particular day would be showing signs of personification. These delusional beliefs are productive deficits, in which there is an exacerbation or production of additional function, while anosognosia itself is a defective disorder in which there is reduction of function (Bottini et al., 2010).

Finally, confabulation can be observed in some individuals with anosognosia. The source of confabulations is not well studied, but they are thought to be an unconscious response to behaviors that

---

SIDEBAR

My first experience with anosognosia was with a patient who had been diagnosed with a right hemisphere tumor. His initial symptoms included getting lost in the hardware store in which he worked and bumping into the wall when walking down a hallway in his house. During a preoperative assessment in which he was asked about the latter problem, he explained: "My wife hangs too many pictures on the wall and I don't like them. So when I'm walking down the hall, I hit them so they fall off the wall." He confabulated an explanation for the symptoms because he was not consciously aware of the unilateral neglect caused by the RH tumor.

the clients cannot fully understand. Clients may produce reasons for not being able to complete tasks, or to explain away other people's concerns (e.g., Nathanson, Nathanson, Bergman, & Gordon, 1952). The confabulations tend to be idiosyncratic, possibly affected by cultural influences and premorbid personality traits (Giacino & Cicerone, 1998; Prigatano, 2010b).

Awareness and the Intact RH

In addition to coining the term "anosognosia" Babinski (1914; translated by Langer & Levine, 2014) suggested that the RH played a role in awareness and control of self-awareness. Similar to the RH dominance for visual attention (i.e., the RH controls attention to both right and left visual fields but the LH controls attention only to the right visual field), he suggested that the RH premotor intention system activates both the left and right sides of the body, whereas the homologous LH system activates only the contralateral right side.

There is a long list of regions within the RH that have been linked to aspects of self-awareness and anosognosia. Anosognosia has been reported as a result to lesions in the premotor and primary motor regions, primary sensory cortex, the dorsolateral prefrontal cortex, insula, and inferior parietal lobe (Berti et al., 2005). Specifically, anosognosia for hemiparesis has been linked to the right frontal-parietal region (Orfei et al., 2007, Pia et al., 2004) and the pars orbitalis in the inferior frontal gyrus (Korttke et al., 2014). Anosognosia for

sensory deficits has been linked to right lenticular and/or thalamic lesions (Bisiach et al., 1986). The right insula also has been suggested to be important for agency and ownership of one's body as well as housing neural representations of the body and mental representations of the self (Pia, Neppi-Modona, Ricci, & Berti, 2004). Reduced awareness of pragmatics, social behavior, and executive function deficits has been linked to damage in the anterior medial prefrontal regions (Orfei et al., 2007). Implicit anosognosia may occur with damage to the anterior insula, deep white matter, basal ganglia, or limbic system structures, but rarely with cortical frontal or parietal lesions (Fotopoulou et al., 2010). Vocat and colleagues (2010) reported that patients with acute anosognosia tended to have lesions in the insula and adjacent subcortical white matter. Accompanying cortical lesions in the premotor area, cingulate, parietal-temporal junction, or medial temporal lobe were present in those patients whose anosognosia persisted into subacute stages of recovery.

Anosognosia and RHD

The true incidence of anosognosia following stroke is unknown, with estimates ranging from 10 to 77% (Orfei et al., 2007). Factors that influence the diagnosis of anosognosia include the various subtypes, spontaneous recovery, the subjectivity of assessment of awareness, and problems related to inconsistent terminology (described above). As with all deficits caused by stroke, spontaneous recovery is possible, especially within the first few weeks poststroke. In one study, 32% of patients with RHD evidenced anosognosia within the first three days after stroke. The incidence decreased to 18% after one week, and to 5% after six months (Vocat et al., 2010). The authors caution, though, that at six months, some of the individuals may have learned the "right" answers to the awareness questions, even if their intrinsic awareness had not changed.

While there seems to be an RH bias for anosognosia (occurring in 17–69% of individuals with RHD and 6–46% of those with LHD; Nurmi & Jehkonen, 2014), the problem is not strictly related to RHD. The incidence of anosognosia caused by LHD appears to have been vastly underestimated for many decades. This is likely due to the theories of RH dominance for awareness as well as the fact that most assessments of awareness depend on verbal report. The latter made it difficult to reliably evaluate awareness in individuals with aphasia. Cocchini, Della Sala, and colleagues (Cocchini, Gregg, Beschin, Dean, & Della Sala, 2010; Della Sala, Cocchini, Beschin, & Cameron, 2009) developed a visual analog scale for assessing awareness of motor and language deficits that could be used with adults with aphasia. Prior to development of this scale, over 50% of potential LHD participants were routinely excluded from studies of anosognosia due to aphasia and an inability to complete structured interviews. With the visual analog scale, Cocchini and colleagues were able to assess 72% of their sample of adults with LHD. They reported that anosognosia for hemiplegia occurs equally often as a result of RHD and LHD.

This pattern of occurrence was replicated by Nurmi and Jehkonen (2014).

The relationship between anosognosia and other cognitive disorders is unclear. Some researchers have reported a relationship between awareness and executive functions (Bottini et al., 2010; Starkstein et al., 2010). In contrast, Vocat et al. (2010) reported that anosognosia was not related to executive function or mood but was related to deficits in proprioception and disorientation. The level of anosognosia does not appear to be related to short-term memory or scores on Raven's progressive matrices (Berti et al., 1996)

In some cases an apparent unawareness is not due to anosognosia itself, but rather to other cognitive deficits that create the appearance of reduced awareness. Clients with short-term memory loss may not be able to retain information about their impairments, and thus forget that they have deficits. This may appear as reduced awareness but is mediated by the memory loss. Similarly, clients with deficits in abstract reasoning may also appear to have anosognosia if they are unable to reason through the consequences of their deficits. A grocery store clerk who has executive function deficits may not be able to conclude that unilateral neglect would affect the way he stocked shelves (Giacino & Cicerone, 1998).

Anosognosia is related to decreased participation in cognitive rehabilitation, poorer prognoses for treatment gains and more restrictive discharge location, reduced functional recovery for activities of daily living, and increased caregiver burden (Jehkonen et al., 2001; Prigatano, 2010b; Vossel, Weiss, Eschenbeck, & Fink,

2012). Given these far-reaching consequences, careful assessment and treatment is needed to reduce the potential effects of anosognosia on participation and quality of life.

Assessment of Awareness

Assessment should include the following: modality specificity; explicit and implicit awareness; the presence of other phenomena or deficits such as unilateral neglect, confabulation, and anosodiaphoria; and differential diagnosis of psychological denial versus anosognosia. Patients' perceptions of the cause of their deficits, the functional implications or consequences of their deficits, their expectations for recovery, and their perceptions of the need for treatment also should be assessed (Orfei et al., 2009). Finally, clinicians should evaluate the level of awareness. Crosson and colleagues (1989) describe three interdependent levels that impact functional activities: intellectual, emergent, and anticipatory awareness. Intellectual awareness is the ability to recognize a deficit as well as its consequences. It encompasses education and knowledge of a deficit as well as recognition of when the deficit may impact success and the consequences of the deficit. Anosognosia, as described in this chapter, would affect intellectual awareness. The next level in Crosson's model is emergent awareness, when a client becomes aware of a deficit during a task when errors or failure occurs. Intellectual awareness is required for emergent awareness: one must be aware a deficit is

present to begin to recognize the effects of the deficit on performance. Differences between knowing and doing can occur in clients with problems in emergent awareness: they can describe their deficits but cannot predict what tasks will be difficult or use a strategy to avoid failure. The highest level is anticipatory awareness. This occurs when a client understands her deficits and can anticipate errors or failures if compensatory measures are not used. Toglia and Kirk (2000) expand upon Crosson's model, highlighting the difference between knowledge of a deficit and online or situational awareness in which self-monitoring occurs. Their expanded model includes aspects of inconsistencies in awareness, described earlier, in which a client can be aware of, and possibly compensate for, some deficits but not others. Additionally, they assert that the ability to self-monitor or self-correct can also be influenced by the task or situation.

Assessment of anosognosia is necessarily subjective and relies on patient report. There is no objective way to determine someone else's level of awareness, particularly for deficits of relatively abstract abilities such as pragmatics and cognition. A variety of questionnaires have been designed for assessing awareness (Table 9–2). The majority of the early assessments were designed to assess awareness of hemiplegia, with some targeting unilateral neglect (see reviews in Orfei et al., 2007, 2009). As the understanding of anosognosia grew, so did the depth and breadth of the questionnaires. There are now quite a few that address awareness of cognitive or pragmatic deficits and have questions that address both implicit and explicit awareness.

Table 9–2. Select Assessments of Anosognosia that Address Cognition, Pragmatics, and/or Neglect

Scale	Authors	Domains Assessed	Reliability*	Validity*
Awareness Questionnaire	Sherer et al., 1998, 2003	Cognition, emotion/ pragmatics, functional implications, implicit awareness, hemiparesis, neglect	OK	Good
Bisiach scale	Bisiach et al., 1986	Hemiplegia, neglect	None	None
Head Injury Behavior Scale (HIBS)	Godfrey, 2003	Emotion/pragmatics, functional implications	OK	OK
Impaired Self-Awareness (ISA) scale	Prigatano & Klonoff, 1998	Cognition	None	OK
Levine Denial of Illness Scale	Levine 1987	Prognosis/compliance	Good	OK
Patient Competency Rating Scale (PCRS)	Prigatano & Klonoff, 1998	Cognition, emotion/ pragmatics, functional implications	Good	OK
PCRS-NR	Borgaro & Prigatano, 2003	Cognition, emotion/ pragmatics, functional implications	OK	OK
Self-Awareness of Deficit Interview (SADI)	Fleming et al., 1996	Cognition, emotion/ pragmatics, functional implications, treatment compliance	Good	OK
Structured Awareness Interview (SAI)	Marcel et al., 2004	Implicit awareness, hemiplegia vision/ neglect	None	None
Visual-Analogue Test for Anosognosia Language	Cocchini et al., 2010	Functional implications, aphasia	OK	None
Visual-Analogue Test for Anosognosia for Motor Impairment	Della Sala et al., 2009	Functional implications, hemiparesis	Good	OK

Note. *Good = moderate–strong estimates of two or more types of reliability/validity; OK = moderate–strong estimates of one type of reliability/validity or mixture of weak and strong estimates; weak = weak estimates of one or more types of reliability/validity; none = no estimates reported. See Appendix for detailed information about reliability and validity.

SIDEBAR

A 58-year-old male, six years post-RH stroke, had a variety of communication and cognitive deficits, including mild unilateral neglect. Over the course of his rehabilitation, he had received many different therapies. He was aware of his unilateral neglect and had received targeted treatment for neglect at several time points. Upon questioning, he would report that he had neglect, that it used to affect his reading but not anymore (this was true), and that he needed to remind himself to look to the left when he couldn't find something. In conversation with his wife, she reported that he commonly has problems finding socks in his sock drawer. He will look through the drawer several times and ask if the socks were in the laundry or had not yet been put away. The majority of times, the socks were actually in the drawer but were pushed over to the left side.

This man showed good intellectual awareness of his deficit and knew the strategies (look to the left), yet was not at the level of anticipatory awareness, with which he would begin scanning his sock drawer from the left side to prevent the error (not finding the socks) from occurring.

Additionally, some include questions for family members or caregivers as well as patients.

The distinction between denial of deficit and anosognosia is critical, as the approach to treatment is different for psychological denial than for a cognitive deficit of awareness. Giacino and Cicerone (1998) espouse the use of a structured interview and close attention to patients' responses to feedback to identify deficits that might be related to psychological denial versus true impairment of awareness (see also Prigatano & Klonoff, 1998; Prigatano & Morrone-Strupinsky, 2010). They also suggest that patients' responses can help distinguish between unawareness due to other cognitive deficits (e.g., memory or abstract reasoning) versus anosognosia.

Clinicians should examine patients' cognitive and affective responses as well as how they use the feedback given. Table 9–3 provides details of the types of responses typical of awareness deficits with different underlying mechanisms.

Treatment of Anosognosia

General Strategies

Specific treatment suggestions and supporting evidence will be provided in the next section; however, several generalizations are provided here, based on the underlying mechanism of unawareness. If the problem is thought to be related to

Table 9–3. Responses to Feedback Based on Mechanism of Unawareness

	Cognitive Deficit (impairments of memory, reasoning)	*Neurologic Injury (anosognosia)*	*Psychological Denial of Deficit*
Cognitive response	Surprise, confusion	Rationalization or minimization	Refute the feedback; may attribute the problem to someone else or to the environment
Affective response	Increased concern	Neutral or blunted response; perplexed; indifferent	Increased arousal and anger (may eventually develop into depression)
Behavioral response	Actively use feedback (although may be transient or inconsistent)	Passive response; may momentarily try to understand	Intolerant of feedback; actively resist it or discount it; irritated, agitated responses

Source: Based on Giacino and Cicerone (1998).

a specific cognitive deficit, then that deficit should be targeted first. For example, if short-term and working memory are impaired, then the patient may not be able to encode and store the information for later retrieval. Increased awareness may not be possible until the memory deficits have been addressed. In contrast, if the problem is due to damage to the awareness networks, then direct treatment of awareness can be used. Finally, if the deficit appears to be one of psychological denial, the best course of action is to refer the patient to a neuropsychologist or related professional who can directly work with the psychological issues.

Treatment Approaches

The majority of the treatment research has been conducted with individuals with ISA resulting from moderate-to-severe TBI,

and much of it comes from the occupational therapy literature. In their review of cognitive treatments, Cicerone and colleagues (2011) concluded that metacognitive training for executive functions, including awareness deficits, should be a practice standard. Schrijnemaekers, Smeets, Ponds, van Heugten, and Rasquin (2013) are more cautious in their recommendations based on their review of 25 studies of moderate-to-strong quality. They indicate that positive results have been found in both task-specific and more general treatments for ISA but that there are too many inconsistencies in the literature to recommend any one treatment over another. One problem, they note, is that few of the studies have a theoretical basis for what components of awareness are being targeted.

A variety of tasks have been used in treatment for anosognosia and ISA. Verbal and visual (e.g., via video recording) forms of feedback are commonly used with the goal of increasing awareness of deficits and consequences of those deficits (e.g., Cheng & Man, 2006). Verbal feedback can be given during a task whenever an error occurs or can be reserved for a review of performance once the task has been completed. Video feedback has the added benefit that the clients can watch their performance after the fact when they can focus on evaluating their performance instead of trying to monitor during the activity. Videos also allow clients to see the errors being made rather than having to accept or rely on the clinician's reports.

Experiential exercises also have been employed. Clinicians select a task that they know will elicit errors due to the client's deficits. Self-regulation and metacognitive strategies are important facets of this treatment to help the client recognize the errors as they occur. The steps for using metacognitive strategies are employed: The client reviews the task, sets goals for completion, and predicts how well he will do. Goverover, Johnston, Toglia, and Deluca (2007) added a self-assessment of how much assistance the client felt he would need to successfully complete the task. Then the client generates strategies for completing the task and selects one. He then employs the strategy and monitors performance during the task. The clinician may add feedback regarding performance as needed to augment the client's self-monitoring. Finally, the client evaluates his performance and compares the results to his initial prediction.

Treatment for anosognosia can be adapted for group settings. Youngjohn and Altmann (1989) described a group treatment in which participants predict their level of performance on a specific task and write the predictions on a board visible to all participants. After task completion the actual scores are written next to the predicted scores and the group engages in discussion about the discrepancies. The authors reported improvements in the accuracy of predictions that were maintained over a one-week period.

Cheng and Man (2006) examined the effectiveness of their Awareness Intervention Programme (AIP) compared with conventional cognitive rehabilitation. The goals of AIP were to increase knowledge of deficits, apply that knowledge to real-world functioning, and practice self-prediction and goal setting. The techniques used in the AIP included predicting, monitoring, and evaluating performance. Clinicians also provided concrete feedback and education about each participant's deficits and the etiology of the deficits. After 40 treatment sessions (twice daily for four weeks), participants in AIP evidenced increased self-awareness, while those in conventional rehabilitation did not. However, there were no differences between groups in functional outcomes, such as activities of daily living.

Although the use of metacognitive strategies is the only practice standard recommended by Cicerone and colleagues (2011), positive gains have been reported from all of the methods described above. Depending on the study, improvements in the following areas have been reported: accuracy of predictions, awareness of deficits, awareness of errors, online monitoring, error management, self-regulation, and performance on functional tasks (Cheng & Man, 2006; Cicerone et al., 2011; Fleming & Ownsworth, 2006; Goverover et al., 2007;

Ownsworth, Fleming, Desbois, Strong, & Kuipers, 2006; Youngjohn & Altman, 1989).

A somewhat novel approach to treatment of ISA is motivational interviewing (Bell et al., 2005; Medley & Powell, 2010; Watkins et al., 2007). Motivational interviewing is based on the principles of nonconfrontation, collaboration, and self-efficacy. It is a client-centered approach designed to increase a client's motivation to change. Bell et al. (2005) reported significant improvements in functional and subjective quality of life following motivational interviewing that targeted problem solving, individual goal setting, and motivation to change. Improvement in mood in stroke survivors also has been reported (Watkins et al., 2007).

Several treatments designed for remediating unilateral neglect have secondary effects on awareness. Ronchi and colleagues (2013) employed caloric vestibular stimulation to treat unilateral neglect in a patient with LHD. The patient exhibited aphasia, apraxia of speech, right-sided personal and extrapersonal neglect as well as anosognosia for both neglect and hemiparesis. The treatment decreased the severity of neglect as well as the anosognosia for hemiparesis. Two days later, the benefits for neglect had disappeared, but the patient remained aware of his hemiparesis. Interestingly, at the follow-up there was new anosodiaphoria for hemiparesis. Essentially, the client became aware of his hemiparesis but was unconcerned about it. In a related study, Beschin, Cocchini, Allen, and Della Sala (2012) provided a series of optokinetic stimulation, prism adaptation, and transcutaneous electrical nerve stimulation (TENS) treatments to five participants with moderate-to-severe neglect and anosognosia for hemiparesis. Each of these treatments has been reported to have transient effects on visuospatial neglect. Participants received one treatment every two days. One participant exhibited improvement in awareness but not neglect following each mode of treatment. Two others exhibited the opposite pattern, with transient improvements in neglect but no change in anosognosia. The remaining two participants showed some change in neglect for some treatments, and slight changes in anosognosia for the others. The results suggest that neglect and anosognosia are separate deficits that may respond to similar treatments.

Conclusions and Implications

Anosognosia is a relatively common consequence of RHD, and can be caused by lesions in various areas of the RH. Clinically, reduced awareness of deficits is a major barrier to participation and progress in treatment. Identifying the underlying cause can aid in planning and conducting treatment. Education, feedback, and experiential learning exercises have all been used with some success.

10

Memory

There is a long history of research on memory processes resulting in various classifications of stages and types of memory. Interested readers are encouraged to read books and reviews by Brandimonte, Einstein, and McDaniel, 1996; Cohen and Conway, 2008; Conway, Jarrold, Kane, Miyake, and Towse, 2007; and Tulving and Craik, 2000. Memory functions can be affected by stroke, although not as commonly as with more diffuse brain injury. There are few memory impairments linked specifically with RHD; however, understanding the various types of memory can be important in diagnosing deficits when they are present and determining relative strengths that can be used to facilitate performance in light of weaknesses in other cognitive domains.

Stages of Memory Processing

There are four generally agreed-upon stages of memory. First is encoding, in which information is attended to and there is an analysis of the material to be remembered. The more attention and thought is given to information during encoding, the more likely it is to be stored and easily retrieved at a later point in time. Deep processing involves thinking about the information, linking it to previously learned information, elaborating upon meaning (semantic encoding), or visualizing the information. Chunking, or combining pieces of information into groups, also can aid in encoding. Encoding is mediated by the frontal lobes that assist with deep processing and strategy use, as well as modality-specific areas (e.g., occipital lobes for visual information, temporal lobes for auditory). Cues established during encoding (e.g., mnemonic devices or links to previously stored information) can be used to facilitate recognition and recall. For example, when introduced to someone new, if you can link the person's name to someone you already know (MacKenzie—that's my niece's name), then that cue can be used to retrieve the name later. Also, repeated accurate retrieval of information will strengthen the storage and facilitate future recall, particularly for

---

SIDEBAR

There are many strategies for increasing the depth of processing and creating cues for retrieval during the encoding phase. Meeting a woman named Karsyn, you could imagine her driving a car (car-Karsyn). Or ask about the spelling and imagine seeing the name with its unusual spelling. Or link the name to another person: think about the ensuing confusion if she was married to Johnny Carson.

---

relatively small chunks of information such as addresses or passwords.

The second stage of memory is consolidation, which is the process of transferring information from temporary to more permanent storage. The consolidation process is vulnerable to interference. Proactive interference occurs when old information interferes with the new information to be stored. Learning to use an Apple phone when your previous model was an Android can create proactive interference, when you continue to look for Android-specific icons or tools. Retroactive interference is the opposite, in which new information interferes with old. Consolidation is mediated primarily by the hippocampi and other medial temporal lobe structures.

Successful consolidation results in storage, which is the third stage of memory. Stored information is held for later use. It is unclear where memories are stored; there is some evidence for storage in the medial temporal lobe (in and around the hippocampus), but also in modality-specific areas. The likelihood of successful storage is strongly related to encoding: the deeper the encoding, the more likely the information will be stored.

The final stage of memory is retrieval, in which previously stored information is activated and recovered. Retrieval can be triggered by either recognition or recall. Recognition occurs when the to-be-remembered information is provided and one must determine if it was seen before. Multiple-choice questions are one way to test recognition memory. Recall occurs when the information is directly retrieved. Recognition is easier than recall, as the information is present and has to be recognized (or judged to be familiar), whereas recall requires searching for and reactivating the information. Failure to retrieve information can occur for several reasons. It may not have been well encoded, causing tenuous links for retrieval. It may not have been stored, in which case it is not available for retrieval. Finally, the cue to retrieve it may not be the right cue, or is not a strong enough cue.

The frontal lobes are primarily responsible for retrieval. Retrieval can be facilitated by executive functions (EFs) such as initiating the search, using the temporal order of memories to retrieve information, and self-monitoring to assess the veracity of memories. As noted earlier, the stages of memory are highly interactive: attention influences encoding, encoding influences storage, and all of the early stages influence the ease of retrieval.

SIDEBAR

An example of an ineffective retrieval cue: My husband states, "That actor was in the movie we saw in the little theater in Pittsburgh." I have no immediate recollection of the particular movie in which I previously saw that particular actor. I scan through memories of the theater, trying to recall what movies we saw at that particular place, but still cannot retrieve it. My husband then adds, "It was the movie about the small town in England." I have an "aha" moment in which I recall the movie, the actor's role, and then remember that we did see that one at that particular theater. This highlights the individuality of episodic memories as well as the differential effectiveness of retrieval cues. To my husband, the theater was a salient cue. For me, that cue was not effective, but rather the theme of the movie was the cue that was linked to the actor.

Classifications of Memory Types

There are several types of memory. One method of classification is based on the amount of information that can be held and the length of time it is stored (Table 10–1). Short-term memory (STM) is a space to store a limited amount of information (approximately 4–7 individual "bits") for a very limited amount of time (a few minutes at most). Information in STM must be constantly rehearsed in order for it to remain in STM. The ability to remember a phone number (often through repetition) long enough to dial it is an example of STM.

Working memory (WM) is also a limited capacity, limited duration storage. What differentiates WM from STM is that in WM, information is not only temporarily stored, but is also undergoing processing.[1] WM thus supports a variety of cognitive processes, such as comprehension and reasoning. Because of this, WM is considered by many to be not simply a memory system, but a component of EF and frontal lobe function. This perspective was explained in more detail in Chapter 8. Working memory also is very closely linked to attentional functions, as described in Chapter 6.

Digit span tasks highlight the difference between STM and WM. Forward digit span, in which a client hears a string of digits and has to repeat them back in the same order, taps simple STM—the information is temporarily held (typically via rehearsal) and then produced. Backward digit span taps WM. In this task, the client

---

[1]Some researchers do not differentiate between STM and WM but consider them to be one memory system that involves both storage and processing. Of these researchers, some use the label STM and others call it WM.

Table 10–1. Types of Memory

Type of Memory	Characteristics
Short-term memory (STM)	Short duration, limited capacity, must be active to prevent loss
Working memory (WM)	Short duration, limited capacity, simultaneous processing and storage
Long-term memory (LTM)	Long duration, unlimited capacity, new information connected with old through associations
	Declarative: conscious memory—can be verbal or visuospatial • Episodic: memories about events (what/where/when) • Semantic: memories about facts/things Nondeclarative: unconscious/implicit memory • Procedural learning • Motor learning/motor memory • Classical conditioning
Metamemory	Understanding or awareness of one's memory abilities
Prospective memory	Remembering to do something in the future

again hears a string of digits but then has to repeat them back in reverse order (e.g., 1-5-2-3-6 → 6-3-2-5-1). The numbers are not only temporarily stored, but also processed to reverse the order.

Baddeley and Hitch's (1994; Baddeley, 2003) model of WM contains four major components: a central executive and three storage systems: the visuospatial sketchpad, the phonological loop, and the episodic buffer. The storage systems temporarily store and encode the information. The visuospatial sketchpad is used for visualizing items, the phonological loop is for verbal rehearsal, and the episodic buffer is for integration across modalities. These three systems are controlled by the central executive. This centralized processor controls attentional processing (focuses or divides attention), resource allocation (how much attention/effort should be directed toward storage versus processing), and selection of the most appropriate strategy (e.g., visualization or verbal rehearsal).

As suggested above, WM is critical for language. During auditory comprehension, listeners must interpret individual words and hold on to them to build a context, and they must be accessible for some amount of time in case reinterpretation is required. Just and Carpenter (1992) developed the WM model of language comprehension and demonstrated that individuals with larger WM capacities were more adept at comprehension of complex sentence structures (Table 10–2). These

Table 10–2. Sentences With Temporary Syntactic Ambiguities Requiring Revision and Good Working Memory Capacity

Garden Path Sentences	Interpretation
The cotton clothing is made of grows in Mississippi.	The cotton // clothing is made of // grows in Mississippi.
While Lynn dressed the baby that was small and cute played in the crib.	While Lynn dressed // the baby that was small and cute // played in the crib.
An impatient shopper pushed through the doors complained to the manager.	An impatient shopper [*who was*] pushed through the doors complained to the manager.

structures include garden path sentences, in which an initial syntactic interpretation must be revised. An example is the sentence, "The man who whistles tunes pianos." Most readers initially interpret the word "tunes" as a noun (he whistles tunes) but then have to revise their interpretation once they read the word "pianos," which does not fit with the syntactic structure. "Tunes" must be reinterpreted as a verb (The man who whistles // tunes pianos). Individuals with larger WM capacities are faster at reinterpretation and correct comprehension of such garden path sentences because they are able to hold the first part of the sentence active in WM so that it is easily accessible when the revision is necessary.

The final type of memory is long-term memory (LTM). Both the capacity and duration of LTM, as far as we know, are unlimited. However, long-term memories can change over time (e.g., Schmolck, Buffalo, & Squire, 2000). LTM is subdivided into content-dependent stores: declarative and nondeclarative. Declarative memories are stores of conscious, explicit knowledge, further divided into semantic and episodic memories. Semantic memories are facts about the world that are not linked to context. Knowing that William the Conqueror began his conquest of England in 1066 is a semantic declarative memory, as is knowing the names of the seven dwarves in the fairy tale Snow White. Episodic memories are memories about personal events. Remembering that you learned about William the Conqueror in your high school world history class is an episodic memory. Episodic memories are unique to each individual. Even if you shared an event with someone else, you each have a different memory colored by your personal knowledge, feelings, and perspectives of that day. Spouses will have different episodic memories of their wedding day. While there is likely to be extensive overlap of various facts or events, the episodic memories will differ. Episodic memories can be used to access semantic memories, and vice versa. According to one model, remembering events from the past can be achieved by recollecting the event and specific details of the event, or can be recollected through a feeling of familiarity: a "knowing" that an event occurred in the past, even in the absence of details of the context (Yonelinas, 2002).

The hippocampus is important for both episodic and semantic memory processes.

There is increasing evidence that for episodic memories, each time a memory is retrieved and then re-stored it is reconsolidated and often changed, updated, and colored by the context in which it was most recently retrieved or possibly elaborated to enhance the seeming importance of the event. Thus, memories that you retrieve often or stories that you repeatedly tell are likely further from the truth than those that have been stored untouched (e.g., Alberini & Ledoux, 2013; Besnard, Caboche, & Laroche, 2012; Hupbach, Gomez, Hardt, & Nadel, 2007; St. Jacques & Schacter, 2013).

The other major store within LTM is nondeclarative memory. These are memories that are not explicit or conscious. Nondeclarative memories are actions and behaviors that have been learned but often are difficult to verbalize. Procedural memories, or knowing how to do certain things, are nondeclarative memories. Motor learning, or learned skill movements (e.g., knowing how to shoot a basketball, type on a keyboard, tie shoe laces) are nondeclarative memories and are strongly linked to motor systems in the brain. Memories for procedures on how to do something or strategies commonly used to reach a goal are also nondeclarative. Classical conditioning or implicit learning of connections between two unrelated events is yet another type of nondeclarative memory. Pavlov's dogs, who began to salivate at the sound of a bell after the bell ringing had consistently and repeatedly preceded the presentation of food, are the archetypal example of classical conditioning. Nondeclarative

memories are often the most robust in the face of brain injury and can be used to facilitate storage and recall when other memory processes are impaired.

Two other forms of memory need to be mentioned. These both consist of a set of processes, and so do not fit into the categories described above. First is prospective memory. This is the ability to remember to do something in the future. It could be remembering to take a vitamin with your next meal, or remembering to call the doctor's office when it reopens after lunch. The second is metamemory. This is a cognitive ability that reflects one's understanding of one's own memory abilities. A client who erroneously believes that he has a good memory for names of new acquaintances would have poor metamemory (as well as a poor declarative store of memory for names).

Localization of Memory Processes

As suggested above, there are a variety of brain regions that are important for different memory types and processes (e.g., Lim & Alexander, 2009; Table 10–3). The hippocampus and surrounding areas of the medial temporal lobe are critical for storage; prefrontal areas are involved in storage and retrieval as well as the use of strategies to enhance encoding; the parietal lobes are involved in retrieval, perhaps related to attentional functions. Additionally, the basal ganglia, cerebellum, and frontal lobes have been implicated in WM processes (Baier et al., 2010; Burgess, Maguire, & O'Keefe, 2002; Buri-

Table 10–3. Regions Associated With Memory Function

Region	Processes	RH	LH
Hippocampus	Storage, episodic memory	X (especially spatial)	X (especially verbal)
Inferior frontal	Working memory, episodic memory	Recollection, familiarity	
Prefrontal region	Encoding, retrieval (episodic and semantic), working memory	Episodic retrieval, confidence in memory judgments, working memory	Episodic and semantic encoding, semantic retrieval
Parietal lobe	Episodic retrieval, experience of remembering	X	X
Basal ganglia	Working memory, declarative retrieval	X	X
Lingual gyrus	Declarative retrieval		X
Cerebellum	Working memory	X	

anova, Mcintosh, & Grady, 2010; Cabeza, Ciaramelli, Olson, & Moscovitch, 2008; Marvel & Desmond, 2010; Tulving, 2002; Wagner, Shannon, Kahn, & Buckner, 2005; Yokoyama et al., 2010). The frontal lobe appears to play a greater role than the parietal lobe in WM processes, even visuospatial WM (Grosdemange et al., 2015; Roussel, Dujardin, Hénon, & Godefroy, 2012).

The RH specifically has been found to be involved more in visual than verbal memory, although this pattern is not universally reported (e.g., Gillespie, Bowen, & Foster, 2006). Right prefrontal regions are important for episodic retrieval (but not storage), WM (particularly with high memory loads), and confidence judgments in one's memory (Lim & Alexander, 2009; Yokoyama et al., 2010).

Memory After Stroke

The vast majority of studies examining memory after a stroke use mixed groups of stroke survivors. Most have unilateral lesions, either LH or RH; others have bilateral or cerebellar damage. Few studies report differences between LHD and RHD participants, thus the ensuing discussion will cover memory deficits related to stroke in general. Specifics related to RHD will be provided as possible given the existing knowledge.

Snaphaan and De Leeuw (2007) conducted a systematic review to explore the prevalence of memory deficits following stroke. Memory deficits occurred in 13 to 50% of stroke survivors in the acute stage of recovery, decreasing to 11 to 31%

after one year poststroke. Memory deficits tended to occur more often after LH versus RH lesions, although white matter lesions in either temporal lobe were related to memory impairments. Similar results were reported by Godefroy, Roussel, Leclerc, and Leys (2009) in terms of verbal episodic memory impairments. These impairments affected up to 40% of their sample of stroke survivors and were more common after LH than RH strokes.

Declarative and Episodic Memory After Stroke

Serial order effects are consistently observed in studies of list learning by healthy adults. The primacy effect occurs when the first few items in a list are remembered better than the others. Better recall of the last few items is called the recency effect. Such temporal (serial) order effects can be affected after stroke, regardless of hemisphere or anterior versus posterior localization (Schoo et al., 2014). Group results indicate that primacy and recency effects are present but are substantially smaller for a poststroke group compared with a control group. In this particular study, up to 40% of the stroke survivors showed no typical serial position effects.

In a study of encoding, storage, and retrieval processes, Campos, Barroso, and De Lara Menezes (2010) reported that stroke survivors were impaired on all three processes compared with a control group. However, the RHD group had more problems with visual encoding, while the LHD group evidenced deficits primarily on verbal storage and retrieval. In this study, potential participants with "serious cognitive disorders" were excluded, but there was no assessment of the presence or severity of either aphasia or unilateral neglect in the participants who were included.

Memory for autobiographical events can be affected by RHD (Batchelor, Thompson, & Miller, 2008). In this study participants were asked to describe important events in their lives. Since the accuracy of the memories could not be verified, the researchers scored the descriptions based on the depth of the description and the details of the time and place. The personal events were compared with descriptions of public events. Personal memories described by the RHD group were less detailed than LHD and non–brain-damaged (NBD) groups. An inspection of individual performance suggested that 40% of the participants with RHD had deficits compared with only 10% of the LHD participants. The problem was not with verbal descriptions, as the same RHD participants described public events just as well as the other groups.

Working Memory After Stroke

Working memory also can be impaired after stroke. Frontal lobe lesions can cause impairments in the function of the major components of WM (phonological loop, visuospatial sketchpad, and central executive; Roussel et al., 2012). In some studies, equal proportions of adults with RHD and LHD have shown deficits on verbal and visual WM (e.g., Grosdemange et al., 2015). However, other studies report greater WM deficits or impairment of central EF after RHD compared with LHD

(Meier et al., 2011; Roussel et al., 2012). In one case, LHD resulted only in verbal WM deficits, while RHD was associated with both verbal and visual WM deficits (Philipose, Alphs, Prabhakaran, & Hillis, 2007).

One possible reason for the apparent equivalence of RH and LH contributions to WM following stroke is the pattern of neural activity in older adults. The HAROLD model of aging (Hemispheric Asymmetry Reduction in Older Adults; Cabeza, 2002) suggests that bilateral processing develops for complex tasks that once were controlled unilaterally. The theory suggests that aging results in bilateral control over WM that was once controlled primarily by the LH (Meier et al., 2012). Thus, studies of memory deficits after stroke are likely to find equal contributions of the right and left hemispheres because the majority of stroke survivors are older, and the expected asymmetry has been supplanted by bilateral control.

Metamemory After Stroke

Impairments in metamemory may be expected given the prevalence of anosognosia, or reduced awareness of deficits that occurs after RHD (see Chapter 9). However, the few studies of metamemory following stroke fail to identify differences depending on laterality of lesions (Barrett, Galletta, Zhang, Masmela, & Adler, 2014; Boosman, van Heugten, Winkens, Heijnen, & Visser-Meily, 2014). Impaired metamemory is more likely to appear as overestimation of memory abilities than underestimation. Additionally, overestimators tended to have deficits in a variety of cognitive domains (e.g., visuopercep-

tion, memory, EF, affect, attention, language, orientation). In contrast, the few individuals who underestimated their performance were more likely to have deficits in affect (Boosman et al., 2014).

Metamemory is a multifaceted concept. Awareness of some memory abilities may be preserved, while others may be impaired. Barrett and colleagues (2014) reported that despite intact awareness of language, EF, and verbal memory abilities, stroke survivors overestimated performance on a medication self-administration task. The participants were accurate in their predictions of relatively simple verbal memory abilities, but awareness of complex task performance was affected. However, the scores were related, such that poorer declarative memory was related to greater overestimation. Impairments of metamemory for prospective memory after stroke also have been reported (Brooks, Rose, Potter, Jayawardena, & Morling, 2004).

Prospective Memory After Stroke

Prospective memory deficits may occur as often as retrospective deficits, affecting approximately 40% of stroke survivors (Kant et al., 2014). They can co-occur with deficits of attention, retrospective memory, EF, and speed of processing (Brooks et al., 2004; Kant et al., 2014; Kim, Craik, Luo, & Ween, 2009).

Brooks et al. (2004) used both virtual reality (VR) and traditional tasks to examine prospective memory following RHD. The VR environment was a small house, and participants were instructed to take items out of the house to be moved to a new house. There were three prospective memory actions, each with a separate trigger: (a) close the door every time you go through the kitchen, (b) alert the experimenter at five-minute intervals, and (c) mark every object that is breakable/fragile. Overall, the RHD group completed fewer activities on the VR task than an NBD control group. The researchers also included traditional prospective memory tasks. At the beginning of the session, the experimenter took a personal item (e.g., wristwatch) from each person and told them to request it when the session was done. Participants were also told to ask for a written description of the study at the end of the session. The RHD and NBD groups were equally accurate at requesting their personal items, but both groups were significantly impaired in remembering to ask for the study material. Similar to this benefit for recall of personally relevant information, prospective memory deficits are less likely to occur in naturalistic compared with experimental tasks (Brooks et al., 2004; Kant et al., 2014). One explanation for this pattern of performance is that the problem lies more in self-initiation of complex processes than prospective memory itself (Kim et al., 2009); those tasks that are personal or naturalistic may be more relevant and less cognitively demanding than contrived or novel tasks.

Memory and Executive Function

Given the role of the frontal lobes in encoding and retrieval, it is not surprising that EF and memory impairments might inter-

act. Individuals with EF deficits at six months poststroke are more likely to have impairments in verbal learning and recall than individuals with intact EF. Additionally, those with EF deficits at six months continued to show memory deficits at two years poststroke, particularly in the areas of verbal learning and immediate visual recall (Turunen et al., 2016).

Assessment of Memory

There are a plethora of tests available for assessing the various types and stages of memory, as well as different modalities (particularly visual and verbal). A select list of assessments is provided in Table 10–4.

Several factors that influence memory performance in stroke survivors include characteristics of the stimuli, the potential for memory tests to evoke anxiety, and the naturalness of the tests. First, word learning can be facilitated by emotionality of words even for adults with RHD who may have decreased emotional processing (Berrin-Wasserman, Winnick, & Borod, 2003). Second, stroke survivors may have greater anxiety over memory tests than adults without brain injury, and anxiety decreases performance on WM tasks (Grosdemange et al., 2015). Third, as noted above, prospective memory performance generally is better on naturalistic or personally relevant tasks compared with experimental tasks (Brooks et al., 2004; Kant et al., 2014; Kim et al., 2009). Particularly in outpatient settings, it may be important to ask for feedback from family members or caregivers regarding a client's prospective memory ability.

Table 10–4. Select Measures of Memory

Test	Authors	Type of Memory	Reliability*	Validity*
Benton Visual Retention Test, 5th ed.	Sivan, 1992	Immediate and delayed visual memory	OK	None
Brief Assessment of Prospective Memory (BAPM)	Man et al., 2011	Prospective memory	Good	OK
California Verbal Learning Test, 2nd ed.	Delis et al., 1983	Verbal learning	OK	Good
Cambridge Prospective Memory Test	Wilson et al., 2005	Prospective memory	Good	Weak
Contextual Memory Test	Toglia, 1993	Metamemory	OK	OK
Corsi Block Tapping Task	Corsi, 1972; Kessels et al., 2000	Visuospatial memory	None	OK
Continuous Visual Memory Test– Revised	Trahan & Larrabee 1997	Visual memory	Good	Good
Everyday Memory Questionnaire– Revised	Royle & Lincoln, 2008	Metamemory	OK	OK
Hopkins Verbal Learning Test– Revised	Brandt & Benedict 2001	Verbal learning	Weak	Good
Memory for Intentions Test (MIST)	Raskin et al., 2010	Prospective memory	Good	Good
Memory Test for Older Adults	Hubley & Tombaugh, 2002	Visual and verbal memory	Weak	Weak
Oxford Cog Screen–Memory Subtests	Demeyere et al., 2015	Orientation; recall recognition episodic	OK	Good
Prospective and Retrospective Memory Questionnaire (PRMQ)	Smith et al., 2000	Prospective and retrospective memory	OK	OK

continues

Table 10–4. *continued*

Test	Authors	Type of Memory	Reliability*	Validity*
Recognition Memory Test	Warrington, 1984	Visual memory	Weak	Weak
Rey Auditory Verbal Learning Test	Schmidt, 1996	Verbal learning	OK	Good
Rey Complex Figure Test and Recognition Trial	Myers & Myers, 1995	Visuospatial ability and visuospatial memory	Good	Good
Rivermead Behavioral Memory Test, 2nd ed. (RBMT)	Wilson et al., 2003	"Everyday" memory	Good	Good
Test of Memory and Learning, 2nd ed.	Reynolds & Voress 2007	Immediate and delayed verbal and nonverbal memory	Good	Good
Three Cities Test	Johnson-Green et al., 2009	Learning and short term memory	None	OK
Wechsler Memory Scales, 4th ed.	Wechsler, 2009	Verbal and visual short-term and working memory	OK	OK

Note. *Good = moderate–strong estimates of two or more types of reliability/validity; OK = moderate–strong estimates of one type of reliability/validity or mix of weak and strong estimates; weak = weak estimates of one or more types of reliability/validity; none = no estimates reported. See Appendix for detailed information about reliability and validity.

Treatment for Memory Deficits

Elliot and Parente (2014) conducted a meta-analysis of 26 studies of memory treatment for participants with either stroke or traumatic brain injury (TBI). Results indicated significant improvements related to memory treatment and that improvements tended to be greater for deficits resulting from to stroke compared with TBI. The memory studies spanned a wide range of types of deficits (verbal memory, prospective memory, WM, etc.) and methods of treatment (systematic instruction, errorless learning, external aids, etc.). While the conclusion that "memory treatment works" is positive, this study cannot answer other questions, such as what kind of treatment works for a specific memory deficit or whether some treatments are more effective than others for either types of deficits or types of clients.

Treatment for Declarative Memory

The results from extensive research on memory training in the 1970 to 1980s with healthy young adults indicated that memory, in general, cannot be improved. Strategies can be learned to improve memory for specific information. Chunking numbers into meaningful groups (e.g., running times, birthdates, zip codes) can facilitate learning of a sequence of random numbers; assigning people and places to different playing cards and creating stories can result in learning the sequence of cards in a random shuffle (e.g., Serena Williams is the Queen of Spades; Denzel Washington is the Jack of Clubs; the 10 of diamonds is Paris, thus that sequence of cards could be remembered as Serena and Denzel meet-

ing in Paris). However, these strategies are task specific and would not aid in remembering someone's name or remembering where you put your car keys. More general strategies, such as mnemonics, visualization, or semantic elaboration can be used to remember a variety of different sets of information, such as grocery lists or names of new acquaintances.

Two recent treatment programs developed specifically for stroke survivors show promising results. Miller and Radford (2014) reported positive results from a group treatment program for adults with memory deficits related to stroke. Ten of the 40 participants had RHD; the other 30 had LHD. The six-week manualized treatment includes education along with internal (repetition, mnemonics) and external (note taking, organizing, photographs, etc.) memory strategies (see Table 10–5 for lists of internal and external strategies). Gains in verbal learning, delayed recall, and functional prospective memory and reports of increased use of strategies

Table 10–5. Internal and External Memory Strategies

Internal Strategies	External Strategies (can be implemented via paper/pencil or electronic device such as computer or smartphone)
Attend to context	Calendars/clocks/alarms
Attend to detail	Diaries/journals
Clustering	Lists
Elaboration	Note taking
Method of loci	Organizational system
Mneumonics	Photographs
Repetition	
Visualization	
Word association	

were observed. Both RHD and LHD participants evidenced similar gains. Participants with lower initial scores made the greatest gains, and greater gains in use of strategies were related to higher levels of education and IQ. The length of time after stroke was inversely related to gains in prospective memory.

Following stroke or brain injury, one approach to treatment is to determine what the person does not remember and what affect that has on his daily functioning and then seek a method for addressing the problem. From the TBI literature, there is reliable evidence for immediate improvements and maintenance of gains from systematic, implicit learning treatments (e.g., spaced retrieval, method of vanishing cues) used to aid in remembering specific pieces of information (Ehlhardt et al., 2008). These include names of people, addresses, locations, or set schedules that do not change frequently.

There are a variety of memory strategies, both internal and external, that can be used with varying efficiency and effectiveness by individual clients (see Table 10–5). It has long been established that deeper encoding enhances the likelihood of storage and later retrieval in healthy adults. Internal strategies generally work because they encourage deeper encoding. This encoding also facilitates verbal memory in adults with stroke and is equally beneficial for RHD and LHD (Berrin-Wasserman et al., 2003). However, such strategies can be cognitively demanding to create, much less remember, and may not be effective for all clients. Strategies must be selected with input from the client and in consideration of the client's other cognitive, sensory, and motor deficits.

Sohlberg and Turkstra (2011) provide a clear, systematic approach to selecting treatment strategies and methods for implementing practice (in a single versus multiple environments; with a single versus multiple stimuli and cues) depending on the client's needs and goals. The following recommendations can be useful in structuring memory treatment (Elkhardt et al., 2005; Sohlberg & Turkstra, 2011):

- Clearly establish the targets of intervention.
  - ☐ Facts? Multistep procedures? Variable schedule items? Consistent schedule items?

- Targets and strategies should be personally relevant and ecologically valid.

- Use task analyses to identify specific steps and targets for training multistep procedures.

- Use errorless learning to minimize errors during acquisition phases of treatment.

- Provide sufficient practice to allow learning of the material or the strategy.

- During acquisition, massed practice (long sessions of intense practice) is generally more effective.

- During maintenance and generalization, distributed practice (multiple, short sessions of practice) is more effective.

- Strategies should be practiced in the environments/settings they will be used in (if the strategy is developed for a single environment, it should be practiced only in that one).

■ Internal strategies are generally more effortful than external and may lead to greater gains if they do not add too much cognitive demand to the task.

Treatment for Visuospatial Memory

Chen and colleagues (Chen, Hartman, Galarza, & DeLuca, 2012) developed a visuospatial memory treatment for adults with RHD based on the idea that such memory deficits were related to a focus on local, rather than global, visual processing (e.g., missing the forest for the trees). They conducted a single training session that provided implicit global processing training. They presented participants with a series of figures based on the Rey–Osterreith figure (Figure 10–1). The task was to trace the portions shown as dotted lines. In the treatment group, the figure was presented in five stages. These began with the global features, with local features added sequentially throughout the stages. The comparison group that was given rote treatment was provided with the entire figure in dotted lines, to be traced all in one step. After the entire figure had been copied, participants were given a blank sheet of paper and asked to recreate the figure. During treatment the participants completed five different figures using the assigned method (global versus rote). Results indicated that the participants given the global training demonstrated better accuracy and organization during

immediate recall, beginning after the third of the five figures. Gains were maintained up to several weeks. These results support the idea that implicit training can facilitate efficiency and accuracy of cognitive processes (e.g., see discussion of Contextual Constraint Treatment, Chapter 4) and that emphasizing a global-to-local processing strategy may be beneficial for improving visual memory.

Treatment for Working Memory

Improvement of WM has been explored in adults with and without brain injury, as well as in children. A meta-analysis of studies of both children and adults with and without clinical diagnoses (including attention deficit hyperactivity disorder, learning difficulties, and stroke) indicated reliable short-term changes in WM tasks after treatment, but no consistent maintenance or generalization of those improvements (Melby-Lervåg & Hulme, 2013).

Studies conducted to examine the physiological effects of WM training have reported changes in cerebral activation in healthy adults (e.g., Olesen, Westerberg, & Klingberg, 2004). Additionally, some studies report differential activation change for training that focuses on manipulation versus storage (Jolles, Grol, Van Buchem, Rombouts, & Crone, 2010), suggesting that these components are controlled by different networks and can be differentially affected by training. Relationships between changes in neural function and meaningful improvement in WM for daily activities have yet to be rigorously explored.

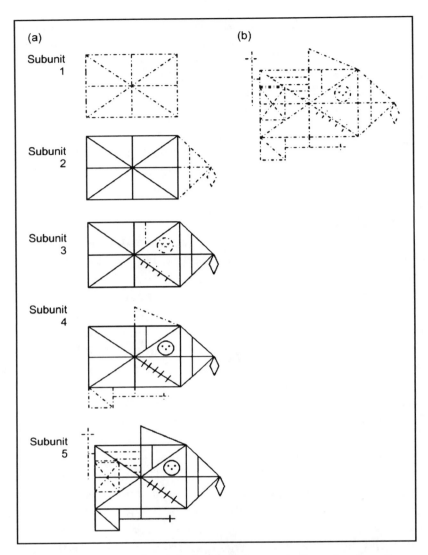

Figure 10–1. Sample global processing training stimulus. From Chen, P., Hartman, A. J., Galarza, C. P., & DeLuca, J. (2012). Global processing training to improve visuospatial memory deficits after right-brain stroke. *Archives of Clinical Neuropsychology, 27*(8), 891–905. Used by permission of Oxford University Press.

Computerized training for cognitive functions generally results in short-term, task-specific changes. The results for WM training are no different. Positive results were reported in two studies of computerized WM training (Lundqvist, Grund-strom, Samuelsson, & Ronnberg, 2010; Westerberg et al., 2007). Both reported generalization to related executive functions as well as functional/occupational changes. However, neither included a control group to determine whether the changes were specific to the WM treatment or were a result of general cognitive activity and placebo effects.

Treatment for Prospective Memory

External memory aids have been repeatedly shown to be effective for decreasing the functional impact of memory deficits caused by TBI (Sohlberg et al., 2007). They are particularly effective for reducing the impact of prospective memory deficits or for keeping track of events that do not occur in a consistent, predictable pattern (Sohlberg & Turkstra, 2011). More evidence is needed to clarify the type of aid(s) that are best for individual clients with different profiles of memory and associated cognitive deficits.

Other Treatments for Memory Deficits

Noninvasive brain stimulation techniques such as transcranial direct current stimulation (tDCS) and repetitive transcranial magnetic stimulation (rTMS) have been used both with healthy adults and clinical populations to improve WM. Generally, stimulation is applied to the left prefrontal region (typically dorsolateral prefrontal cortex). In a systematic review and meta-analysis, Russowsky and Vanderhasselt (2014) reported immediate positive changes in response time (both tDCS and rTMS) and accuracy (rTMS only). Questions regarding the generalization of gains to related tasks and to functional abilities have yet to be answered.

Exercise programs have been shown to improve verbal memory (Rand, Eng, Liu-Ambrose, & Tawashy, 2010) and WM (Liu-Ambrose & Eng, 2014) and may be a useful complement to cognitive rehabilitation (see Chapter 8).

Conclusions

Memory deficits have received less attention than other cognitive problems associated with RHD. Deficits in working memory, recall of episodic memories, metamemory, and prospective memory all have been reported after RHD, although they may be fairly similar to memory deficits following LHD. Treatments designed for adults with TBI are likely to be useful, including internal and external strategies and external memory aids.

Appendix
Psychometrics for Select Assessments

Table A–1. Select Assessment Batteries for RHD (see Table 2–5)

Test	Authors	Areas Assessed	Reliability	Validity
Burns Brief Inventory	Burns, 1997	RH Inventory: visuospatial skills, prosody, abstract language. Complex Neuropathology inventory: orientation, memory, attention.	Test-retest reliability: $r > .70$ for most task sets Internal consistency: $\alpha = .74–.97$	Construct validity: factor analysis indicated several task sets loaded on multiple factors
Mini Inventory of Right Brain Injury–2 (MIRBI)	Pimental & Knight, 2000	Visual processing, unilateral neglect, reading/writing, nonliteral language, emotion/affect, conversation, general behavior	Inter/intrarater reliability: $r = .98$ for set of 8 raters Internal consistency: $\alpha = .84$	Construct validity: factor analysis identified 4 factors, but 21 of 27 items all loaded on one factor Convergent validity: $r > .70$ with related measures of cognition Discriminant: reported differential performance of adults with RHD, LHD, and controls
Montreal Evaluation of Communication–English version (MEC)	Joanette et al., 2015	Prosody, nonliteral language, conversation, pragmatic inference, discourse, lexico-semantics, awareness of deficits	Interrater reliability: $r > .8$ for all but conversation and emotional prosody production/repetition (based on French and Brazilian data) Internal consistency: $\alpha > .70$ for all but indirect speech subtest	Construct: agreement between SLP giving the MEC and a second SLP engaged in conversation and a communication screening questionnaire. Discriminant: reported 25/25 adults with RHD evidenced deficits on 4+ MEC tasks, 20/25 identified as having a communication disorder in conversation with SLP

Test	Authors	Areas Assessed	Reliability	Validity
Rehab Institute of Chicago (RIC) Evaluation of Communication Problems in Right Hemisphere Dysfunction–3*	Halper, Cherney, & Burns, 2010	Visual scanning and tracking, writing, pragmatics, nonliteral language	Intrarater: $r > .9$ on all subtests for 2 trained raters; $r > .9$ for 3 of 6, and $r = .51–.78$ for 3 subtests for untrained rater Internal consistency: within subtests, correlations between items and total scores ranged $r = .72–.85$ behavioral; $r = .58–.85$ pragmatics; $r = .02–.52$ writing; $r = .14–.62$ metaphors	Construct: Rasch analysis indicated item separation reliability $r = .89–.91$ for behavioral observation, pragmatic communication, and writing
Right Hemisphere Language Battery, 2nd ed. (RHLB)	Bryan, 1994	Lexical semantics, nonliteral language, humor, inferences, prosody	Test-retest: $r = .62–.83$ for individual subtests; Interrater reliability: $r = .89$ for discourse subtest Internal consistency: correlations between subtests and total $r = .57–.77$	Construct: adults with RHD made more errors across subtests than adults with LHD or controls.
Ross Information Processing Assessment–Revised (RIPA–R)	Ross-Swain, 1996	Memory, problem solving, auditory processing	Interrater reliability $r = .99$ for 3 raters on one assessment Internal consistency: $\alpha = .70$ overall; 9/10 subtests $\alpha = .86–.94$	Construct validity: authors claim test measures 10 different components of cognition, but factor analyses identified 1–3.

Notes. α = Cronbach's alpha; LHD = left hemisphere brain damage; RHD = right hemisphere brain damage.
*RIC–3 appears to be the same as RIC–R (new psychometrics were not provided for RIC–3).

Table A–2. Select Cognitive Screening Tools (see Table 2–6)

Name	Authors	Scope of Test	Reliability	Validity
Cognistat: The Neurobehavioral Cognitive Status Examination	Kiernan et al., 1987	Memory, language, construction, calculations, and reasoning	None (reported as inappropriate for test design)	No meaningful measures of validity
Cognitive–Linguistic Quick Test	Helm-Estabrooks, 2001	Attention, memory, executive functions, language, and visuospatial skills	Test-retest: $r = .03–.81$ for individual tasks; $r = .61–.90$ for domains; Inter/intrarater: only 1 task and 2 domains had reliability coefficients greater than $r = .80$	Construct: factor analysis supported the 5 domain structure Discriminant: limited evidence of differential performance by adults with neurological damage compared with controls
Mini Mental State Exam	Folstein, Folstein, & McHugh, 1975	Orientation, memory, language, visuospatial processing	Test-retest: ICC = 0.94–99 Internal consistency: $\alpha = 0.36–0.57$	Construct: correlations between clinical and normative samples $r = 0.61–91$ Convergent: area under ROC curve for MMSE similar to related Cognitive Performance Scale (MMSE = 0.88, CPS = 0.87) Discriminant: differential performance between control and dementia groups Sensitivity to cognitive impairment in nursing home residents = 0.97; specificity = 0.59

Name	Authors	Scope of Test	Reliability	Validity
Montreal Cognitive Assessment (MoCA)–Canadian/ English version	Nasreddine et al., 2005	Orientation, memory, language, visuospatial processing	Test–retest reliability: r = .92 Parallel form reliability: no significant difference in scores on French and English versions	Convergent: r > .79 correlations with similar cognitive screenings Discriminant: sensitivity for MCI = 90%; AD group = 100%; specificity = 87%
Neuropsychological Assessment Battery (NAB)–screening module	Pulsipher et al., 2013	Attention, memory, language, visuospatial, executive function	Internal consistency: domain areas α = 0.24–.75 Test–retest: r = .74 for total scores; corrected stability coefficients for domain areas range from r = 0.3–0.71 for all but shape learning (.11) and visual discrimination (.16) Inter/intrarater: r = 0.83–1.0 Internal consistency: α = 0.20–0.87	Content: total screening significantly correlated with domain areas (r = .16 to .45); factor analysis indicated 5 expected factors. Convergent: r = .46–.65 total screening score and related cognitive screen Discriminative: sensitivity 95%; specificity 44%–75% for domain areas

continues

Table A–2. *continued*

Name	Authors	Scope of Test	Reliability	Validity
The Oxford Cognitive Screen	Demeyere et al., 2015	Apraxia, unilateral neglect, memory, language, exec function, and number abilities	Test-retest: combined score ICC = 0.547; subtests range .33–.78	Convergent: significant correlations between individual subtests and related cognitive measures (all r > .45 except object symmetry, number writing & executive function (all r = .32–.44) Discriminant: sensitivity for individual subtests range from 45%–95%; specificity for individual subtests range from 70%–98%.
Scales of Cognitive and Communicative Ability for Neurorehabilitation	Milman & Holland, 2012	Problem solving, language, memory	Test-retest: r = .78 to .96 Internal consistency: subtest α = .66 to .91; total score α = .95.	Content: item discrimination coefficient = .41; item difficulty coefficient = .72 Convergent: significant correlations (r = .73 to .98) with related measures of cognition, language, and memory Discriminant: effect size = .82 discriminating impaired from nonimpaired

Notes. AD = Alzheimer's disease; FIM = Functional Independence Measure; ICC = intraclass correlation coefficient; MCI = mild cognitive impairment.

Table A–3. Select Assessment Measures of Pragmatics (see Table 3–8)

Test	Authors	Areas Assessed	Reliability	Validity
Behaviourally Referenced Rating System of Intermediate Social Skills (BRISS)*	Wallander et al., 1985	Verbal and nonverbal skills used in conversational interaction and collaborative decision making; heterosocial interactions	Interrater: .53–.92 Intrarater: .6–.9 (with 24 hours of training)	Construct: 70% of correlations between BRISS scores and peer ratings were significant. Discriminant: 88% sensitivity; 67% specificity
Communication Performance Scale	Ehrlich & Barry, 1989	Conversational interaction	Interrater .75–.98; Intrarater .70–.97	Construct: nonsignificant correlations with linguistic tasks (repetition and auditory comprehension); moderate inter-item correlations ($r > .5$) between eye gaze and initiation; and sentence formation and coherence suggesting differentiation between linguistic and nonlinguistic skills
LaTrobe Communication Questionnaire	Douglas et al., 2000, 2007	Perceived communication ability in relation to quantity, quality, relation, and manner	Test-retest for self-report $r = .76$ Internal consistency: total score $\alpha = .86$	Construct: factor analysis indicated 7 factors (inhibitory control, conversational fluency, attentional control, task management, eye contact, rate control, and tone of voice)
Pragmatic Protocol	Prutting & Kirchner, 1987	Linguistic, paralinguistic and nonverbal communication	Interrater reliability: $r > .90$ after 8–10 hours of training	None

continues

Table A–3. *continued*

Test	Authors	Areas Assessed	Reliability	Validity
Profile of Pragmatic Impairment in Communication**	Linscott et al., 1996; Hays et al., 2004	Conversational interactions; content, style, organization, etc.	interrater reliabitliy .75–.88 TBI; .60–.77 for 6/9 subscales with AD (subject matter, quality, and social style = unreliable); generalizability coefficients .86–.94 for all but previous 3 subsets	concurrent validity TBI study: correlations between group and scores *r* = .58–.97 Alzheimers study: *r* = .75–.85 with relevant subsections of the Pragmatic Protocol; General participation + CETI *r* = .84
Social Communication Skills Questionnaire	McGann et al., 1997	Conversation, including expressing and responding to opinions	None	None

Notes. *Assessed almost exclusively with males with moderate–severe TBI; heterosocial interactions created by having participants with TBI interact with a female confederate trained to be minimally responsive.

**Formerly known as the Profile of Functional Impairment in Communication (PFIC). CETI, Communicative Effectiveness Index.

Table A–4. Select Assessments of Attention (see Table 6–2)

Test	Authors	Domains Assessed	Reliability	Validity
Brief Test of Attention	Schretlen et al., 1996, 1997	Auditory divided attention	Test-retest: $r = .7$ Internal consistency: control group $r = .80$ total test; $r = .65–.69$ for alternative forms; control+clinical group $r = .82$ total test, $r = .81–.82$ for alternative forms Parallel forms: controls $r = .65$; controls+clinical group $r = .79$	Construct: factor analysis indicated 3 factors: attentional ability (significant loading), general/verbal mental ability (moderate loading); psychomotor speed and perception (low–moderate loading) Concurrent: moderate–strong correlations with related memory and executive function tasks (e.g., digit span, Trail Making Test, Stroop) Discriminant: differential performance of patients with Huntington's disease compared with controls; no difference between patients with amnesia and controls
Moss Attention Rating Scale	Hart et al., 2006	Observation of behaviors indicative of attention deficits	None	Construct: significant difference in slopes across disciplines. Interpreted as a cognitive index of disability, not a physical index

continues

Table A–4. *continued*

Test	Authors	Domains Assessed	Reliability	Validity
Paced Auditory Serial Addition Task (PASAT)	Gronwall, 1977	Divided and sustained attention; working memory, speed of processing	Test-retest: minimal practice effects noted Internal consistency: $\alpha = .9$; split-half reliability $r = .96$	Concurrent: significant correlations with digit span, working memory, fluid and nonverbal intelligence, and speed of processing measures Discriminant: differential performance of individuals with brain injury compared with controls
Rating Scale of Attentional Behavior	Ponsford & Kinsella, 1991	Observational rating of behaviors indicative of attentional deficits	Intrarater $r = .9$ interrater $r = .5$ (SLP vs. OT) Internal consistency: $\alpha > .9$	Construct: principal component analyses indicated 2–3 factors (attention, psychomotor slowing, ability to focus) Concurrent: moderate significant correlations with related measures of attention
Ruff Selective Attention Test	Ruff & Allen, 1992	Sustained and selective visual attention	Test-retest: $r = .73–.97$, practice effects noted Internal consistency: adequate split-half reliability	Construct: factor analysis indicated 3 factors (speed of visual processing, controlled processing, and automatic processing) Concurrent: significant correlations with visual learning, visual STM; not significantly correlated with measures of attention, learning, and memory

Test	Authors	Domains Assessed	Reliability	Validity
Sustained Attention to Response Task	Robertson et al., 1997	Sustained attention	Test-retest: $r = .76$	Concurrent: significant, moderate correlations with related sustained attention tasks Discriminant: differential performance between patient and control groups
Symbol Digit Modalities Test	Smith 1973, 1991	Divided visual attention, processing speed	Test-retest: $r = .7–.8$; practice effects noted for same form; no practice effects for alternative forms	Construct: scores not significantly related to age, education, or gender
Test of Everyday Attention	Robertson et al., 1994	Visual selective attention/speed, attention switching, sustained attention, auditory-verbal working memory	Test-retest: $r = .59–.86$; dual decrement subtest $r = .41$ for stroke patients Parallel forms: $r = .41–90$	Construct: factor analysis indicated 4 factors (visual selective attention/speed, attentional switching, sustained attention, auditory-verbal working memory); differentiation of types of attention deficits (sustained, selective, divided, and alternating attention) Discriminant: differential performance of adults with TBI compared with controls

Notes. OT = occupational therapist; SLP = speech-language pathologist; TBI = traumatic brain injury.

Table A–5. Select Assessments of Unilateral Neglect (see Table 7–4)

Scale	Authors	Domains Assessed	Reliability	Validity
Apples Test (part of Birmingham Cognitive Screen; BCoS)	Bickerton et al., 2011	Peripersonal egocentric and allocentric visuospatial neglect	Test-retest: $r = 89$ egocentric neglect; $r = .94$ allocentric neglect	Concurrent: $r = .9$ egocentric with star cancellation Discriminant: 100% sensitivity, 59% specificity using Star cancellation as "gold standard"
Balloons Test	Edgeworth et al., 1998	Extrapersonal, viewer-centered, visuospatial neglect	Test-retest: $r = .64$ generalized inattention; $r = .71$ lateralized inattention	Concurrent: $r = .78$ with BIT; $r = .67$ with CBS Discriminant: 83% agreement on identification of visual neglect; sensitive to patients with neglect who compensate in real-world activities
Behavioural Inattention Test (BIT)	Wilson et al., 1987	Peripersonal viewer centered visuospatial neglect	Test-retest: $r = .99$ Inter/intrarater: $r = .99$ Parallel form: $r = .91$ Internal consistency: significant correlation between total score and subtest scores	Content: $r = .92$ behavioral and conventional subtests; Concurrent: $r = .67$ behavioral score and clinician assessment; moderate–strong significant correlations with relevant subtests of other neglect measures. Discriminant: 48% sensitivity; 85% specificity
Catherine Bergego Scale (CBS)	Azouvi et al., 1996, 2003	Personal, peripersonal, and extrapersonal neglect	Internal consistency: significant correlation between total score and items (except eating)	Concurrent: significant moderate–large correlations with paper/pencil tasks; significant correlations with wheelchair collisions, FIM scores and anosognosia. Discriminant: sensitivity 77%–96%; most sensitive items: limb awareness, dressing, collisions

Scale	Authors	Domains Assessed	Reliability	Validity
Comb & Razor Test	Beschin & Robertson 1997	Personal neglect	Test-retest: $r = .94$	Discriminant: sensitivity = 59% specificity = 64%; differential performance of controls, RHD with neglect and RHD without neglect
Gap Detection Task	Ota et al., 2001 Marsh & Hillis, 2008	Peripersonal viewer- and stimulus-centered visuospatial neglect	Test-retest: $r = .75$ performance scores; $r = .100$ identification of egocentric vs. allocentric neglect	Construct: rates of incidence similar to that of other neglect measures
Line Bisection Test	Schenkenberg et al., 1980	Peripersonal, viewer-centered, visuospatial neglect	Test-retest: ranges $r = .84–.97$; more consistent for severe neglect	Construct: moderate correlations with lesions to temporal, parietal, and occipital lobes. Concurrent: low–moderate correlations with cancellation tasks Discriminant: differentiates patients with diffuse or RH lesions from LH lesions and controls; does not discriminate RHD from LHD in acute phases; sensitivity = 76%
Vest Test	Glocker, Bittl, & Kerkhoff, 2006	Personal neglect	Test-retest: $r = .79$ Internal consistency: $\alpha = .96$	Concurrent: $r = .31–.61$ with fluff test; $r = .80$ with CBS Discriminant: sensitivity = 80% for RH personal (body) neglect; specificity = 92%.
Wheelchair Collision Test	Qiang et al., 2005	Extrapersonal visuospatial neglect	Test-retest: $r = .68–.97$	Discriminant: $r = .72$ with CBS

Notes. FIM = Functional Independence Measure; egocentric neglect = viewer-centered neglect; allocentric neglect = stimulus/object-centered neglect.

Table A–6. Select Measures of Executive Function (see Table 8–2)

Scale	Authors	Domains Assessed	Reliability	Validity
Behavioral Assessment of the Dysexecutive Syndrome (BADS)	Wilson et al., 1996	Organization, planning, problem solving, self-monitoring	Test-retest reliability: practice effect apparent	Convergent validity: $r > .5$ correlations with related cognitive assessments for adults with Alzheimer's disease. Discriminant validity: sensitivity and specificity both = 83%
Behavior Rating Inventory of Executive Function (BRIEF)–Adult version	Roth et al., 2005	Self-regulation in natural environment	Test-retest reliability: $r > .82$ Interrater reliability: $r = 0.44$–0.68 between self- and informant reports. Internal consistency: $\alpha = 0.73$–0.90 for self-report $\alpha = 0.80$–0.93 for informant report	Construct validity: expert rating of whether each item belonged in its assigned scale: range 35% agreement (self-monitor scale) to 98% agreement (emotional control scale). Factor analysis: self report form correlation 0.78 (73% of variance) and informant report factor correlation was .79 (81% of variance). Concurrent validity: $r > .34$ correlations with related cognitive assessments
Brixton-Spatial Anticipation Test	Burgess & Shallice, 1997	Rule derivation and shifting, fluid ability	Test-retest reliability: $r = .71$ Internal consistency: split-half reliability $\alpha = 0.62$	Construct validity: total scores correlated with related cognitive assessments ($r > .40$). Discriminant validity: differential performance of patients with anterior vs. posterior lesions

Scale	Authors	Domains Assessed	Reliability	Validity
Delis-Kaplan Executive Function System	Delis et al., 2001	Nine separate tests of executive function: Word Context test, Sorting test, Twenty Questions test, Tower test, Color-Word Interference test, Verbal Fluency test, Design Fluency test, Trail Making test, Proverb test	Internal consistency: varied by subtest, $\alpha = .32-.9$; Generally low SEM	Convergent: small correlations with CVLT and WCST
Dysexecutive Questionnaire (DEX)	Burgess et al., 1998; Wilson et al., 1996	Intentionality, inhibition, executive memory, affect	None	Convergent validity: $r > .35$ correlations between significant other scores and other cognitive measures. Discriminant validity: sensitivity 49%, specificity 71%
Functional Assessment of Verbal Reasoning and Executive Strategies (FAVRES)	McDonald, 2005	Verbal reasoning, executive function	Interrater: $r > .9$	Discriminant: sensitivity 88%; specificity 83%; group with acquired brain injury scored significantly lower than control group
Frontal Systems Behavior Scale	Grace & Malloy, 2001	Intentionality and disinhibition	Internal consistency: $\alpha > .72$ family and self-rating forms	Construct validity: factor analysis confirmed 83% of items loaded to hypothesized factors; but only explained 41% of variance. Convergent validity: $r = .41$ with neuropsychological inventory for adults with dementia

continues

Table A–6. *continued*

Scale	Authors	Domains Assessed	Reliability	Validity
Hayling Sentence Completion Test	Burgess & Shallice, 1997	Response inhibition, fluid ability	Test-retest reliability: $r > 0.60$ Internal consistency: $\alpha = 0.62–0.76$	Construct validity: converging data regarding lesion-symptom matching from imaging studies Discriminant validity: specificity effect size 0.37; differential performance of patients with anterior vs. posterior lesions on inhibition task
Iowa Gambling Task (IGT)	Bechara et al., 1994	Executive function, decision making, and emotional signals	None	Convergent validity: scores moderately correlated with related cognitive measures
MicroCog: Assessment of Cognitive Functioning, 2004 Edition	Powell et al., 2004	Computerized assessment of attention, memory, EF, reaction time, speed of processing, general cognitive functioning	Internal consistency: $\alpha = .83$ to .95	Construct validity: factor analysis supported hypothesized structure. Discriminant validity: Sensitivity = 65%–89%; specificity = 65%–94%
Multiple Errands Test	Shallice & Burgess, 1991	Strategy allocation, planning	Interrater: $r = 0.71–0.88$ Internal consistency: $\alpha = 0.77$	Convergent validity: $r = -0.93$ correlated to Zoo map; $r = 0.76–0.80$ instrumental activities of daily living. Discriminant validity: 82%–85% sensitivity; 95% specificity

Scale	Authors	Domains Assessed	Reliability	Validity
Naturalistic Action Test	Schwarz et al., 2002	Planning, sequencing, and strategy allocation	Test retest reliability: $r = 0.66$ Interrater reliability: kappa > .7 Internal consistency: $\alpha > .75$	Concurrent validity: $r > .60$ correlations with other cognitive measures (processing speed, visual attention, working memory, and FIM scores). Discriminant validity: 85.7% sensitive (dementia); 87% specific (controls)
Revised Strategy Application Test	Levine et al., 2000	Executive function and strategy allocation	None	Discriminant validity: adults with RHD scored lower than control group. Concurrent validity: $r = 40$ correlation with Sickness Impact Profile
Ruff Figural Fluency Test (RFFT)	Ruff, 1996	"Cognitive fluency"–shift, cognitive set, planning strategies, executive ability	Test-retest reliability: $r = 0.76$ (but practice effect observed) Interrater reliability: $r = .66–93$	Construct validity: factor analysis suggested loading planning flexibility factor. Discriminant validity: 85% sensitive (right frontal dysfunction)
Tower of Hanoi	Newell & Simon, 1972	Planning	Internal consistency: split-half reliability 0.87, $\alpha = 0.9$, inter-item correlations $r = 0.68–0.81$	Convergent validity: $r = .37$ correlation with Tower of London

continues

Table A–6. *continued*

Scale	Authors	Domains Assessed	Reliability	Validity
Tower of London	Shallice, 1982	Planning	Test-retest reliability: $r = .80$ for pediatric sample with attention deficit disorder. Internal consistency: split-half correlation $r = 0.72$ controls; $r = 0.83$ mild cognitive impairment	Convergent validity: $r > .40$ correlation with related cognitive measures. Discriminant validity: adults with cognitive deficits consistently score lower than controls
Trail Making Test	Reitan, 1958	Attention, planning, working memory	None	Discriminant validity: sensitivity 33.7%; specificity 76%. Poorer performance on Trails A, B, and B–A by adults with brain injury compared with controls
Wisconsin Card Sorting Test (WCST)	Heaton et al., 1993	Switching/perseveration	Interrater reliability $r > .91$ Intrarater reliability $r > .83$ Internal consistency: principle component accounts for at least 66% of variance	Construct validity: speed of processing accounted for greatest variance in multiple regression, suggesting WCST assesses processing speed. Discriminant validity: low specificity, impacted by age

Notes. α = Cronbach's alpha; CVLT = California Verbal Learning Test; FIM = Functional Independence Measure; MoCA = Montreal Cognitive Assessment (Nasreddine et al., 2005).

Table A–7. Select Assessments of Anosognosia that Address Cognition, Pragmatics, and/or Neglect (see Table 9–2)

Scale	Authors	Domains Assessed	Reliability	Validity
Awareness Questionnaire (AQ)	Sherer et al.,1998, 2003	Cognition, emotion/ pragmatics, functional implications. Implicit awareness, hemiparesis, neglect	Internal consistency: total score $\alpha > .85$; cognitive and behavioral/affective factors $\alpha > .75$ for patient and family; motor/sensory factor $\alpha > .55$ for patient and family	Construct: factor analysis indicated 3 factors (cognitive; behavioral/affective and motor/ sensory); clinician + family scores $r = .44$. Convergent: significant correlations with PCRS total scores (all $r > .35$); significant correlations between discrepancy scores of AQ and PCRS (all $r > .5$)
Bisiach scale	Bisiach et al., 1986	Hemiplegia, neglect	None	None
Head Injury Behavior Scale (HIBS)	Godfrey, 2003	Emotion/pragmatics, functional implications	Internal consistency: $r > .47$ within subtests; emotional and behavioral regulation $\alpha > .85$	Construct: factor analysis indicated 2 factors (emotional and behavioral)
Impaired Self-Awareness (ISA) scale	Prigatano & Klonoff, 1998	Cognition	Inter/intrarater: Severity of impaired self-awareness ratings $r = .25$ (NS); denial of disability severity rating $r = .82$	Discriminant validity *Differentiation between patients with ISA and denial of disability

continues

Table A–7. *continued*

Scale	Authors	Domains Assessed	Reliability	Validity
Levine Denial of Illness Scale	Levine, 1987	Prognosis/compliance	Interrater: individual items $r = .65$; total score $r = .78$ Internal consistency: $\alpha = .76$	Convergent: significant correlations with anxiety, depression and severity measures as well as progress notes mentioning awareness (all $r > .35$)
Patient Competency Rating Scale (PCRS)	Prigatano & Fordyce, 1986; Prigatano & Altman, 1990	Cognition, emotion/pragmatics, functional implications	Interrater: whole test $r > .8$; patient and relative ratings $r > .95$	Convergent: significant correlations with AQ total scores (all $r > .35$); higher agreement within rating groups (patients, clinicians, families) than between groups; significant correlations between discrepancy scores of AQ and PCRS (all $r > .5$)
Patient Competency Rating Scale for inpatient NeuroRehabilitation (PCRS-NR)	Borgaro & Prigatano, 2003	Cognition, emotion/pragmatics, functional implications	Internal consistency: total scale $\alpha = .82$ emotional, interpersonal and cognitive function factors $\alpha > .78$	Construct: factor analysis indicated 3 factors (emotional, interpersonal, and cognitive) Discriminant: correlations with unrelated constructs ranged from $r = .06$ to .27
Self-Awareness of Deficit Interview (SADI)	Fleming et al., 1996	Cognition, emotion/pragmatics, functional implications, treatment compliance	Interrater reliability $r > .9$ for whole test and $r > .85$ for subtests	Correlations between SADI and other 2 awareness questionnaires $r > .5$

Scale	Authors	Domains Assessed	Reliability	Validity
Structured Awareness Interview (SAI)	Marcel et al., 2004	Implicit awareness, hemiplegia vision/neglect	None	None
Visual-Analogue Test for Anosognosia Language	Cocchini et al., 2010	Functional implications, aphasia	Test-retest reliability $r > .9$ for personal and professional caregivers; $r = .84$ for patients	None
Visual-Analogue Test for Anosognosia for Motor Impairment	Della Salla et al., 2009	Functional implications, hemiparesis	Test-retest reliability $r > .9$ for caregivers; $r = .83$ for patients Internal consistency: $\alpha = .93$ for upper limb; .84 lower limb	Discriminant validity: sensitivity of items ranged from 73% to 90.5%

Notes. α = Cronbach's alpha; NS = nonsignificant.

227

Table A–8. Select Measures of Memory (see Table 10–4)

Test	Authors	Type of Memory	Reliability	Validity
Benton Visual Retention Test, 5th edition	Sivan, 1992	Immediate and delayed visual memory	Test-retest: $r = .53-.77$ Interrater: $r = .85-.98$	None
Brief Assessment of Prospective Memory (BAPM)	Man et al., 2011	Prospective memory	Test-retest: ICC = .76 for IADL and .66 for BADL Internal consistency: total score $\alpha = .83-.90$; IADL $\alpha = .76$; BADL $\alpha = .69-78$	Convergent: correlation $r = .9$ with CAPM
California Verbal Learning Test, 2nd edition	Delis et al., 2000	Verbal learning	Test-retest: $r = 0.82$ Internal consistency: overall sample $r > .8$, but some individual age/gender groups were unacceptably low	Construct: Factor analysis indicated 6 factors (learning strategy, acquisition rate, serial position effect, discriminability, and learning interference) Convergent: $r = .63-.86$ with first edition Discriminant: specificity 91%, sensitivity 74%
Cambridge Prospective Memory Test	Wilson et al., 2005	Prospective memory	Test-retest: tau-b correlation of 0.64 (practice effects observed) Interrater: $r = 0.998$ Parallel form: no significant differences in scores across forms	Convergent: small but significant correlations ($r = .38$) with related memory tests

Test	Authors	Type of Memory	Reliability	Validity
Contextual Memory Test	Toglia, 1993	Metamemory	Test-retest: incomplete information Parallel form: parallel form $r = 0.73$–0.81	Convergent: correlations $r = .7$–$.8$ with related memory tests Discriminant: hit rate .87–.91
Corsi Block Tapping Task	Corsi, 1972; Kessels et al., 2000	Visuospatial memory	None	Construct: factor analysis identified 2 factors (verbal and spatial working memory); forward and backward tasks equivalent in terms of difficulty Discriminant: adults with AD or RHD perform more poorly than controls.
Continuous Visual Memory Test–Revised	Trahan & Larrabee 1997	Visual memory	Test-retest: $r = .85$ total score; .76 delayed recognition Internal consistency: split-half reliability $r = .8$–.98	Construct: factor analysis indicated 4 factors: information and vocabulary (17.7% of variance), visual/nonverbal cognitive caption (11.1% of variance), verbal learning and memory (11% of variance), visual memory (8.1% of variance) Discriminant: specificity 0.99%, sensitivity 0.25%; differential performance by adults with RHD and LHD
Everyday Memory Questionnaire–Revised	Royle & Lincoln, 2008	Metamemory	Internal consistency: $\alpha = .91$	Content: factor analyses indicated 5–7 factors including memory, retrieval, and attention Discriminant: differential scores for adults with MS and CVA

continues

Table A–8. *continued*

Test	Authors	Type of Memory	Reliability	Validity
Hopkins Verbal Learning Test–Revised	Brandt & Benedict 2001	Verbal learning	Test-retest: $r = .74$ for total recall; $r = .39$ for retention	Construct: factor analysis supports theoretical framework Concurrent: moderate, significant correlations with related memory tests (e.g., $r = 0.65$–0.77 for Wechsler Memory Scales) Discriminant: correctly classifies 85%–90% of adults with Alzheimer's dementia
Memory for Intentions Test (MIST)	Raskin et al., 2010	Prospective memory	Test-retest: $r = .78$ (15 day period) Inter/intrarater: $r = .81$–.97 Internal consistency: $\alpha = .93$; Spearman Brown split-half $r = .97$ Subscales $\alpha = .54$ to .64.	Concurrent: $r = .80$ with relevant subtests of RBMT; no significant correlation with MMSE
Memory Test for Older Adults	Hubley & Tombaugh, 2002	Visual and verbal memory	Inter/intrarater: .81–.97 for long version; .70–.99 for short version Internal consistency: long version: $\alpha = .68$–.87 total acquisition; $\alpha = .24$–.81 retention; short version: $\alpha = .35$–.76 total acquisition; $\alpha = .30$–.72 retention	Discriminant: differential performance by controls and adults with dementia difficult to interpret due to small sample sizes

Test	Authors	Type of Memory	Reliability	Validity
Oxford Cog Screen–Memory Subtests	Riddoh et al., 2015	Orientation; recall recognition episodic	Test-retest: ICC r = .49–.77 for memory subsections	Construct: scores on 2 memory subtests significantly correlated with each other and with praxis and number subtests; language is not as large a confounding factor as for other memory tests Convergent: r = .44–.70 with related memory tests Discriminant: orientation: ranges 52%–68% sensitivity and 87%–92% specificity
Prospective and Retrospective Memory Question-naire (PRMQ)	Smith et al., 2000	Prospective and retrospective memory	Internal consistency: α = 0.89 total score; α = 0.84 prospective; α = 0.80 retrospective	Construct: factor analysis confirmed 3 structures: general memory, prospective and retrospective memory
Recognition Memory Test	Warrington, 1984	Visual memory	Test-retest: r = .81 for faces Parallel form: r = .41 for words; r = .53 for faces	Concurrent: moderate correlations with related memory tests; no significant relationships to verbal reasoning, visual problem solving, verbal fluency, or intelligence
Rey Auditory Verbal Learning Test	Schmidt, 1996	Verbal learning	Test-retest: r = 0.76 for immediate recall; r = 0.89 delayed recall; r = 0.87 recognition interrater r = 0.94	Construct: 98.4% of variance accounted for via factor analysis Discriminant: significant correlations with related visuospatial and memory tests; nonsignificant correlation with language test; 58%–78% specificity depending on measure (copy, recall, and recognition)

continues

Table A–8. *continued*

Test	Authors	Type of Memory	Reliability	Validity
Rey Complex Figure Test and Recognition Trial	Myers & Myers, 1995	Visuospatial ability and visuospatial memory	Test-retest: r = .75–.88 Interrater: r = .94	Construct: 98.4% of variance accounted for via factor analysis Convergent: moderate–strong correlations with related memory measures; no significant correlation with language measure Discriminant: sensitivity: copy/time to copy: 58% correctly classified immediate and delayed recall: 61% correctly; recall and recognition: 78% correctly classified. Poor differentiation of patients with psychiatric diagnoses vs. brain injury; sensitive to brain injury vs. malingering
Rivermead Behavioral Memory Test, 2nd edition (RBMT)	Wilson et al., 2003	"Everyday" memory	Interrater: r = 0.87 Parallel forms: 0.57–0.86	Construct: factor analysis indicated all items loaded on a single factor Convergent: r = .44 correlations with observer questionnaire; significant correlation with related memory test and tests of new learning Discriminant: differential performance by adults with brain injury and controls

Test	Authors	Type of Memory	Reliability	Validity
Test of Memory and Learning, 2nd edition	Reynolds & Voress 2007	Immediate and delayed verbal and nonverbal memory	Test-retest: r = .81–.93 core indexes; r = .68–.94 supplementary indices Inter/intrarater: r > .9 for all subtests and indices Internal consistency: α > .9 for core and supplementary indices	Construct: factor analysis indicated strong correlations between subtests Convergent: moderate–strong correlation with related memory test
Three Cities Test	Johnson-Green et al., 2009	Learning and short term memory	None	Convergent: significant correlation with MMSE, functional recovery, and length of hospitalization
Wechsler Memory Scales, 4th edition	Wechsler, 2009	Verbal and visual short-term and working memory	Test-retest: r = .59–.77 (adult), r = .69–.81 (older adult) Internal consistency: α = .74–.99	Construct: factor analyses indicated and 2 factors in the older adults version (auditory and visual memory); third factor (visual working memory) in adult version Convergent: moderate correlations with related memory tests; significant correlation with measures of daily living skills Discriminant: patients with severe TBI perform more poorly than mild–moderate TBI

Notes. α = Crohnbach's alpha; AD = Alzheimer's disease; CVA = cerebrovascular accident; MS = multiple sclerosis; RHD = right hemisphere brain damage.

References

Abbott, J. D., Wijerante, T., Hughes, A., Perre, D., & Lindell, A. K. (2014a). The influence of left and right hemisphere brain damage on configural and featural processing of affective faces. *Laterality, 19*(4), 455–472.

Abbott, J. D., Wijeratne, T., Hughes, A., Perre, D., & Lindell, A. K. (2014b). The perception of positive and negative facial expressions by unilateral stroke patients. *Brain and Cognition, 86*, 42–54. http://doi.org/10.1016/j.bandc.2014.01.017

Adamit, T., Maeir, A., Ben Assayag, E., Bornstein, N. M., Korczyn, A. D., & Katz, N. (2015). Impact of first-ever mild stroke on participation at 3 and 6 month post-event: The TABASCO study. *Disability and Rehabilitation, 37*(8), 667–673. http://doi.org/10.3109/09638288.2014.923523

Adolphs, R., Damasio, H., & Tranel, D. (2002). Neural systems for recognition of emotional prosody: A 3-D lesion study. *Emotion, 2*(1), 23–51. http://doi.org/10.1037//1528-3542.2.1.23

Agis, D., Goggins, M. B., Oishi, K., Oishi, K., Davis, C., Wright, A., . . . Hillis, A. E. (2016). Picturing the size and site of stroke with an expanded National Institutes of Health Stroke Scale. *Stroke,* STROKEAHA.115.012324. http://doi.org/10.1161/STROKEAHA.115.012324

Agosta, S., Herpich, F., Miceli, G., Ferraro, F., & Battelli, L. (2014). Contralesional rTMS relieves visual extinction in chronic stroke. *Neuropsychologia, 62*(1), 269–276. http://doi.org/10.1016/j.neuropsychologia.2014.07.026

Alberini, C. M., & Ledoux, J. E. (2013). Memory reconsolidation. *Current Biology, 23*(17), R746–R750. http://doi.org/10.1016/j.cub.2013.06.046

Alderman, N., Evans, J. J., Emslie, H., Wilson, B. W., & Burgess, P. W. (1996). Zoo Map Test. In B. A. Wilson, N. Alderman, P. W., Burgess, H. Emslie, & J. J. Evans (Eds.), *Behavioural Assessment of the Dysexecutive Syndrome.* Bury St. Edmunds, UK: Thames Valley Test Co.

Alho, K., Salmi, J., Koistinen, S., Salonen, O., & Rinne, T. (2015). Top-down controlled and bottom-up triggered orienting of auditory attention to pitch activate overlapping brain networks. *Brain Research, 1626*, 136–145. http://doi.org/10.1016/j.brainres.2014.12.050

Allen, C. C., & Ruff, R. M. (2007). Differential impairment of patients with right versus left hemisphere lesions on the Ruff-Light Trail Learning Test. *Applied Neuropsychology, 14*(3), 141–6. http://doi.org/10.1080/09084280701508192

Alpers, G. W. (2008). Eye-catching: Right hemisphere attentional bias for emotional pictures. *Laterality, 13*(2), 158–178. http://doi.org/10.1080/13576500701779247

Alvarez, J. A., & Emory, E. (2006). Executive function and the frontal lobes: A meta-analytic review. *Neuropsychology Review, 16*(1), 17–42. http://doi.org/10.1007/s11065-006-9002-x

American Speech-Language-Hearing Association. (2016). Code of ethics [Ethics]. Available from http://www.asha.org/policy

Anand, R., Chapman, S. B., Rackley, A., Keebler, M., Zientz, J., & Hart, J. (2011). Gist reasoning training in cognitively normal seniors. *International Journal of Geriatric Psychiatry*, 26(9), 961–968. http://doi.org/10.1002/gps.2633

Anderson, B., Mennemeier, M., & Chatterjee, A. (2000). Variability not ability: Another basis for performance decrements in neglect. *Neuropsychologia2*, 38, 785–796. http://doi.org/10.1016/S0028-3932(99)00137-2

Andrade, K., Kas, A., Valabrègue, R., Samri, D., Sarazin, M., Habert, M.-O., . . . Bartolomeo, P. (2012). Visuospatial deficits in posterior cortical atrophy: Structural and functional correlates. *Journal of Neurology, Neurosurgery, and Psychiatry*, 83(9), 860–863. http://doi.org/10.1136/jnnp-2012-302278

Andy, O. J., & Bhatnagar, S. C. (1984). Right-hemispheric language evidence from cortical stimulation. *Brain and Language*, 23(1), 159–166. http://doi.org/10.1016/0093-934X(84)90014-2

Antonucci, G., Guariglia, C., Judica, A., Magnotti, L., Paolucci, S., Pizzamiglio, L., . . . Zoccolotti, P. (1995). Effectiveness of neglect rehabilitation in a randomized group study. *Journal of Clinical and Experimental Neuropsychology*, 17, 383–389.

Aparicio-López, C., García-Molina, A., García-Fernández, J., Lopez-Blazquez, R., Enseñat-Cantallops, A., Sánchez-Carrión, R., . . . Roig-Rovira, T. (2015). Cognitive rehabilitation with right hemifield eye-patching for patients with sub-acute stroke and visuospatial neglect: A randomized controlled trial. *Brain Injury*, 29(4), 501–507. http://doi.org/10.3109/02699052.2014.995230

Appelros, P. (2007). Prediction of length of stay for stroke patients. *Acta Neurologica Scandinavica*, 116(1), 15–19. http://doi.org/10.1111/j.1600-0404.2006.00756.x

Appelros, P., Karlsson, G. M., & Hennerdal, S. (2007). Anosognosia versus unilateral neglect. Coexistence and their relations to age, stroke severity, lesion site and cognition. *European Journal of Neurology*, 14(1), 54–59. http://doi.org/10.1111/j.1468-1331.2006.01544.x

Appelros, P., Nydevik, I., Karlsson, G. M., Thorwalls, A., & Seiger, A. (2003). Assessing unilateral neglect: Shortcomings of standard test methods. *Disability and Rehabilitation*, 25(9), 473–479. http://doi.org/10.1080/0963828031000071714

Appelros, P., Nydevik, I., Karlsson, G. M., Thorwalls, A., & Seiger, A. (2004). Recovery from unilateral neglect after right-hemisphere stroke. *Disability and Rehabilitation*, 26(8), 471–477. http://doi.org/10.1080/09638280410001663058

Arcara, G., Lacaita, G., Mattaloni, E., Passarini, L., Mondini, S., Beninca, P., & Semenza, C. (2012). Is "hit and run" a single word? The processing of irreversible binomials in neglect dyslexia. *Frontiers in Psychology*, 3, 1–11. http://doi.org/10.3389/fpsyg.2012.00011

Arene, N. U., & Hillis, A. E. (2007). Rehabilitation of unilateral spatial neglect and neuroimaging. *Eura Medicophysiology*, 43(2), 255–269.

Aron, A. R., Robbins, T. W., & Poldrack, R. A. (2004). Inhibition and the right inferior frontal cortex. *Trends in Cognitive Sciences*, 8(4), 170–177. http://doi.org/10.1016/j.tics.2004.02.010

Asanowicz, D., Marzecová, A., Jaśkowski, P., & Wolski, P. (2012). Hemispheric asymmetry in the efficiency of attentional networks. *Brain and Cognition*, 79(2), 117–128. http://doi.org/10.1016/j.bandc.2012.02.014

Austin, M. W., Ploughman, M., Glynn, L., & Corbett, D. (2014). Aerobic exercise effects on neuroprotection and brain repair following stroke: A systematic review and perspective. *Neuroscience Research*, 87, 8–15. http://doi.org/10.1016/j.neures.2014.06.007

Awh, E., & Jonides, J. (2001). Overlapping mechanisms of attention and spatial working memory. *Trends in Cognitive Sciences*, 5(3), 119–126.

Azouvi, P., Bartolomeo, P., Beis, J., Perennou, D., Pradat-Diehl, P., & Rousseaux, M. (2006). A battery of tests for the quantitative assessment of unilateral neglect. *Restorative Neurology and Neuroscience, 24*, 273–285.

Azouvi, P., Marchal, F., Samuel, C., Morin, L., Renard, C., Louis-Dreyfus, A., . . . Bergego, C. (1996). Functional consequences and awareness of unilateral neglect: Study of an evaluation scale. *Neuropsychological Rehabilitation, 6*(2), 133–150. http://doi.org/10.1080/713755501

Azouvi, P., Samuel, C., Bernati, T., Bartolomeo, P., Beis, J., Chokron, S., . . . Perennou, D. (2002). Sensitivity of clinical and behavioural tests of spatial neglect after right hemisphere stroke. *Journal of Neurology, Neurosurgery & Psychiatry, 73*, 160–167. http://doi.org/doi:10.1136/jnnp.73.2.160

Baddeley, A. (2003). Working memory: Looking back and looking forward. *Nature Reviews, 4*(October), 829–839. http://doi.org/10.1038/nrn1201

Baddeley, A. D., & Hitch, G. J. (1994). Developments in the concept of working memory. *Neuropsychology, 8*(4), 485–493. http://doi.org/10.1037/0894-4105.8.4.485

Baheux, K., Yoshizawa, M., Seki, K., & Handa, Y. (2006). Virtual reality pencil and paper tests for neglect: A protocol. *Cyberpsychology & Behavior: The Impact of the Internet, Multimedia and Virtual Reality on Behavior and Society, 9*(2), 192–195. http://doi.org/10.1089/cpb.2006.9.192

Baheux, K., Yoshizawa, M., Tanaka, A., Seki, K., & Handa, Y. (2005). Diagnosis and rehabilitation of hemispatial neglect patients with virtual reality technology. *Technology and Health Care, 13*, 245–260.

Bahrainwala, Z. S., Hillis, A. E., Dearborn, J., & Gottesman, R. F. (2014). Neglect performance in acute stroke is related to severity of white matter hyperintensities. *Cerebrovascular Diseases (Basel, Switzerland), 37*(3), 223–230. http://doi.org/10.1159/000357661

Baier, B., Karnath, H.-O., Dieterich, M., Birklein, F., Heinze, C., & Mu, N. G. (2010). Keeping memory clear and stable—The contribution of human basal ganglia and prefrontal cortex to working memory. *The Journal of Neuroscience, 30*(29), 9788–9792. http://doi.org/10.1523/JNEUROSCI.1513-10.2010

Bailey, M. J., Riddoch, M. J., & Crome, P. (2002). Treatment of visual neglect in elderly patients with stroke: A single-subject series using either a scanning and cueing strategy or a left-limb activation strategy. *Physical Therapy, 82*(8), 782–797.

Balaban, N., Friedmann, N., & Ariel, M. (2016a). The effect of theory of mind impairment on language: Referring after right hemisphere damage. *Aphasiology, 7038*(1066), 1–38. http://doi.org/10.1080/02687038.2015.1137274

Balaban, N., Friedmann, N., & Ziv, M. (2016b). Theory of mind impairment after right hemisphere damage. *Aphasiology, 7038*(March), 1–33. http://doi.org/10.1080/02687038.2015.1137275

Baldassarre, A., Ramsey, L., Hacker, C. L., Callejas, A., Astafiev, S. V., Metcalf, N. V., . . . Corbetta, M. (2014). Large-scale changes in network interactions as a physiological signature of spatial neglect. *Brain, 137*(12), 3267–3283. http://doi.org/10.1093/brain/awu297

Barker-Collo, S. L., Feigin, V. L., Lawes, C. M. M., Parag, V., & Senior, H. (2010). Attention deficits after incident stroke in the acute period: Frequency across types of attention and relationships to patient characteristics and functional outcomes. *Topics in Stroke Rehabilitation, 17*(6), 463–476. http://doi.org/10.1310/tsr1706-463

Barker-Collo, S., Feigin, V., Lawes, C., Senior, H., & Parag, V. (2010). Natural history of attention deficits and their influence on functional recovery from acute stages to 6 months after stroke. *Neuroepidemiology, 35*(4), 255–262. http://doi.org/10.1159/000319894

Barnes, S., & Armstrong, E. (2010). Conversation after right hemisphere brain damage: Motivations for applying conversation analysis. *Clinical Linguistics & Phonetics*, *24*(1), 55–69. http://doi.org/10.3109/02699200903349734

Barnett, S. D., Heinemann, A. W., Libin, A., Houts, A. C., Gassaway, J., Sen-Gupta, S., . . . Brossart, D. F. (2012). Small N designs for rehabilitation research. *The Journal of Rehabilitation Research and Development*, *49*(1), 175. http://doi.org/10.1682/JRRD.2010.12.0242

Baron, C., Goldsmith, T., & Beatty, P. W. (1999). Family and clinician perceptions of pragmatic communication skills following right hemisphere stroke. *Topics in Stroke Rehabilitation*, *5*(4), 55–64. http://doi.org/10.1310/78XM-RVMK-NNJ1-3NV9

Barrett, A. M., Buxbaum, L. J., Coslett, H. B., Edwards, E., Heilman, K. M., Hillis, A. E., . . . Robertson, I. H. (2006). Cognitive rehabilitation interventions for neglect and related disorders: Moving from bench to bedside in stroke patients. *Journal of Cognitive Neuroscience*, *18*(7), 1223–1236. http://doi.org/10.1162/jocn.2006.18.7.1223

Barrett, A. M., Galletta, E. E., Zhang, J., Masmela, J. R., & Adler, U. S. (2014). Stroke survivors over-estimate their medication self-administration (MSA) ability, predicting memory loss. *Brain Injury*, *28*(10), 1328–1333. http://doi.org/10.3109/02699052.2014.915984

Bartels-Tobin, L. R., & Hinckley, J. J. (2005). Cognition and discourse production in right hemisphere disorder. *Journal of Neurolinguistics*, *18*(6), 461–477. http://doi.org/10.1016/j.jneuroling.2005.04.001

Bartolo, A., Benuzzi, F., Nocetti, L., Baraldi, P., & Nichelli, P. (2006). Humor comprehension and appreciation: An FMRI study. *Journal of Cognitive Neuroscience*, *18*(1998), 1789–1798. http://doi.org/10.1162/jocn.2006.18.11.1789

Bartolomeo, P., & Chokron, S. (1999). Left unilateral neglect or right hyperattention? *Neurology*, *53*, 2023–2027. http://doi.org/10.1212/WNL.53.9.2023

Bartolomeo, P., & Chokron, S. (2002). Orienting of attention in left unilateral neglect.

Neuroscience and Biobehavioral Reviews, *26*(2), 217–234. http://doi.org/10.1016/S0149-7634(01)00065-3

Bartolomeo, P., Siéroff, E., Decaix, C., & Chokron, S. (2001). Modulating the attentional bias in unilateral neglect: The effects of the strategic set. *Experimental Brain Research*, *137*(3–4), 432–444. http://doi.org/10.1007/s002210000642

Bartolomeo, P., Thiebaut De Schotten, M., & Doricchi, F. (2007). Left unilateral neglect as a disconnection syndrome. *Cerebral Cortex*, *17*(11), 2479–2490. http://doi.org/10.1093/cercor/bhl181

Batchelor, S., Thompson, E. O., & Miller, L. A. (2008). Retrograde memory after unilateral stroke. *Cortex*, *44*(2), 170–178. http://doi.org/10.1016/j.cortex.2006.05.003

Baum, S. R., & Pell, M. D. (1999). The neural bases of prosody: Insights from lesion studies and neuroimaging. *Aphasiology*, *13*(8), 581–608.

Baum, S. R., Pell, M. D., Leonard, C. L., & Gordon, J. K. (2001). Using prosody to resolve temporary syntactic ambiguities in speech production: Acoustic data on brain-damaged speakers. *Clinical Linguistics & Phonetics*, *15*(6), 441–456.

Bechara, A. (1994). *Iowa Gambling Task.* Lutz, FL: Psychological Assessment Resources.

Becker, E., & Karnath, H.-O. (2007). Incidence of visual extinction after left versus right hemisphere stroke. *Stroke*, *38*(12), 3172–3174.

Beeman, M. (1993). Semantic processing in the right hemisphere may contribute to drawing inferences from discourse. *Brain and Language*, *44*, 80–120.

Beeman, M. (1998). Coarse semantic coding and discourse comprehension. In M. Beeman & Chiarello, C. (Ed.), *Right Hemisphere Language Comprehension: Perspectives from Cognitive Neuroscience* (pp. 255–284). Book Section, Mahwah, NJ: Lawrence Erlbaum.

Beeson, P. M., & Robey, R. R. (2006). Evaluating single-subject treatment research: Lessons learned from aphasia literature. *Neuropsychology Review*, *16*(4), 161–169. http://doi.org/10.1007/s11065-006-9013-7.

Behrmann, M., Black, S., McKeeff, T., & Barton, J. (2002). Oculographic analysis of word reading in hemispatial neglect. *Physiology & Behavior*, *77*(4–5), 613–619. http://doi .org/10.1016/S0031-9384(02)00896-X

Bélanger, N., Baum, S. R., & Titone, D. (2009). Use of prosodic cues in the production of idiomatic and literal sentences by individuals with right- and left-hemisphere damage. *Brain and Language*, *110*(1), 38–42. http:// doi.org/10.1016/j.bandl.2009.02.001

Bell, K. R., Temkin, N. R., Esselman, P. C., Doctor, J. N., Bombardier, C. H., Fraser, R. T., . . . Dikmen, S. (2005). The effect of a scheduled telephone intervention on outcome after moderate to severe traumatic brain injury: A randomized trial. *Archives of Physical Medicine & Rehabilitation*, *86*(5), 851–856. http:// doi.org/10.1016/j.apmr.2004.09.015

Ben-David, B. M., Shakuf, V., & van Lieshout P. H. H. M. (2017). T- RES Test for Rating of Emotions in Speech. An English and Hebrew resource of validated digital audio recordings to assess identification of emotion in spoken language [data set] Retrieved from https://idc-primo.hosted.exlibris group.com:443/972IDC_INST_V1:IDC: 972IDC_INST_ALMA1139384700003105&p refLang=en_US

Ben-Yishay, Y. (1996). Reflections on the evolution of the therapeutic milieu concept. *Neuropsychological Rehabilitation*, *6*, 327–343. http://doi.org/10.1080/713755514

Ben-Yishay, Y., & Diller, L. (2011). *Handbook of holistic neuropsychological rehabilitation: Outpatient rehabilitation of traumatic brain injury.* New York, NY: Oxford University Press.

Berrin-Wasserman, S., Winnick, W. A., & Borod, J. C. (2003). Effects of stimulus emotionality and sentence generation on memory for words in adults with unilateral brain damage. *Neuropsychology*, *17*(3), 429–438. http:// doi.org/10.1037/0894-4105.17.3.429

Berryhill, M. E., Chein, J., & Olson, I. R. (2012). At the intersection of attention and memory: The mechanistic role of the posterior parietal lobe in working memory. *Neuropsychologia*,

49(5), 1306–1315. http://doi.org/10.1016/j .neuropsychologia.2011.02.033.At

Berryhill, M. E., Wencil, E. B., Coslett, H. B., & Olson, I. R. (2010). A selective working memory impairment after transcranial direct current stimulation to the right parietal lobe. *Neuroscience Letters*, *479*, 312–316. http://doi.org/10.1016/j.neulet.2010.05.087

Berti, A., Bottini, G., Gandola, M., Pia, L., Smania, N., Stracciari, A., . . . Paulesu, E. (2005). Shared cortical anatomy for motor awareness and motor control. *Science*, *309*(5733), 488–491. Retrieved from http://www.jstor .org/stable/3843342

Berti, A., Ladavas, E., & Della Corte, M. (1996). Anosognosia for hemiplegia, neglect dyslexia, and drawing neglect: Clinical findings and theoretical considerations. *Journal of the International Neuropsychological Society*, *2*, 426–440.

Berti, A., & Pia, L. (2006). Understanding motor awareness through normal and pathological behavior. *Current directions in Psychological Science*, *15*, 245–250.

Berti, A., Rizzolatti, G., & Umana, F. (1987). Visual processing without awareness: Evidence from unilateral neglect. *Journal of Cognitive Neuroscience*, *4*(4), 345–351.

Beschin, N., Cazzani, M., Cubelli, R., Della Sala, S., & Spinazzola, L. (1996). Ignoring left and far: An investigation of tactile neglect. *Neuropsychologia*, *34*(1), 41–49.

Beschin, N., Cocchini, G., Allen, R., & Della Sala, S. (2012). Anosognosia and neglect respond differently to the same treatments. *Neuropsychological Rehabilitation*, *22*(4), 550–562. http://doi.org/10.1080/09602011.2012 .669353

Beschin, N., & Robertson, I. H. (1997). Personal versus extrapersonal neglect: A group study of their dissociation using a reliable clinical test. *Cortex*, *33*(2), 379–384.

Besnard, A., Caboche, J., & Laroche, S. (2012). Reconsolidation of memory: A decade of debate. *Progress in Neurobiology*, *99*(1), 61–80. http://doi.org/10.1016/j.pneurobio .2012.07.002

Beume, L. A., Kaller, C. P., Hoeren, M., Kloppel, S., Kuemmerer, D., Glauche, V., . . . Umarova, R. (2015). Processing of bilateral versus unilateral conditions: Evidence for the functional contribution of the ventral attention network. *Cortex*, *66*, 91–102. http://doi.org/10.1016/j.cortex.2015.02.018

Bickerton, W. L., Samson, D., Williamson, J., & Humphreys, G. W. (2011). Separating forms of neglect using the Apples Test: Validation and functional prediction in chronic and acute stroke. *Neuropsychology*, *25*(5), 567–580. http://doi.org/10.1037/a0023501

Bihrle, A. M., Brownell, H. H., & Powelson, J. A. (1986). Comprehension of humorous and nonhumorous materials by left and right brain-damaged patients. *Brain and Cognition*, *5*(4), 399–411. http://doi.org/10.1016/0278-2626(86)90042-4

Bisiach, E., Cornacchia, L., Sterzi, R., & Vallar, G. (1984). Disorders of perceived auditory lateralization after lesions of the right hemisphere. *Brain*, *107*, 37–52. http://doi.org/10.1093/brain/107.1.37

Bisiach, E., & Luzzatti, C. (1978). Unilateral neglect of representational space. *Cortex*, *14*, 129–133.

Bisiach, E., Mcintosh, R. D., Dijkerman, H. C., McClements, K. I., Colombo, M., & Milner, A. D. (2004). Visual and tactile length matching in spatial neglect. *Cortex*, *40*, 651–657.

Bisiach, E., & Rusconi, M. L. (1990). Breakdown of perceptual awareness in unilateral neglect. *Cortex*, *26*(4), 643–649. http://doi.org/10.1016/S0010-9452(13)80313-9

Bisiach, E., Vallar, G., Perani, D., Papagno, C., & Berti, A. (1986). Unawareness of disease following lesions of the right hemisphere: Anosognosia for hemiplegia and anosognosia for hemianopia. *Neuropsychologia*, *24*(4), 471–482.

Blake, M. L. (2003). Affective language and humor appreciation after right hemisphere brain damage. *Seminars in Speech and Language*, *24*(2), 107–119. http://doi.org/10.1055/s-2003-38902

Blake, M. L. (2006). Clinical relevance of discourse characteristics after right hemisphere brain damage. *American Journal of Speech-Language Pathology*, *15*(3), 256–267. http://doi.org/10.1044/1058-0360(2006/024)

Blake, M. L. (2007). Perspectives on treatment for communication deficits associated with right hemisphere brain damage. *American Journal of Speech-Language Pathology*, *16*(4), 331–342. http://doi.org/10.1044/1058-0360(2007/037)

Blake, M. L. (2009a). Inferencing processes after right hemisphere brain damage: Effects of contextual bias. *Journal of Speech, Language, and Hearing Research: JSLHR*, *52*(2), 373–384. http://doi.org/10.1044/1092-4388(2009/07-0012)

Blake, M. L. (2009b). Inferencing processes after right hemisphere brain damage: Maintenance of inferences. *Journal of Speech, Language, and Hearing Research: JSLHR*, *52*(2), 359–372. http://doi.org/10.1044/1092-4388(2009/07-0012)

Blake, M. L. (2016). Cognitive communication deficits associated with right hemisphere brain damage. In M. L. Kimbarow (Ed.), *Cognitive communication disorders* (2nd ed., pp. 119–168). San Diego, CA: Plural.

Blake, M. L., Duffy, J. R., Myers, P. S., & Tompkins, C. A. (2002). Prevalence and patterns of right hemisphere cognitive/communicative deficits: Retrospective data from an inpatient rehabilitation unit. *Aphasiology*, *16*(4–6), 537–547. http://doi.org/10.1080/02687030244000194

Blake, M. L., & Freeland, T. (May, 2014). *There's more than one way to skin a cat: Teaching novel idioms*. Presented at Clinical Aphasiology Conference, St. Simon's Island, GA.

Blake, M. L., Frymark, T., & Venedictov, R. (2013). An evidence-based systematic review on communication treatments for individuals with right hemisphere brain damage. *American Journal of Speech-Language Pathology*, *22*(2), 146–160. http://doi.org/10.1044/1058-0360(2012/12-0021)b

Blake, M. L., & Lesniewicz, K. (2005). Contextual bias and predictive inferencing in adults with and without right hemisphere brain damage. *Aphasiology, 19*(3–5), 423–434. http://doi.org/10.1080/02687030444000868

Blake, M. L., Tompkins, C. A., Scharp, V. L., Meigh, K. M., & Wambaugh, J. (2015). Contextual Constraint Treatment for coarse coding deficit in adults with right hemisphere brain damage: Generalisation to narrative discourse comprehension. *Neuropsychological Rehabilitation, 25*(1), 15–52. http://doi.org/10.1080/09602011.2014.932290

Blonder, L. X., Pettigrew, L. C., & Kryscio, R. J. (2012). Emotion recognition and marital satisfaction in stroke. *Journal of Clinical and Experimental Neuropsychology, 34*(6), 634–642. http://doi.org/10.1080/13803395.2012.667069

Bloom, R. L., Borod, J. C., Obler, L. K., & Gerstman, L. J. (1992). Impact of emotional content on discourse production in patients with unilateral brain damage. *Brain and Language, 42*(2), 153–164. http://doi.org/10.1016/0093-934X(92)90122-U

Bloom, R. L., Borod, J. C., Obler, L. K., & Koff, E. (1990). A preliminary characterization of lexical emotional expression in right and left brain-damaged patients. *International Journal of Neuroscience, 55*(2–4), 71–80. http://doi.org/10.3109/00207459008985952

Boers, F., Eyckmans, J., & Stengers, H. (2007). Presenting figurative idioms with a touch of etymology: More than mere mnemonics? *Language Teaching Research, 11*(1), 43–62. http://doi.org/10.1177/1362168806072460

Bohrn, I. C., Altmann, U., & Jacobs, A. M. (2012). Looking at the brains behind figurative language—a quantitative meta-analysis of neuroimaging studies on metaphor, idiom, and irony processing. *Neuropsychologia, 50*(11), 2669–2683. http://doi.org/10.1016/j.neuropsychologia.2012.07.021

Bonnelle, V., Leech, R., Kinnunen, K. M., Ham, T. E., Beckmann, C. F., De Boissezon, X., . . . Sharp, D. J. (2011). Default mode network connectivity predicts sustained attention deficits after traumatic brain injury. *The Journal of Neuroscience, 31*(38), 13442–13451. http://doi.org/10.1523/JNEUROSCI.1163-11.2011

Bookheimer, S. (2002). Functional MRI of language: New approaches to understanding the cortical organization of semantic processing. *Annual Review of Neuroscience, 25,* 151–188. http://doi.org/10.1146/annurev.neuro.25.112701.142946

Boosman, H., van Heugten, C. M., Winkens, I., Heijnen, V. A, & Visser-Meily, J. M. A. (2014). Awareness of memory functioning in patients with stroke who have a good functional outcome. *Brain Injury, 9052*(7), 1–6. http://doi.org/10.3109/02699052.2014.888763

Borgaro, S. R., & Prigatano, G. P. (2003). Modification of the Patient Competency Rating Scale for use on an acute neurorehabilitation unit: The PCRS-NR. *Brain Injury, 17*(10), 847–853. http://doi.org/10.1080/0269905031000089350

Borod, J. C. (1993). Cerebral mechanisms underlying facial, prosodic, and lexical emotional expression: A review of neuropsychological studies and methodological issues. *Neuropsychology, 7*(4), 445–463. http://doi.org/10.1037/0894-4105.7.4.445

Borod, J. C., Andelman, F., Obler, L. K., Tweedy, J. R., & Welkowitz, J. (1992). Right hemisphere specialization for the identification of emotional words and sentences: Evidence from stroke patients. *Neuropsychologia, 30*(9), 827–844.

Borod, J. C., Bloom, R. L., Brickman, A. M., Nakhutina, L., & Curko, E. A. (2002). Emotional processing deficits in individuals with unilateral brain damage. *Applied Neuropsychology, 9*(1), 23–36. http://doi.org/10.1207/S15324826AN0901_4

Borod, J. C., Koff, E., Lorch, M. P., & Nicholas, M. (1985). Channels of emotional expression in patients with unilateral brain damage. *Archives of Neurology, 42*(4), 345–348. http://doi.org/10.1001/archneur.1985.0406 0040055011

Borod, J. C., Pick, L. H., Hall, S., Sliwinski, M., Madigan, N., Obler, L. K., . . . Tabert, M. H. (2000). Relationships among facial, prosodic, and lexical chnnels of emotional perceptual processing. *Cognition and Emotion, 14*(2), 193–211.

Borod, J. C., Rorie, K. D., Haywood, C. S., Andelman, F., Obler, L. K., Welkowitz, J., . . . Tweedy, J. R. (1996). Hemispheric specialization for discourse reports of emotional experiences: Relationships to demographic, neurological, and perceptual variables. *Neuropsychologia, 34*(5), 351–359. http://doi .org/10.1016/0028-3932(95)00131-X

Borod, J. C., Rorie, K. D., Pick, L. H., Bloom, R. L., Andelman, F., Campbell, A. L., . . . Sliwinski, M. (2000). Verbal pragmatics following unilateral stroke: Emotional content and valence. *Neuropsychology, 14*(1), 112–124. http://doi.org/10.1037//0894-4105.14.1.112

Borod, J. C., Welkowitz, J., & Obler, L. K. (1992). New York Emotion Battery. Unpublished.

Borovsky, A., Kutas, M., & Elman, J. L. (2013). Getting it right: Word learning across the hemispheres. *Neuropsychologia, 51*(5), 825–837. http://doi.org/10.1016/j.neuropsycho logia.2013.01.027

Bottini, G., Paulesu, E., Gandola, M., Pia, L., Invernizzi, P., & Berti, A. (2010). Anosognosia for hemiplegia and models of motor control: Insights from lesional data. In G. P. Prigatano (Ed.), *The study of anosognosia* (pp. 17–38). New York, NY: Oxford University Press.

Bouaffre, S., & Faita-Ainseba, F. (2007). Hemispheric differences in the time-course of semantic priming processes: Evidence from event-related potentials (ERPs). *Brain and Cognition, 63*(2), 123–135. http://doi .org/10.1016/j.bandc.2006.10.006

Bour, A., Rasquin, S., Limburg, M., & Verhey, F. (2011). Depressive symptoms and executive functioning in stroke patients: A follow-up study. *International Journal of Geriatric Psychiatry, 26*(7), 679–686. http:// doi.org/10.1002/gps.2581

Bourgeois, M. S., & Hickey, E. (2009). *Dementia: From diagnosis to management—A functional approach.* New York, NY: Taylor & Francis.

Bowen, A., Hazelton, C., Pollock, A., & Lincoln, N. B. (2013). Cognitive rehabilitation for spatial neglect following stroke. *Cochrane Database of Systematic Reviews* (7). http:// doi.org/10.1002/14651858.CD003586.pub3

Bowen, A., McKenna, K., & Tallis, R. C. (1999). Reasons for variability in the reported rate of occurrence of unilateral spatial neglect after stroke. *Stroke, 30*(6), 1196–1202. http:// doi.org/10.1161/01.STR.30.6.1196

Bowers, D., Blonder, L., & Heilman, K. (1991). The Florida Affect Battery. *Center for Neuropsychological Studies Cognitive Neuroscience Laboratory.* University of Florida. Retrieved from http://neurology.ufl.edu/files/2011/ 12/Florida-Affect-Battery-Manual.pdf

Braden, C., Hawley, L., Newman, J., Morey, C., Gerber, D., & Harrison-Felix, C. (2010). Social communication skills group treatment: A feasibility study for persons with traumatic brain injury and comorbid conditions. *Brain Injury, 24*(11), 1298–1310. http:// doi.org/10.3109/02699052.2010.506859

Brady, M., Armstrong, L., & Mackenzie, C. (2005). Further evidence on topic use following right hemisphere brain damage: Procedural and descriptive discourse. *Aphasiology, 19*(8), 731–747. http://doi.org/ 10.1080/02687030500141430

Brady, M., Armstrong, L., & Mackenzie, C. (2006). An examination over time of language and discourse production abilities following right hemisphere brain damage. *Journal of Neurolinguistics, 19*(4), 291–310. http://doi. org/10.1016/j.jneuroling.2005.12.001

Brady, M., Mackenzie, C., & Armstrong, L. (2003). Topic use following right hemisphere brain damage during three semistructured conversational discourse samples. *Aphasiology, 17*(9), 881–904. http://doi .org/10.1080/02687030344000292

Braga, R. M., Wilson, L. R., Sharp, D. J., Wise, R. J. S., & Leech, R. (2013). Separable networks for top-down attention to auditory nonspatial and visuospatial modalities. *Neuro-*

Image, 74, 77–86. http://doi.org/10.1016/j .neuroimage.2013.02.023

Brandimonte, M., Einstein, G. O., & McDaniel, M. A. (Eds.). (1996). *Prospective memory: Theory and applications.* New York, NY: Psychology Press.

Brandt, J., & Benedict, R. H. B. (2001). *Hopkins Verbal Learning Test–Revised.* Lutz, FL: Psychological Assessment Resources.

Brasure, M., Lamberty, G. J., Sayer, N. A., Nelson, N. W., MacDonald, R., Ouelette, J., . . . Wilt, Ti. J. (2012). *Multidisciplinary postacute rehabilitation for moderate to severe traumatic brain injury in adults.* (Prepared by the Minnesota Evidence-based Practice Center under Contract No. 290-2007-10064-I.) AHRQ Publication No. 12-EHC101-EF. Rockville, MD: Agency for Healthcare Research and Quality. http://www.effectivehealthcare.ahrq.gov/reports/final.cfm

Braun, M., Traue, H. C., Frisch, S., Deighton, R. M., & Kessler, H. (2005). Emotion recognition in stroke patients with left and right hemispheric lesion: Results with a new instrument—the FEEL Test. *Brain and Cognition, 58*(2), 193–201. http://doi.org/10.1016/j.bandc.2004.11.003

Bressler, S. L., Tang, W., Sylvester, C. M., Shulman, G. L., & Corbetta, M. (2008). Top-down control of human visual cortex by frontal and parietal cortex in anticipatory visual spatial attention. *Journal of Neuroscience, 28*(40), 10056–10061. http://doi.org/10.1523/JNEUROSCI.1776-08.2008

Broeren, J., Samuelsson, H., Stibrant-Sunnerhagen, K., Blomstrand, C., & Rydmark, M. (2007). Neglect assessment as an application of virtual reality. *Acta Neurologica Scandinavica, 116*(3), 157–163. http://doi.org/10.1111/j.1600-0404.2007.00821.x

Brooks, B. M., Rose, F. D., Potter, J., Jayawardena, S., & Morling, A. (2004). Assessing stroke patients' prospective memory using virtual reality. *Brain Injury, 18*(4), 391–401. http://doi.org/10.1080/02699050310001619855

Brookshire, R. H., & Nicholas, L. E. (1997). *Discourse Comprehension Test.* Minneapolis, MN: BRK.

Brott, T., Adams, H. P., Olinger, C. P., Marler, J. R., Barsan, W. G., Biller, J., . . . Walker, M. (1989). Measurements of acute cerebral infarction: A clinical examination scale. *Stroke, 20*(7), 864–870. http://doi.org/10.1161/01.STR.20.7.864

Brownell, H. H., Carroll, J. J., Rehak, A., & Wingfield, A. (1992). The use of pronoun anaphora and speaker mood in the interpretation of conversational utterances by right hemisphere brain-damaged patients. *Brain and Language, 43*(1), 121–147. http://doi.org/10.1016/0093-934X(92)90025-A

Brownell, H., & Lundgren, K. (2015). Selective training of theory of mind in traumatic brain injury: A series of single subject training studies. *The Open Behavioral Science Journal, 9*(1), 1–11. http://doi.org/10.2174/1874230001509010001

Brownell, H., & Martino, G. (1998). Deficits in inference and social cognition: The effects of right hemisphere brain damage on discourse. In M. Beeman & C. Chiarello (Eds). *Right hemisphere language comprehension: Perspectives from cognitive neuroscience* (pp. 309–328). Mahwah, NJ: Lawrence Erlbaum.

Brownell, H. H., Michel, D., Powelson, J., & Gardner, H. (1983). Surprise but not coherence: Sensitivity to verbal humor in right-hemisphere patients. *Brain and Language, 18*(1), 20–27. http://doi.org/10.1016/0093-934X(83)90002-0

Brownell, H. H., Potter, H. H., & Bihrle, A. M. (1986). Inference deficits in right brain–damaged patients. *Brain and Language, 27,* 310–321.

Brownell, H. H., Simpson, T. L., Bihrle, A. M., Potter, H. H., & Gardner, H. (1990). Appreciation of metaphoric alternative word meanings by left and right brain-damaged patients. *Neuropsychologia, 28*(4), 375–383. http://doi.org/10.1016/0028-3932(90)90063-T

Brozzoli, C., Demattè, M. L., Pavani, F., Frassinetti, F., & Farnè, A. (2006). Neglect and extinction: Within and between sensory modalities. *Restorative Neurology and Neuroscience, 24*(4–6), 217–232.

Brunila, T., Lincoln, N., Lindell, A., Tenovou, O., & Hämäläinen, H. (2002). Experiences of combined visual training and arm activation in the rehabilitation of unilateral visual neglect: A clinical study. *Neuropsychological Rehabilitation, 12,* 27–40.

Brush, J. A., Calkins, M. P., Bruce, C., & Sanford, J. A. (2012). *Environment and Communication Assessment Toolkit for Dementia Care (ECAT).* Baltimore, MD: Health Professions Press.

Brush, J., Sanford, J., Fleder, H., Bruce, C., & Calkins, M. (2011). Evaluating and modifying the communication environment for people with dementia. *Perspectives on Gerontology, 16*(2), 32–40. http://doi.org/10.1044/gero16.2.32

Buckner, R. L., Andrews-Hanna, J. R., & Schacter, D. L. (2008). The brain's default network: Anatomy, function, and relevance to disease. *Annals of the New York Academy of Sciences, 1124,* 1–38. http://doi.org/10.1196/annals.1440.011

Burgess, C., & Chiarello, C. (1996). Neurocognitive mechanisms underlying metaphor comprehension and other figurative language. *Metaphor and Symbolic Activity, 11*(1), 67–84.

Burgess, N., Maguire, E. A., & O'Keefe, J. (2002). The human hippocampus and spatial and episodic memory. *Neuron, 35,* 625–641.

Burgess, P. W., Alderman, N., Forbes, C., Costello, A., Coates, L. M., Dawson, D. R., . . . Channon, S. (2006). The case for the development and use of "ecologically valid" measures of executive function in experimental and clinical neuropsychology. *Journal of the International Neuropsychological Society: JINS, 12*(2), 194–209. http://doi.org/10.1017/S1355617706060310

Burgess, P. W., Alderman, N., Wilson, B. A., Evans, J. J., & Emslie, H. (1996). *The Dysexecutive Questionnaire.* Bury St. Edmunds, UK: Thames Valley Test Company.

Burgess, P. W., & Shallice, T. (1997). *The Hayling and Brixton Tests.* Oxford, UK: Pearson Assessment.

Burianova, H., Mcintosh, A. R., & Grady, C. L. (2010). A common functional brain network for autobiographical, episodic, and semantic memory retrieval. *NeuroImage, 49,* 865–874. http://doi.org/10.1016/j.neuroimage.2009.08.066

Butler, B. C., Eskes, G. A., & Vandorpe, R. A. (2004). Gradients of detection in neglect: Comparison of peripersonal and extrapersonal space. *Neuropsychologia, 42,* 346–358. http://doi.org/10.1016/j.neuropsychologia.2003.08.008

Butler, B. C., Lawrence, M., Eskes, G. A., & Klein, R. (2009). Visual search patterns in neglect: Comparison of peripersonal and extrapersonal space. *Neuropsychologia, 47*(3), 869–878. http://doi.org/10.1016/j.neuropsychologia.2008.12.020

Buxbaum, L. J., Ferraro, M. K., Veramonti, T., Farne, A., Whyte, J., Ladavas, E., . . . Coslett, H. B. (2004). Hemispatial neglect: Subtypes, neuroanatomy, and disability. *Neurology, 62,* 749–756. doi:10.1037/t02229-000

Byrnes, J. P. (1996). *Cognitive development and learning in instructional contexts.* Boston, MA: Allyn & Bacon

Cabeza, R. (2002). Hemispheric asymmetry reduction in older adults: The HAROLD model. *Psychology and Aging, 17*(1), 85–100. http://doi.org/10.1037/0882-7974.17.1.85

Cabeza, R., Ciaramelli, E., Olson, I. R., & Moscovitch, M. (2008). The parietal cortex and episodic memory: An attentional account. *Nature Reviews, 9,* 613–626. http://doi.org/10.1038/nrn2459

Calvo, M. G., & Beltrán, D. (2014). Brain lateralization of holistic versus analytic processing of emotional facial expressions. *NeuroImage, 92,* 237–247. http://doi.org/10.1016/j.neuroimage.2014.01.048

Calvo, M. G., & Castillo, M. D. (1996). Predictive inferences occur on-line, but with delay: Convergence of naming and reading times. *Discourse Processes, 22,* 57–78.

Campos, T. F., Barroso, M. T. M., & De Lara Menezes, A. A. (2010). Encoding, storage and retrieval processes of the memory and the implications for motor practice in stroke patients. *NeuroRehabilitation, 26*(2), 135–142. http://doi.org/10.3233/NRE-2010-0545

Cannizzaro, M. S., & Coelho, C. A. (2002). Treatment of story grammar following traumatic brain injury: A pilot study. *Brain Injury, 16*(12), 1065–1073. http://doi.org/10.1080/02699050210155230

Cappa, S. F., Benke, T., Clarke, S., Rossi, B., Stemmer, B., & Heugten, C. M. (2005). EFNS guidelines on cognitive rehabilitation: Report of an EFNS task force. *European Journal of Neurology, 12*(9), 665–680. http://doi.org/10.1111/j.1468-1331.2005.01330.x

Caramazza, A., & Hillis, A. E. (1990). Levels of representation, co-ordinate frames, and unilateral neglect. *Cognitive Neuropsychology, 7*(5–6), 391–445. http://doi.org/10.1080/02643299008253450

Cardillo, E. R., Watson, C. E., Schmidt, G. L., Kranjec, A., & Chatterjee, A. (2012). From novel to familiar: Tuning the brain for metaphors. *NeuroImage, 59*(4), 3212–3221. http://doi.org/10.1016/j.neuroimage.2011.11.079

Cazzoli, D., Müri, R. M., Hess, C. W., & Nyffeler, T. (2010). Treatment of hemispatial neglect by means of rTMS—A review. *Restorative Neurology and Neuroscience, 28*(4), 499–510. http://doi.org/10.3233/RNN-2010-0560

Champagne-Lavau, M., & Joanette, Y. (2009). Pragmatics, theory of mind and executive functions after a right-hemisphere lesion: Different patterns of deficits. *Journal of Neurolinguistics, 22*(5), 413–426. http://doi.org/10.1016/j.jneuroling.2009.02.002

Chan, E., Khan, S., Oliver, R., Gill, S. K., Werring, D. J., & Cipolotti, L. (2014). Underestimation of cognitive impairments by the Montreal Cognitive Assessment (MoCA) in an acute stroke unit population. *Journal of the Neurological Sciences, 343*(1-2), 176–179. http://doi.org/10.1016/j.jns.2014.05.005

Chantraine, Y., Joanette, Y., & Ska, B. (1998). Conversational abilities in patients with right hemisphere damage. *Journal of Neurolinguistics, 11*(1-2), 21–32.

Chapman, S. B., & Gamino, J. F. (2008). *Strategic Memory and Reasoning Training (SMART).* Dallas, TX: Center for Brain Health.

Chapman, S. B., & Mudar, R. A. (2014). Enhancement of cognitive and neural functions through complex reasoning training: evidence from normal and clinical populations. *Frontiers in Systems Neuroscience, 8*(April), 69. http://doi.org/10.3389/fnsys.2014.00069

Charbonneau, S., Scherzer, B., Aspirot, D., & Cohen, H. (2003). Perception and production of facial and prosodic emotions by chronic CVA patients. *Neuropsychologia, 41*(5), 605–613. http://doi.org/10.1016/S0028-3932(02)00202-6

Chatterjee, A. (1994). Picturing unilateral spatial neglect: Viewer versus object centred reference frames. *Journal of Neurology, Neurosurgery & Psychiatry, 57,* 1236–1240. http://doi.org/doi:10.1136/jnnp.57.10.1236

Cheang, H. S., & Pell, M. D. (2006). A study of humour and communicative intention following right hemisphere stroke. *Clinical Linguistics & Phonetics, 20*(6), 447–462. http://doi.org/10.1080/02699200050013 5684

Chechlacz, M., Gillebert, C. R., Vangkilde, S. A, Petersen, A., & Humphreys, G. W. (2015). Structural variability within frontoparietal networks and individual differences in attentional functions: An approach using the theory of visual attention. *Journal of Neuroscience, 35*(30), 10647–10658. http://doi.org/10.1523/JNEUROSCI.0210-15.2015

Chechlacz, M., Rotshtein, P., Demeyere, N., Bickerton, W. L., & Humphreys, G. W. (2014). The frequency and severity of extinction after stroke affecting different vascular territories. *Neuropsychologia, 54*(1), 11–17. http://doi.org/10.1016/j.neuropsychologia.2013.12.016

Chemerinski, E., & Robinson, R. G. (2000). The neuropsychiatry of stroke. *Psychosomatics, 41,* 5–14. http://doi.org/10.4088/JCP.v61 n0212a

Chen, A. J. W., Novakovic-Agopian, T., Nycum, T. J., Song, S., Turner, G. R., Hills, N. K., . . . D'Esposito, M. (2011). Training of goal-directed attention regulation enhances control over neural processing for individuals with brain injury. *Brain, 134*(5), 1541–1554. http://doi.org/10.1093/brain/awr067

Chen, P., Hartman, A. J., Galarza, C. P., & DeLuca, J. (2012). Global processing training to improve visuospatial memory deficits after right-brain stroke. *Archives of Clinical Neuropsychology, 27*(8), 891–905. http://doi.org/10.1093/arclin/acs089

Chen, P., Hreha, K., Fortis, P., Goedert, K. M., & Barrett, A. M. (2012). Functional assessment of spatial neglect: A review of the Catherine Bergego Scale and an introduction of the Kessler Foundation Neglect Assessment Process. *Topics in Stroke Rehabilitation, 19*(5), 423–435. http://doi.org/10.1310/tsr1905-423.Functional

Cheng, S. K. W., & Man, D. W. K. (2006). Management of impaired self-awareness in persons with traumatic brain injury. *Brain Injury, 20*(6), 621–628. http://doi.org/10.1080/02699050600677196

Cherney, L. R., Drimmer, D. P., & Halper, A. S. (1997). Informational content and unilateral neglect: A longitudinal investigation of five subjects with right hemisphere damage. *Aphasiology, 11*(4/5), 351–363. http://doi.org/10.1080/02687039708248476

Chica, A. B., Thiebaut de Schotten, M., Toba, M., Malhotra, P., Lupiáñez, J., & Bartolomeo, P. (2012). Attention networks and their interactions after right-hemisphere damage. *Cortex, 48*(6), 654–663. http://doi.org/10.1016/j.cortex.2011.01.009

Chokron, S., Colliot, P., Bartolomeo, P., Rhein, F., Eusop, E., Vassel, P., & Ohlmann, T. (2002). Visual, proprioceptive and tactile performance in left neglect patients. *Neuropsychologia, 40*(12), 1965–1976. http://doi.org/10.1016/S0028-3932(02)00047-7

Cicerone, K. D. (2005). Methodological issues in evaluating the effectiveness of cognitive rehabilitation. In P. W. Halligan & D. T. Wade (Eds.), *Effectiveness of rehabilitation for cognitive deficits* (pp. 43–58). New York, NY: Oxford University Press.

Cicerone, K. D., Langenbahn, D. M., Braden, C., Malec, J. F., Kalmar, K., Fraas, M., . . .

Ashman, T. (2011). Evidence-based cognitive rehabilitation: Updated review of the literature from 2003 through 2008. *Archives of Physical Medicine and Rehabilitation, 92*(4), 519–530. http://doi.org/10.1016/j.apmr.2010.11.015

Cicerone, K., Levin, H., Malec, J., Stuss, D., & Whyte, J. (2006). Cognitive rehabilitation interventions for executive function: Moving from bench to bedside in patients with traumatic brain injury. *Journal of Cognitive Neuroscience, 18*(7), 1212–1222. http://doi.org/10.1162/jocn.2006.18.7.1212

Cimino, C. R., Verfaellie, M., Bowers, D., & Heilman, K. M. (1991). Autobiographical memory: Influence of right hemisphere damage in emotionality and specificity. *Brain and Cognition, 15*, 106–118. http://doi.org/10.1016/0278-2626(91)90019-5

Citron, F. M. M., Gray, M. A., Critchley, H. D., Weekes, B. S., & Ferstl, E. C. (2014). Emotional valence and arousal affect reading in an interactive way: Neuroimaging evidence for an approach-withdrawal framework. *Neuropsychologia, 56*(1), 79–89. http://doi.org/10.1016/j.neuropsychologia.2014.01.002

Cocchini, G., Beschin, N., Cameron, A., Fotopoulou, A., & Della Sala, S. (2009). Anosognosia for motor impairment following left brain damage. *Neuropsychology, 23*(2), 223–230. http://doi.org/10.1037/a0014266

Cocchini, G., Beschin, N., & Della Sala, S. (2012). Assessing anosognosia: A critical review. *Acta Neuropsyologica, 10*(3), 419–443.

Cocchini, G., Beschin, N., Fotopoulou, A., & Della Sala, S. (2010). Explicit and implicit anosognosia or upper limb motor impairment. *Neuropsychologia, 48*(5), 1489–1494. http://doi.org/10.1016/j.neuropsychologia.2010.01.019

Cocchini, G., Gregg, N., Beschin, N., Dean, M., & Della Sala, S. (2010). Vata-L: Visual-Analogue Test Assessing Anosognosia for Language Impairment. *The Clinical Neuropsychologist, 24*(8), 1379–1399. http://doi.org/10.1080/13854046.2010.524167

Coelho, C., Ylvisaker, M., & Turkstra, L. S. (2005). Nonstandardized assessment approaches for individuals with traumatic brain injuries. *Seminars in Speech & Language*, *26*(4), 223–241. http://doi.org/10 .1055/s-2005-922102

Cohen, G., & Conway, M. (Eds.). (2008). *Memory in the real world* (3rd ed.). New York, NY: Psychology Press.

Collins, M. (1999). Differences in semantic category priming in the left and right cerebral hemispheres under automatic and controlled processing conditions. *Neuropsychologia*, *37*(9), 1071–1085. http://doi.org/10 .1016/S0028-3932(98)00156-0

Constantinidou, F., Wertheimer, J. C., Tsanadis, J., Evans, C., & Paul, D. R. (2012). Assessment of executive functioning in brain injury: Collaboration between speech-language pathology and neuropsychology for an integrative neuropsychological perspective. *Brain Injury*, *26*(13-14), 1549–1563. http://doi.org/10.3109/02699052.2012.69 8786

Conti, J., Sterr, A., Brucki, S. M. D., & Conforto, A. B. (2015). Diversity of approaches in assessment of executive functions in stroke: Limited evidence? *eNeurologicalSci*, *1*(1), 12–20. http://doi.org/10.1016/j.ensci .2015.08.002

Convento, S., Russo, C., Zigiotto, L., & Bolognini, N. (2016). Transcranial electrical stimulation in post-stroke cognitive rehabilitation. *European Psychologist*, *21*(1), 55–64. http://doi.org/10.1027/1016-9040/a000238

Conway, A. R. A., Jarrold, C., Kane, M. J., Miyake, A., & Towse, J. N. (Eds.). (2007). *Variation in working memory*. New York, NY: Oxford University Press.

Cooper, C. L., Phillips, L. H., Johnston, M., Radlak, B., Hamilton, S., & McLeod, M. J. (2014). Links between emotion perception and social participation restriction following stroke. *Brain Injury*, *28*(1), 122–126. http:// doi.org/10.3109/02699052.2013.848379

Corbetta, M., Kincade, J. M., & Shulman, G. L. (2001). Neural systems for visual orienting and their relationships to spatial working memory. *Journal of Cognitive Neuroscience*, *14*(2), 508–523.

Corballis, M. C. (2014). Left brain, right brain: Facts and fantasies. *PLoS Biology*, *12*(1), e1001767. http://doi.org/10.1371/journal .pbio.1001767

Corbetta, M., Patel, G., & Shulman, G. L. (2008). The reorienting system of the human brain: From environment to theory of mind. *Neuron*, *58*(3), 306–324. http://doi.org/10.1016/ j.neuron.2008.04.017

Corsi, P. M. (1972). *Human memory and the medial temporal region of the brain* (Unpublished doctoral dissertation). McGill University, Montreal, Canada.

Côté, H., Payer, M., Giroux, F., & Joanette, Y. (2007). Towards a description of clinical communication impairment profiles following right-hemisphere damage. *Aphasiology*, *21*(6–8), 739–749. http://doi.org/10.1080/ 02687030701192331

Coulson, S., Federmeier, K. D., Van Petten, C., & Kutas, M. (2005). Right hemisphere sensitivity to word- and sentence-level context: Evidence from event-related brain potentials. *Journal of Experimental Psychology. Learning, Memory, and Cognition*, *31*(1), 129–147. http://doi.org/10.1037/0278-7393.31.1.129

Coulson, S., & Van Petten, C. (2002). Conceptual integration and metaphor: An event-related potential study. *Memory & Cognition*, *30*(6), 958–968. http://doi.org/10.3758/BF 03195780

Coulson, S., & Van Petten, C. (2007). A special role for the right hemisphere in metaphor comprehension? ERP evidence from hemifield presentation. *Brain Research*, *1146*, 128–145. http://doi.org/10.1016/j.brainres.2007 .03.008

Coulson, S., & Williams, R. F. (2005). Hemispheric asymmetries and joke comprehension. *Neuropsychologia*, *43*(1), 128–141. http://doi.org/10.1016/j.neuropsychologia .2004.03.015

Crinion, J. T. (2016). Transcranial direct current stimulation as a novel method for enhancing aphasia treatment effects. *European Psychologist, 21*(1), 65–77. http://doi.org/10.1027/1016-9040/a000254

Critchley, E. M. R. (1991). Speech and the right hemisphere. *Behavioural Neurology, 4*(3), 143–151. http://doi.org/http://dx.doi.org/10.3233/BEN-1991-4302

Crooke, P. J., & Olswang, L. B. (2015). Practice-based research: Another pathway for closing the research-practice gap. *Journal of Speech, Language, and Hearing Research, 58*, S1871–S1882. http://doi.org/10.1044/2015_JSLHR-L-15-0243

Crosson, B., Barco, P. P., Velozo, C. A., Bolesta, M. M., Cooper, P. V., Werts, D., & Brobeck, T. C. (1989). Awareness and compensation in postacute head injury rehabilitation. *Journal of Head Trauma Rehabilitation, 4*(3), 46–54.

Cubelli, R., Guiducci, A., & Consolmagno, P. (2000). Afferent dysgraphia after right cerebral stroke: An autonomous syndrome? *Brain and Cognition, 44*(3), 629–644. http://doi.org/10.1006/brcg.2000.1239

Dahlberg, C. A., Cusick, C. P., Hawley, L. A., Newman, J. K., Morey, C. E., Harrison-Felix, C. L., & Whiteneck, G. G. (2007). Treatment efficacy of social communication skills training after traumatic brain injury: A randomized treatment and deferred treatment controlled trial. *Archives of Physical Medicine and Rehabilitation, 88*(12), 1561–1573. http://doi.org/10.1016/j.apmr.2007.07.033

Daini, R., Albonico, A., Malaspina, M., Martelli, M., Primativo, S., & Arduino, L. S. (2013). Dissociation in optokinetic stimulation sensitivity between omission and substitution reading errors in neglect dyslexia. *Frontiers in Human Neuroscience, 7*(September), 1–10. http://doi.org/10.3389/fnhum.2013.00581

Dalton, P., & Fraenkel, N. (2012). Gorillas we have missed: Sustained inattentional deafness for dynamic events. *Cognition, 124*(3), 367–372. http://doi.org/10.1016/j.cognition.2012.05.012

Damasio, A. R. (1996). The somatic marker hypothesis and the possible functions of the prefrontal cortex. *Philosophical Transactions: Biological Sciences, 351*(1346), 1413–1420.

Damasio, A. R., Tranel, D., & Damasio, H. C. (1991). Somatic markers and the guidance of behavior: Theory and preliminary testing. In H. S. Levin, H. M. Eisenberg, & A. L. Benton (Eds.), *Frontal lobe function and dysfunction* (pp. 217–229). New York, NY: Oxford University Press.

Damschroder, L. J., Aron, D. C., Keith, R. E., Kirsh, S. R., Alexander, J. A., & Lowery, J. C. (2009). Fostering implementation of health services research findings into practice: A consolidated framework for advancing implementation science. *Implementation Science, 4*(50), 40–55. http://doi.org/10.1186/1748-5908-4-50

Dará, C., Bang, J., Gottesman, R. F., & Hillis, A. E. (2014). Right hemisphere dysfunction is better predicted by emotional prosody impairments as compared to neglect. *Journal of Neurology and Translational Neuroscience, 2*(1), 1037–1051.

Dará, C., Kirsch-Darrow, L., Ochfeld, E., Slenz, J., Agranovich, A., Vasconcellos-Faria, A., . . . Kortte, K. B. (2012). Impaired emotion processing from vocal and facial cues in frontotemporal dementia compared to right hemisphere stroke. *Neurocase, 19*(6), 521–529.

Davidson, R. J. (1984). Affect, cognition and hemispheric specialization. In C. E. Izard, J. Kagan, & R. Zajonc (Eds.), *Emotions, cognition and behavior.* New York, NY: Cambridge University Press.

Davis, M. H. (1980a). Interpersonal Reactivity Index. *JSAS Catalog of Selected Documents in Psychology, 10*(1980), 14–15. http://doi.org/10.1037/t01093-000

Davis, M. H. (1980b). A multidimensional approach to individual differences in empathy. *JSAS Catalog of Selected Documents in Psychology, 10*, 85. http://doi.org/10.1017/CBO9781107415324.004

Davis, M. H. (1983). Measuring individual differences in empathy: Evidence for a multidimensional approach. *Journal of Personality and Social Psychology, 44*(1), 113–126. http://doi.org/10.1037/0022-3514.44.1.113

de Aguiar, V., Paolazzi, C. L., & Miceli, G. (2015). tDCS in post-stroke aphasia: The role of stimulation parameters, behavioral treatment and patient characteristics. *Cortex, 63,* 296–316. http://doi.org/10.1016/j.cortex.2014.08.015

DeGutis, J. M., & Van Vleet, T. M. (2010). Tonic and phasic alertness training: A novel behavioral therapy to improve spatial and non-spatial attention in patients with hemispatial neglect. *Frontiers in Human Neuroscience, 4,* 1–17. http://doi.org/10.3389/fnhum.2010.00060

de Haan, B., Karnath, H.-O., & Driver, J. (2012). Mechanisms and anatomy of unilateral extinction after brain injury. *Neuropsychologia, 50*(6), 1045–1053. http://doi.org/10.1016/j.neuropsychologia.2012.02.015

de Haan, B., Stoll, T., & Karnath, H. O. (2015). Early sensory processing in right hemispheric stroke patients with and without extinction. *Neuropsychologia, 73,* 141–150. http://doi.org/10.1016/j.neuropsychologia.2015.05.011

Delis, D. C., Kaplan, E., & Kramer, J. H. (2001). *Delis-Kaplan Executive Function System (D-KEFS).* San Antonio, TX: Pearson.

Delis, D. C., Kramer, J. H., Kaplan, E., & Ober, B. A. (1983). *California Verbal Learning Test.* San Antonio, TX: Pearson.

Delis, D. C., Wapner, W., Gardner, H., & Moses, J. A. J. (1983). The contribution of the right hemisphere to the organization of paragraphs. *Cortex, 19*(1), 43–50.

Della Sala, S., Cocchini, G., Beschin, N., & Cameron, A. (2009). VATA-M: Visual-Analogue Test assessing anosognosia for motor impairment. *The Clinical Neuropsychologist, 23*(3), 406–427. http://doi.org/10.1080/13854040802251393

Demaree, H. A, Everhart, D. E., Youngstrom, E. A, & Harrison, D. W. (2005). Brain lateralization of emotional processing: Historical roots and a future incorporating "dominance." *Behavioral and Cognitive Neuroscience Reviews, 4*(1), 3–20. http://doi.org/10.1177/1534582305276837

Demeyere, N., Riddoch, M. J., Slavkova, E. D., Bickerton, W.-L., & Humphreys, G. W. (2015). The Oxford Cognitive Screen (OCS): Validation of a Stroke-Specific Short Cognitive Screening Tool. *Psychological Assessment, 27*(3), 883–894. http://doi.org/10.1037/pas0000082

Diaz, M. T., Barrett, K. T., & Hogstrom, L. J. (2011). The influence of sentence novelty and figurativeness on brain activity. *Neuropsychologia, 49*(3), 320–330. http://doi.org/10.1016/j.neuropsychologia.2010.12.004

Dickson, D. S., & Federmeier, K. D. (2014). Hemispheric differences in orthographic and semantic processing as revealed by event-related potentials. *Neuropsychologia, 64,* 230–239. http://doi.org/10.1016/j.neuropsychologia.2014.09.037

Dietz, M. J., Friston, K. J., Mattingley, J. B., Roepstorff, A., & Garrido, M. I. (2014). Effective connectivity reveals right-hemisphere dominance in audiospatial perception: Implications for models of spatial neglect. *The Journal of Neuroscience: The Official Journal of the Society for Neuroscience, 34*(14), 5003–5011. http://doi.org/10.1523/JNEUROSCI.3765-13.2014

Di Legge, S., Fang, J., Saposnik, G., & Hachinksi, V. (2005). The impact of lesion side on acute stroke treatment. *Neurology, 65*(1), 81–86. http://doi.org/10.1212/01.wnl.0000167608.94237.aa

Di Monaco, M., Schintu, S., Dotta, M., Barba, S., Tappero, R., & Gindri, P. (2011). Severity of unilateral spatial neglect is an independent predictor of functional outcome after acute inpatient rehabilitation in individuals with right hemispheric stroke. *Archives of Physical Medicine and Rehabilitation, 92*(8), 1250–1256. http://doi.org/10.1016/j.apmr.2011.03.018

Dodd, S.-J., & Epstein, I. (2012). *Practice-based research for social work: A guide for reluctant researchers.* New York, NY: Routledge.

Dolcos, F., Rice, H. J., & Cabeza, R. (2002). Hemispheric asymmetry and aging: Right hemisphere decline or asymmetry reduction. *Neuroscience and Biobehavioral Reviews*, *26*(7), 819–825. http://doi.org/10.1016/S0149-7634(02)00068-4

Dong, Y., Sharma, V. K., Chan, B. P. L., Venketasubramanian, N., Teoh, H. L., Seet, R. C. S., . . . Chen, C. (2010). The Montreal Cognitive Assessment (MoCA) is superior to the Mini-Mental State Examination (MMSE) for the detection of vascular cognitive impairment after acute stroke. *Journal of the Neurological Sciences*, *299*(1-2), 15–18. http://doi.org/10.1016/j.jns.2010.08.051

Donnelly, K. M., Allendorfer, J. B., & Szaflarski, J. P. (2011). Right hemispheric participation in semantic decision improves performance. *Brain Research*, *1419*, 105–116. http://doi.org/10.1016/j.brainres.2011.08.065

Dougall, D., Poole, N., & Agrawal, N. (2015). Pharmacotherapy for chronic cognitive impairment in traumatic brain injury. *The Cochrane Database of Systematic Reviews*, *12*(12), CD009221. http://doi.org/10.1002/14651858.CD009221.pub2

Douglas, J. M., Bracy, C. A., & Snow, P. C. (2007). Exploring the factor structure of the La Trobe Communication Questionnaire: Insights into the nature of communication deficits following traumatic brain injury. *Aphasiology*, *21*(12), 1181–1194. http://doi.org/10.1080/02687030600980950

Douglas, J. M., O'Flaherty, C. A., & Snow, P. C. (2000). Measuring perception of communicative ability: the development and evaluation of the La Trobe communication questionnaire. *Aphasiology*, *14*(3), 251–268. http://doi.org/10.1080/026870300401469

Driver, J., & Mattingley, J. B. (1998). Parietal neglect and visual awareness. *Nature Neuroscience*, *1*, 17–22.

Duecker, F., Formisano, E., & Sack, A. T. (2013). Hemispheric differences in the voluntary control of spatial attention: Direct evidence for a right-hemispheric dominance within frontal cortex. *Journal of Cognitive Neuroscience*, *25*(8), 1332–1342. http://doi.org/10.1162/jocn_a_00402

Duff, M. C., Hengst, J. A., Tranel, D., & Cohen, N. J. (2008). Collaborative discourse facilitates efficient communication and new learning in amnesia. *Brain and Language*, *106*(1), 41–54. http://doi.org/10.1162/jocn.2009.21066.

Duff, M. C., Mutlu, B., Byom, L., & Turkstra, L. S. (2012). Beyond utterances: Distributed cognition as a framework for studying discourse in adults with acquired brain injury. *Seminars in Speech and Language*, *33*(1), 44–54. http://doi.org/10.1055/s-0031-1301162

Duffin, J. T., Collins, D. R., Coughlan, T., O'Neill, D., Roche, R. A., & Commins, S. (2012). Subtle memory and attentional deficits revealed in an Irish stroke patient sample using domain-specific cognitive tasks. *Journal of Clinical and Experimental Neuropsychology*, *34*(8), 864–875. http://doi.org/10.1080/13803395.2012.690368

Duffy, J. R. (2013). *Motor speech disorders: Substrates, differential diagnosis, and management* (3rd ed.). St. Louis, MO: Elsevier.

Dvash, J., & Shamay-Tsoory, S. G. (2014). Theory of Mind and empathy as multidimensional constructs. *Topics in Language Disorders*, *34*(4), 282–295. http://doi.org/10.1097/TLD.0000000000000040

Edgeworth, J., Robertson, I. H., & McMillan, T. M. (1998). *The Balloons Test*. Oxford, UK: Pearson Assessment.

Egan, G. J. (1990). Assessment of emotional processing in right and left hemisphere stroke patients: A validation study of the Perception of Emotions Test (POET). *Dissertation Abstracts International*, *51*(2–B), 1035.

Ehlhardt, L. A, Sohlberg, M. M., Kennedy, M., Coelho, C., Ylvisaker, M., Turkstra, L., & Yorkston, K. (2008). Evidence-based practice guidelines for instructing individuals with neurogenic memory impairments: what have we learned in the past 20 years? *Neuropsychological Rehabilitation*, *18*(March

2015), 300–342. http://doi.org/10.1080/09602010701733190

Ehrlich, J., & Barry, P. (1989). Rating communication behaviours in the head-injured adult. *Brain Injury, 3*(2), 193–198.

Eisenson, J. (1962). Language and intellectual modifications associated with right cerebral damage. *Language and Speech, 5*(2), 49–53. http://doi.org/10.1177/002383096200500201

Elfenbein, H. A., & Ambady, N. (2002). On the universality and cultural specificity of emotion recognition: A meta-analysis. *Psychological Bulletin, 128*(2), 203–235. http://doi.org/10.1037//0033-2909.128.2.203

Elliott, M., & Parente, F. (2014). Efficacy of memory rehabilitation therapy: A meta-analysis of TBI and stroke cognitive rehabilitation literature. *Brain Injury: [BI], 9052*(12), 1–7. http://doi.org/10.3109/02699052.2014.934921

Ellis, A. W., Young, A. W., & Flude, B. M. (1987). "Afferent dysgraphia" in a patient and in normal subjects. *Cognitive Neuropsychology, 4*(4), 465–486.

Elsner, B., Kugler, J., Pohl, M., & Mehrholz, J. (2013). Transcranial direct current stimulation (tDCS) for improving aphasia in patients after stroke (Review). *Cochrane Lib., 6*(5). http://doi.org/10.1002/14651858.CD009760.pub3.www.cochranelibrary.com

Erickson, T. D., & Mattson, M.E. (1981). From words to meaning: A semantic illusion. *Journal of Verbal Learning and Verbal Behavior, 20,* 540–555.

Ethofer, T., Bretscher, J., Gschwind, M., Kreifelts, B., Wildgruber, D., & Vuilleumier, P. (2012). Emotional voice areas: Anatomic location, functional properties, and structural connections revealed by combined fMRI/DTI. *Cerebral Cortex, 22*(1), 191–200. http://doi.org/10.1093/cercor/bhr113

Ethofer, T., Kreifelts, B., Wiethoff, S., Wolf, J., Grodd, W., Vuilleumier, P., & Wildgruber, D. (2008). Differential influences of emotion, task, and novelty on brain regions underlying the processing of speech melody. *Journal of Cognitive Neuroscience, 21*(7), 1255–1268.

Eviatar, Z., & Just, M. A. (2006). Brain correlates of discourse processing: An fMRI investigation of irony and conventional metaphor comprehension. *Neuropsychologia, 44*(12), 2348–2359. http://doi.org/10.1016/j.neuropsychologia.2006.05.007

Fan, Y., Duncan, N. W., de Greck, M., & Northoff, G. (2011). Is there a core neural network in empathy? An fMRI based quantitative meta-analysis. *Neuroscience and Biobehavioral Reviews, 35*(3), 903–911. http://doi.org/10.1016/j.neubiorev.2010.10.009

Federmeier, K. D. (2007). Thinking ahead: The role and roots of prediction in language comprehension. *Psychophysiology, 44*(4), 491–505. http://doi.org/10.1111/j.1469-8986.2007.00531.x.Thinking

Federmeier, K. D., & Kutas, M. (1999). Right words and left words: Electrophysiological evidence for hemispheric differences in meaning processing. *Cognitive Brain Research, 8*(3), 373–392. http://doi.org/10.1016/S0926-6410(99)00036-1

Federmeier, K. D., & Kutas, M. (2002). Picture the difference: Electrophysiological investigations of picture processing in the two cerebral hemispheres. *Neuropsychologia, 40*(7), 730–747. http://doi.org/10.1016/S0028-3932(01)00193-2

Feinberg, T. E., Roane, D. M., & Ali, J. V. (2000). Illusory limb movements in anosognosia for hemiplegia. *Journal of Neurology, Neurosurgery & Psychiatry, 68,* 511–513.

Ferré, P., Fonseca, R. P., Ska, B., & Joanette, Y. (2012). Communicative clusters after a right-hemisphere stroke: Are there universal clinical profiles? *Folia Phoniatrica et Logopaedica: Official Organ of the International Association of Logopedics and Phoniatrics (IALP), 64*(4), 199–207. http://doi.org/10.1159/000340017

Ferreres, A., Abusamra, V., Cuitino, M., Côté, H., Ska, B., & Joanette, Y. (2007). *Protocolo MEC: Protocolo para la Evaluacion de la Communicacion de Montreal.* Neuropsi e. Buenos Aires.

Ferstl, E. C., Neumann, J., Bogler, C., & von Cramon, D. Y. (2008). The extended language network: A meta-analysis of neuroimaging studies on text comprehension. *Human Brain Mapping, 29*(5), 581–593. http://doi.org/10.1002/hbm.20422

Filley, C. M. (2002). The neuroanatomy of attention. *Seminars in Speech & Language, 23*(2), 89–98. http://doi.org/10.1055/s-2002-24985

Fincher-Kiefer, R. (1996). Encoding differences between bridging and predictive inferences. *Discourse Processes, 22*, 225–246.

Fink, J. N. (2005). Underdiagnosis of right-brain stroke: Comment. *The Lancet, 366*, 349–351.

Fink, J. N., Selim, M. H., Kumar, S., Silver, B., Linfante, I., Caplan, L. R., & Schlaug, G. (2002). Is the Association of National Institutes of Health Stroke Scale Scores and acute magnetic resonance imaging stroke volume equal for patients with right- and left-hemisphere ischemic stroke? *Stroke, 33*(4), 954–958. http://doi.org/10.1161/01.STR.0000013069.24300.1D

Fleming, J. M., & Ownsworth, T. (2006). A review of awareness interventions in brain injury rehabilitation. *Neuropsychological Rehabilitation, 16*(4), 474–500. http://doi.org/10.1080/09602010500505518

Fleming, J. M., Strong, J., & Ashton, R. (1996). Self-awareness of deficits in adults with traumatic brain injury: How best to measure? *Brain Injury, 10*(1), 1–15.

Fleming, V. B., & Harris, J. L. (2008). Complex discourse production in mild cognitive impairment: Detecting subtle changes. *Aphasiology, 22*(7-8), 729–740. http://doi.org/10.1080/02687030701803762

Foerch, C., Misselwitz, B., Sitzer, M., Berger, K., Steinmetz, H., & Neumann-Haefelin, T. (2005). Difference in recognition of right and left hemispheric stroke. *The Lancet, 366*, 392–393.

Folstein, M. F., Folstein, S. E., & McHugh, P. R. (1975). "Mini-Mental State": A practical method for grading the cognitive state of patients for the clinician. *Journal of Psychiatric Research, 12*(3), 189–198. http://doi.org/10.1016/0022-3956(75)90026-6

Fonseca, R. P., Guimarães Fachel, J. M., Fagundes Chaves, M. L., Liedtke, F. V., & Pimenta Parente, M. A. (2007). Right hemisphere damage communication processing in adults evaluated by the Brazilian Protocole. *Dementia & Neuropsychologia, 3*, 266–275.

Fotopoulou, A., Pernigo, S., Maeda, R., Rudd, A., & Kopelman, M. A. (2010). Implicit awareness in anosognosia for hemiplegia: Unconscious interference without conscious re-representation. *Brain, 133*, 3564–3577. http://doi.org/10.1093/brain/awq233

Fox, M. D., Snyder, A. Z., Vincent, J. L., Corbetta, M., Van Essen, D. C., & Raichle, M. E. (2005). The human brain is intrinsically organized into dynamic, anticorrelated functional networks. *Proceedings of the National Academy of Sciences, 102*(27), 9673–9678. http://doi.org/10.1073/pnas.0504136102

Fridriksson, J., Hubbard, H. I., & Hudspeth, S. G. (2012). Transcranial brain stimulation to treat aphasia: A clinical perspective. *Seminars in Speech & Language, 33*, 188–202. http://doi.org//dx.doi.org/10.1055/s-0032-1320039

Friedmann, N., & Gvion, A. (2014). Compound reading in Hebrew text-based neglect dyslexia: The effects of the first word on the second word and of the second on the first. *Cognitive Neuropsychology, 31*(1–2), 106–122. http://doi.org/10.1080/02643294.2014.884059

Froming, K., Levy, M., Schaffer, S., & Ekman, P. (2006). *The Comprehensive Affect Testing System.* Psychology Software Inc.

Frühholz, S., Gschwind, M., & Grandjean, D. (2015). Bilateral dorsal and ventral fiber pathways for the processing of affective prosody identified by probabilistic fiber tracking. *NeuroImage, 109*, 27–34. http://doi.org/10.1016/j.neuroimage.2015.01.016

Fujii, T., Fukatsu, R., Kimura, I., Saso, S.-I., & Kogure, K. (1991). Unilateral spatial neglect in visual and tactile modalities. *Cortex, 27*, 339–343.

Funk, J., Finke, K., Müller, H. J., Preger, R., & Kerkhoff, G. (2010). Systematic biases in the tactile perception of the subjective vertical in patients with unilateral neglect and the influence of upright vs. supine posture. *Neuropsychologia, 48*, 298–308. http://doi.org/10.1016/j.neuropsychologia.2009.09.018

Gabbatore, I., Sacco, K., Angeleri, R., Zettin, M., Bara, B. G., & Bosco, F. M. (2014). Cognitive pragmatic treatment: A rehabilitative program for traumatic brain injury individuals. *Journal of Head Trauma Rehabilitation, 30*(5), E14–E28. http://doi.org/10.1097/HTR.0000000000000087

Gainotti, G. (2010). The role of automatic orienting of attention towards ipsilesional stimuli in non-visual (tactile and auditory) neglect: A critical review. *Cortex, 46*, 150–160. http://doi.org/10.1016/j.cortex.2009.04.006

Gainotti, G. (2012). Unconscious processing of emotions and the right hemisphere. *Neuropsychologia, 50*(2), 205–218. http://doi.org/10.1016/j.neuropsychologia.2011.12.005

Galletta, E. E., Campanelli, L., Maul, K. K., & Barrett, A. M. (2014). Assessment of neglect dyslexia with functional reading materials. *Topics in Stroke Rehabilitation, 21*(1), 75–86.

Gandour, J., Ponglorpisit, S., Khunadorn, F., Dechongkit, S., Boongird, P., & Satthamnuwong, N. (2000). Note: Speech timing in Thai left- and right-hemisphere-damaged individuals. *Cortex, 36*, 281–288. http://doi.org/http://dx.doi.org/10.1016/S0010-9452(08)70529-X

Garbarini, F., Piedimonte, A., Dotta, M., Pia, L., & Berti, A. (2013). Dissociations and similarities in motor intention and motor awareness: The case of anosognosia for hemiplegia and motor neglect. *Journal of Neurology, Neurosurgery, and Psychiatry, 84*(4), 416–419. http://doi.org/10.1136/jnnp-2012-302838

Gardner, H., & Brownell, H. H. (1986). *The Right Hemisphere Communication Battery.* Boston, MA: Psychology Service.

Gardner, H., & Denes, G. (1973). Connotative judgments by aphasic patients on a pictorial adaptation of the semantic differential. *Cortex, 9*(2), 183–196. http://doi.org/http://dx.doi.org/10.1016/S0010-9452(73)80027-9

Garrod, S. C., O'Brien, E. J., Morris, R. K., & Rayner, K. (1990). Elaborative inferencing as an active or passive process. *Journal of Experimental Psychology: Learning, Memory, and Cognition, 16*, 250–257.

Gazzaley, A., & Nobre, A. C. (2012). Top-down modulation: Bridging selective attention and working memory. *Trends in Cognitive Sciences, 16*(2), 129–135. http://doi.org/10.1016/j.tics.2011.11.014

Gernsbacher, M. A. (1990). *Language comprehension as structure building.* Hillsdale, NJ: Erlbaum.

Gernsbacher, M. A. (1996). The structure-building framework: What it is, what it might also be, and why. In B. K. Britton & A. C. Graesser (Eds.), *Models of understanding text comprehension.* Mahwah, NJ: Erlbaum.

Geschwind, N. (1965). Disconnexion syndromes in animals and man. *Brain, 88*(3), 585–644.

Giacino, J. T., & Cicerone K. D. (1998). Varieties of deficit unawareness after brain injury. *Journal of Head Trauma Rehabilitation, 13*(5), 1–15.

Gillen, R., Tennen, H., & McKee, T. (2005). Unilateral spatial neglect: Relation to rehabilitation outcomes in patients with right hemisphere stroke. *Archives of Physical Medicine and Rehabilitation, 86*, 763–767.

Gillespie, D. C., Bowen, A., & Foster, J. K. (2006). Memory impairment following right hemisphere stroke: A comparative meta-analytic and narrative review. *The Clinical Neuropsychologist, 20*(1), 59–75. http://doi.org/10.1080/13854040500203308

Giora, R., & Fein, O. (1999). Irony comprehension: The graded salience hypothesis. *Humor, 12*(4), 425–436.

Giora, R., Zaidel, E., Soroker, N., Batori, G., & Kasher, A. (2000). Differential effects of right- and left-hemisphere damage on understanding sarcasm and metaphor. *Metaphor and Symbol, 15*(1-2), 63–83.

Glocker, D., Bittl, P., & Kerkhoff, G. (2006). Construction and psychometric properties of a novel test for body representational neglect (Vest Test). *Restorative Neurology and Neuroscience, 24*(4–6), 303–317.

Glucksberg, S. (1998). Understanding metaphors. *Current Directions in Psychological Science, 7*(2), 39–43. http://doi.org/10.1111/1467-8721.ep13175582

Godefroy, O., Roussel, M., Leclerc, X., & Leys, D. (2009). Deficit of episodic memory: Anatomy and related patterns in stroke patients. *European Neurology, 61*(4), 223–229. http://doi.org/10.1159/000197107

Godfrey, H. P. D., Harnett, M. A, Knight, R. G., Marsh, N. V, Kesel, D. A, Partridge, F. M., & Robertson, R. H. (2003). Assessing distress in caregivers of people with a traumatic brain injury (TBI): A psychometric study of the Head Injury Behaviour Scale. *Brain Injury, 17*(5), 427–435. http://doi.org/10.1080/0269905031000066201

Goedert, K. M., Chen, P., Botticello, A., Masmela, J. R., Adler, U., & Barrett, A. M. (2012). Psychometric evaluation of neglect assessment reveals motor-exploratory predictor of functional disability in acute-stage spatial neglect. *Archives of Physical Medicine and Rehabilitation, 93*(1), 137–142. http://doi.org/10.1016/j.apmr.2011.06.036

Goedert, K. M., Zhang, J. Y., & Barrett, A. M. (2015). Prism adaptation and spatial neglect: The need for dose-finding studies. *Frontiers in Human Neuroscience, 9*(April), 243. http://doi.org/10.3389/fnhum.2015.00243

Goldstein, G., & Shelly, C. (1981). Does the right hemisphere age more rapidly than the left? *Journal of Clinical Neuropsychology, 3*(1), 65–78. http://doi.org/10.1080/01688638108403114

Goldstein, S., Naglieri, J. A., Princiotta, D., & Otero, T. M. (2014). Introduction: A history of executive functioning as a theoretical and clinical construct. In S. Goldstein & J. A. Naglieri (Eds), *Handbook of executive functioning* (pp. 3–12). New York, NY: Springer.

Gonzalez-Liencres, C., Shamay-Tsoory, S. G., & Brüne, M. (2013). Towards a neuroscience of empathy: Ontogeny, phylogeny, brain mechanisms, context and psychopathology. *Neuroscience and Biobehavioral Reviews, 37*(8), 1537–1548. http://doi.org/10.1016/j.neubiorev.2013.05.001

Gootjes, L., Bouma, A., Van Strien, J. W., Scheltens, P., & Stam, C. J. (2006). Attention modulates hemispheric differences in functional connectivity: Evidence from MEG recordings. *NeuroImage, 30*(1), 245–253. http://doi.org/10.1016/j.neuroimage.2005.09.015

Gorelick, P. B., & Ross, E. D. (1987). The aprosodias: Further functional-anatomical evidence for the organisation of affective language in the right hemisphere. *Journal of Neurology, Neurosurgery, and Psychiatry, 50*(5), 553–560. http://doi.org/10.1136/jnnp.50.5.553

Gottesman, R. F., Kleinman, J. T., Davis, C., Heidler-Gary, J., Newhart, M., & Hillis, A. E. (2010). The NIHSS-plus: Improving cognitive assessment with the NIHSS. *Behavioural Neurology, 22*(1-2), 11–15. http://doi.org/10.3233/BEN-2009-0259

Gouldthorp, B., & Coney, J. (2009a). The sensitivity of the right hemisphere to contextual information in sentences. *Brain and Language, 110*(2), 95–100. http://doi.org/10.1016/j.bandl.2009.05.003

Gouldthorp, B., & Coney, J. (2009b). Message-level processing of contextual information in the right cerebral hemisphere. *Neuropsychologia, 47*(2), 473–480. http://doi.org/10.1016/j.neuropsychologia.2008.10.001

Goverover, Y., Johnston, M. V, Toglia, J., & Deluca, J. (2007). Treatment to improve self-awareness in persons with acquired brain injury. *Brain Injury, 21*(9), 913–923. http://doi.org/10.1080/02699050701553205

Grabowska, A., Marchewka, A., Seniów, J., Polanowska, K., Jednoróg, K., Królicki, L., . . . Członkowska, A. (2011). Emotionally negative stimuli can overcome attentional deficits in patients with visuo-spatial hemineglect. *Neuropsychologia, 49*(12), 3327–3337. http://doi.org/10.1016/j.neuropsychologia.2011.08.006

Grace, J., & Malloy, P. F. (2001). *FrSBe Frontal System Behaviour Scale*. Lutz, FL: Psychological Assessment Resources.

Grandjean, D., Sander, D., Lucas, N., Scherer, K. R., & Vuilleumier, P. (2008). Effects of emotional prosody on auditory extinction for voices in patients with spatial neglect. *Neuropsychologia, 46*(2), 487–496. http://doi.org/10.1016/j.neuropsychologia.2007.08.025

Grant, D. A., & Berg, E. A. (1981). *Wisconsin Card Sorting Test (WCST)*. PAR.

Green, J. J., Doesburg, S. M., Ward, L. M., & McDonald, J. J. (2011). Electrical neuroimaging of voluntary audiospatial attention: Evidence for a supramodal attention control network. *Journal of Neuroscience, 31*(10), 3560–3564. http://doi.org/10.1523/JNEUROSCI.5758-10.2011

Green, L. W. (2009). Making research relevant: If it is an evidence-based practice, where's the practice-based evidence? *Family Practice, 25*(May), 20–24. http://doi.org/10.1093/fampra/cmn055

Greicius, M. D., Krasnow, B., Reiss, A. L., & Menon, V. (2003). Functional connectivity in the resting brain: A network analysis of the default mode hypothesis. *Proceedings of the National Academy of Sciences, 100*(1), 253–258. http://doi.org/10.1073/pnas.0135058100\r0135058100 [pii]

Griffin, R., Friedman, O., Ween, J., Winner, E., Happé, F., & Brownell, H. H. (2006). Theory of mind and the right cerebral hemisphere: Refining the scope of impairment. *Laterality, 11*(3), 195–225. http://doi.org/10.1080/13576500500450552

Grimsen, C., Hildebrandt, H., & Fahle, M. (2008). Dissociation of egocentric and allocentric coding of space in visual search after right middle cerebral artery stroke. *Neuropsychologia, 46*(3), 902–914. http://doi.org/10.1016/j.neuropsychologia.2007.11.028

Gronwall, D. M. (1977). Paced auditory serial-addition task: A measure of recovery from concussion. *Perceptual and Motor Skills, 44*(2), 367–373. http://doi.org/10.2466/pms.1977.44.2.367

Grosdemange, A., Monfort, V., Richard, S., Toniolo, A. M., Ducrocq, X., & Bolmont, B. (2015). Impact of anxiety on verbal and visuospatial working memory in patients with acute stroke without severe cognitive impairment. *Journal of Neurology, Neurosurgery, and Psychiatry, 86*(5), 513–519. http://doi.org/10.1136/jnnp-2014-308232

Guilbert, A., Clément, S., Senouci, L., Pontzeele, S., Martin, Y., & Moroni, C. (2016). Auditory lateralisation deficits in neglect patients. *Neuropsychologia, 85*, 177–183. http://doi.org/10.1016/j.neuropsychologia.2016.03.024

Gur, R. C., Packer, I. K., Hungerbuhler, J. P., Reivich, M., Obrist, W. D., Amarnek, W. S., & Sackeim, H. A. (1980). Differences in the distribution of gray and white matter in human cerebral hemispheres. *Science, 207*(4436), 1226–1228. Retrieved from http://www.jstor.org/stable/1683339

Guranski, K., & Podemski, R. (2015). Emotional prosody expression in acoustic analysis in patients with right hemisphere ischemic stroke. *Neurologia I Neurochirurgia Polska, 49*(2), 113–120. http://doi.org/10.1016/j.pjnns.2015.03.004

Habekost, T., & Rostrup, E. (2006). Persisting asymmetries of vision after right side lesions. *Neuropsychologia, 44*(6), 876–895. http://doi.org/10.1016/j.neuropsychologia.2005.09.002

Habekost, T., & Rostrup, E. (2007). Visual attention capacity after right hemisphere lesions. *Neuropsychologia, 45*(7), 1474–1488. http://doi.org/10.1016/j.neuropsychologia.2006.11.006

Haeske-Dewick, H. C., Canavan, A. G., & Hömberg, V. (1996). Directional hyperattention in tactile neglect within grasping space. *Journal of Clinical and Experimental*

Neuropsychology, 18(5), 724–732. http://doi.org/10.1080/01688639608408295

Hald, L. A., Steenbeek-Planting, E. G., & Hagoort, P. (2007). The interaction of discourse context and world knowledge in online sentence comprehension. Evidence from the N400. *Brain Research, 1146*(1), 210–218. http://doi.org/10.1016/j.brainres.2007.02.054

Happé, F., Brownell, H. H., & Winner, E. (1999). Acquired "theory of mind" impairments following stroke. *Cognition, 70,* 211–240.

Harciarek, M., Heilman, K. M., & Jodzio, K. (2006). Defective comprehension of emotional faces and prosody as a result of right hemisphere stroke: Modality versus emotion-type specificity. *Journal of the International Neuropsychological Society: JINS, 12*(6), 774–781. http://doi.org/10.1017/S1355617706061121

Hargrove, P., Anderson, A., & Jones, J. (2009). A critical review of interventions targeting prosody. *International Journal of Speech-Language Pathology, 11*(4), 298–304. http://doi.org/10.1080/17549500902969477

Harris, J. L., Kiran, S., Marquardt, T. P., & Fleming, V. B. (2008). Communication Wellness Check-Up ©: Age-related changes in communicative abilities. *Aphasiology, 22*(7–8), 813–825. http://doi.org/10.1080/02687030701818034

Hart, T., Whyte, J., Ellis, C., & Chervoneva, I. (2009). Construct validity of an attention rating scale for traumatic brain injury. *Neuropsychology, 23*(6), 729–735. http://doi.org/http://dx.doi.org.ezproxy.lib.uh.edu/10.1037/a0016153

Hartley, L. L. (1995). *Cognitive-communicative abilities following brain injury.* San Diego, CA: Singular Thomson Learning.

Harvey, M., & Rossit, S. (2012). Visuospatial neglect in action. *Neuropsychologia, 50*(6), 1018–1028. http://doi.org/10.1016/j.neuropsychologia.2011.09.030

Hasher, L. (2007). Inhibition: Attentional regulation of cognition. In H. L. Roediger, Y.

Dudai, & S. M. Fitzpatrick (Eds.), *Science of memory concepts* (pp. 291–294). New York, NY: Oxford University Press.

Hasher, L., & Zacks, R. T. (1988). Working memory, comprehension, and aging: A review and a new view. In G. H. Bower (Ed.), *Psychology of learning & motivation* (pp. 193–225). San Diego, CA: Academic Press.

Hays, S.-J., Niven, B. E., Godfrey, H. P. D., & Linscott, R. J. (2004). Clinical assessment of pragmatic language impairment: A generalisability study of older people with Alzheimer's disease. *Aphasiology, 18*(8), 693–714. http://doi.org/10.1080/02687030444000183

He, B. J., Snyder, A. Z., Vincent, J. L., Epstein, A., Shulman, G. L., & Corbetta, M. (2007). Breakdown of functional connectivity in frontoparietal networks underlies behavioral deficits in spatial neglect. *Neuron, 53*(6), 905–918. http://doi.org/10.1016/j.neuron.2007.02.013

Head, J., Neumann, E., Helton, W. S., & Shears, C. (2013). Novel word processing. *The American Journal of Psychology, 126*(3), 323–333.

Heath, R. L., & Blonder, L. X. (2003). Conversational humor among stroke survivors. *Humor, 16*(1), 91–106.

Heath, R. L., & Blonder, L. X. (2005). Spontaneous humor among right hemisphere stroke survivors. *Brain and Language, 93*(3), 267–276. http://doi.org/10.1016/j.bandl.2004.10.006

Hedna, V. S., Bodhit, A. N., Ansari, S., Falchook, A. D., Stead, L., Heilman, K. M., & Waters, M. F. (2013). Hemispheric differences in ischemic stroke: Is left-hemisphere stroke more common? *Journal of Clinical Neurology (Seoul, Korea), 9*(2), 97–102. http://doi.org/10.3988/jcn.2013.9.2.97

Heilman, K. M. (1991). Anosognosia: Possible neuropsychological mechanisms. In G. P. Prigatano & D. L. Schacter (Eds.), *Awareness of deficit after brain injury: Clinical and theoretical issues* (pp. 53–62). New York, NY: Oxford University Press.

Heilman, K. M., Bowers, D., Valenstein, E., & Watson, R. T. (1986). The right hemisphere: Neuropsychological functions. *Journal of Neurosurgery, 64*(5), 693–704.

Heilman, K. M., & Harciarek, M. (2010). Anosognosia and anosodiaphoria of weakness. In G. P. Prigatano (Ed.), *The study of anosognosia* (pp. 89–112). New York, NY: Oxford University Press.

Heilman, K. M., & Van Den Abell, T. (1980). Right hemisphere dominance for attention: The mechanism underlying hemispheric asymmetries of inattention (neglect). *Neurology, 30*(3), 327–330.

Helffenstein, D. A., & Wechsler, F. S. (1982). The use of Interpersonal Process Recall (IPR) in the remediation of interpersonal and communication skill deficits in the newly brain-injured. *Clinical Neuropsychology, 4*(3), 139–143.

Hesse, M. D., Sparing, R., & Fink, G. R. (2011). Ameliorating spatial neglect with non-invasive brain stimulation: From pathophysiological concepts to novel treatment strategies. *Neuropsychological Rehabilitation, 21*(5), 676–702.

Hillis, A. E. (2006). Rehabilitation of unilateral spatial neglect: New insights from magnetic resonance perfusion imaging. *Archives of Physical Medicine and Rehabilitation, 87*(12 Suppl.), 43–49. http://doi.org/10.1016/j.apmr.2006.08.331

Hillis, A. E. (2014). Inability to empathize: Brain lesions that disrupt sharing and understanding another's emotions. *Brain: A Journal of Neurology, 137*(Pt 4), 981–997. http://doi.org/10.1093/brain/awt317

Hillis, A. E., Newhart, M., Heidler, J., Barker, P. B., Herskovits, E. H., & Degaonkar, M. (2005). Anatomy of spatial attention: Insights from perfusion imaging and hemispatial neglect in acute stroke. *Journal of Neuroscience, 25*, 3161–3167. doi:10.1523/JNEUROSCI.4468-04.2005

Hillis, A. E., & Tippett, D. C. (2014). Stroke recovery: Surprising influences and residual consequences. *Advances in Medicine*, 1–10. http://doi.org/10.1144/2014/378263

Hird, K., & Kirsner, K. (2003). The effect of right cerebral hemisphere damage on collaborative planning in conversation: An analysis of intentional structure. *Clinical Linguistics & Phonetics, 17*(4–5), 309–315. http://doi.org/10.1080/0269920031000080037

Hochstenbach, J., Mulder, T., Limbeek, J. Van, & Donders, R. (1998). Cognitive decline following stroke: A comprehensive study of cognitive decline following stroke. *Journal of Clinical and Experimental Neuropsychology, 20*(4), 503–517.

Holland, R., & Crinion, J. (2012). Can tDCS enhance treatment of aphasia? *Aphasiology, 26*(9), 1169–1191. http://doi.org/10.1080/02687038.2011.616925

Hopper, T. (2007). The ICF and dementia. *Seminars in Speech and Language, 28*(4), 273–282. http://doi.org/10.1055/s-2007-986524

Horn, S., & Gassaway, J. (2010). Practice based evidence: Incorporating clinical heterogeneity and patient-reported outcomes for comparative effectiveness research. *Medical Care, 48*(6), 17–22. http://doi.org/10.1097/MLR.0b013e3181d57473

Howick, J., Chalmers, I., Glasziou, P., Greenhalgh, T., Heneghan, C., Liberati, A., . . . Thornton, H. (2011). *The 2011 Oxford CEBM levels of evidence: Introductory document. Oxford Centre for Evidence-Based Medicine* (Vol. 1). Retrieved from http://www.cebm.net/index.aspx?o=5653

Huang, S., Seidman, L. J., Rossi, S., & Ahveninen, J. (2013). Distinct cortical networks activated by auditory attention and working memory load. *NeuroImage, 83*, 1098–1108. http://doi.org/10.1016/j.neuroimage.2013.07.074

Hubley, A. M., & Tombaugh, T. N. (2002). *Memory Test for Older Adults*. North Tonawanda, NY: MultiHealth Systems.

Humphreys, G. W., Bickerton, W.-L., Samson, D., & Riddoch, M. J. (2012). *BCoS Cognition Screen*. Hove, UK: Psychology Press.

Hupbach, A., Gomez, R., Hardt, O., & Nadel, L. (2007). Reconsolidation of episodic memories: A subtle reminder triggers integration of new information. *Learning & Memory*, 14(1-2), 47–53. http://doi.org/10.1101/lm.365707

Hupp, J. M., & Jungers, M. K. (2013). Beyond words: Comprehension and production of pragmatic prosody in adults and children. *Journal of Experimental Child Psychology*, 115(3), 536–551. https://doi.org/10.1016/j.jecp.2012.12.012

Husain, M., Mattingley, J. B., Rorden, C., Kennard, C., & Driver, J. (2000). Distinguishing sensory and motor biases in parietal and frontal neglect. *Brain*, 123, 1643–1659.

Hyndman, D., Pickering, R. M., & Ashburn, A. (2007). The influence of attention deficits on functional recovery post stroke during the first 12 months after discharge from hospital. *Journal of Neurology, Neurosurgery & Psychiatry*, 79(6), 656–663. http://doi.org/10.1136/jnnp.2007.125609

Institute of Medicine (IOM). (2011). *Cognitive rehabilitation therapy for traumatic brain injury: Evaluating the evidence* (R. Koehler, E. Wilhelm, & I. Shoulson, Eds.). Washington, DC: The National Academies Press. http://doi.org/10.1016/S0140-6736(11)61632-2

Iredale, J. M., Rushby, J. A, McDonald, S., Dimoska-Di Marco, A., & Swift, J. (2013). Emotion in voice matters: Neural correlates of emotional prosody perception. *International Journal of Psychophysiology*, 89(3), 483–490. http://doi.org/10.1016/j.ijpsycho.2013.06.025

Iturria-Medina, Y., Perez Fernandez, A., Morris, D. M., Canales-Rodriguez, E. J., Haroon, H. A., Garcia Penton, L., . . . Melie-Garcia, L. (2011). Brain hemispheric structural efficiency and interconnectivity rightward asymmetry in human and nonhuman primates. *Cerebral Cortex*, 21, 56–67. http://doi.org/10.1093/cercor/bhq058

Jacobs, S., Brozzoli, C., & Farnè, A. (2012). Neglect: A multisensory deficit? *Neuropsychologia*, 50(6), 1029–1044. http://doi.org/10.1016/j.neuropsychologia.2012.03.018

Jehkonen, M., Ahonen, J.-P., Dastidar, P., Koivisto, A.-M., Laippala, P., Vilkki, J., & Molnar, G. (2001). Predictors of discharge to home during the first year after right hemisphere stroke. *Acta Neurologica Scandinavica*, 104(3), 136–141. http://doi.org/10.1034/j.1600-0404.2001.00025.x

Jenkinson, P. M., Edelstyn, N. M. J., Drakeford, J. L., & Ellis, S. J. (2009). Reality monitoring in anosognosia for hemiplegia. *Consciousness and Cognition*, 18(2), 458–470. http://doi.org/10.1016/j.concog.2008.12.005

Jenkinson, P. M., Preston, C., & Ellis, S. J. (2011). Unawareness after stroke: a review and practical guide to understanding, assessing, and managing anosognosia for hemiplegia. *Journal of Clinical and Experimental Neuropsychology*, 33(10), 1079–1093. http://doi.org/10.1080/13803395.2011.596822

Joanette, Y., Ska, B., & Côté, H. (2004). *Protocole Montréal d'Evaluation de la Communication*. Isbergues, France: Ortho Edition.

Joanette, Y., Ska, B., Côté, H., Ferré, P., LaPointe, L., Coppens, P., & Small, S. (2015). *Montreal Protocol for the Evaluation of Communication (MEC)*. Sydney, Australia: ASSBI Resources.

Johnson-Greene, D., Touradji, P., & Emmerson, L. C. (2009). The Three Cities Test: Preliminary validation of a short bedside memory test in persons with acute stroke. *Topics in Stroke Rehabilitation*, 16(5), 321–329.

Jolles, D. D., Grol, M. J., Van Buchem, M. A., Rombouts, S. A. R. B., & Crone, E. A. (2010). Practice effects in the brain: Changes in cerebral activation after working memory practice depend on task demands. *NeuroImage*, 52(2), 658–668. http://doi.org/10.1016/j.neuroimage.2010.04.028

Jones, H. N., Shrivastav, R., Wu, S. S., Plowman-Prine, E. K., & Rosenbek, J. C. (2009). Fundamental frequency and intensity mean and variability before and after two behavioral treatments for aprosodia. *Journal of Medical Speech-Language Pathology*, 17(1), 45–53.

Jorge, R. E. (2010). Emotional awareness among brain-damaged patients. In G. P. Prigatano (Ed.), *The study of anosognosia* (pp. 333–356). New York, NY: Oxford University Press.

Jorgensen, H. S., Nakayama, H., Pedersen, P. M., Kammersgaard, L. P., Raaschou, H. O., & Olsen, T. S. (1999). Epidemiology of stroke-related disability: The Copenhagen Stroke Study. *Clinics in Geriatric Medicine, 15*(4), 785–799.

Jorgensen, M., & Togher, L. (2009). Narrative after traumatic brain injury: A comparison of monologic and jointly-produced discourse. *Brain Injury, 23*(9), 727–740. http://doi.org/10.1080/02699050903133954

Joseph, R. M., Fricker, Z., & Keehn, B. (2015). Activation of frontoparietal attention networks by non-predictive gaze and arrow cues. *Social Cognitive and Affective Neuroscience, 10*(2), 294–301. http://doi.org/10.1093/scan/nsu054

Just, M. A., & Carpenter, P. A. (1992). A capacity theory of comprehension: Individual differences in working memory. *Psychological Review, 99*(1), 122–149. http://doi.org/10.1037/0033-295X.99.1.122

Kahlaoui, K., Scherer, L. C., & Joanette, Y. (2008). The right hemisphere's contribution to the processing of semantic relationships between words. *Linguistics and Language Compass, 2*(4), 550–568. http://doi.org/10.1111/j.1749-818X.2008.00065.x

Kammersgaard, L. P., Jørgensen, H. S., Reith, J., Nakayama, H., Pedersen, P. M., & Olsen, T. S. (2004). Short- and long-term prognosis for very old stroke patients. The Copenhagen Stroke Study. *Age and Ageing, 33*(2), 149–154. http://doi.org/10.1093/ageing/afh052

Kandhadai, P., & Federmeier, K. D. (2008). Summing it up: Semantic activation processes in the two hemispheres as revealed by event-related potentials. *Brain Research, 1233*, 146–159. http://doi.org/10.1016/j.brainres.2008.07.043

Kang, E. K., Kim, Y. K., Sohn, H. M., Cohen, L. G., & Paik, N. J. (2011). Improved picture naming in aphasia patients treated with cathodal tDCS to inhibit the right Broca's homologue area. *Restorative Neurology and Neuroscience, 29*(3), 141–152. http://doi.org/10.3233/RNN-2011-0587

Kanne, S. M. (2002). The role of semantic, orthographic, and phonological prime information in unilateral visual neglect. *Cognitive Neuropsychology, 19*, 245–261. http://doi.org/10.1080/02643290143000178

Kant, N., van den Berg, E., van Zandvoort, M. J. E., Frijns, C. J. M., Kappelle, L. J., & Postma, A. (2014). Functional correlates of prospective memory in stroke. *Neuropsychologia, 60*(1), 77–83. http://doi.org/10.1016/j.neuropsychologia.2014.05.015

Kaplan, J. A., Brownell, H. H., Jacobs, J. R., & Gardner, H. (1990). The effects of right hemisphere damage on the pragmatic interpretation of conversational remarks. *Brain and Language, 38*, 315–333.

Kaplan, E., Goodglass, H., & Weintraub, S. (2001). *Boston Naming Test*. Austin, TX: Pro-Ed.

Karnath, H.-O. (2015). Spatial attention systems in spatial neglect. *Neuropsychologia, 75*, 61–73. http://doi.org/10.1016/j.neuropsychologia.2015.05.019

Karnath, H.-O., & Baier, B. (2010). Anosognosia for hemiparesis and hemiplegia: Disturbed sense of agency and body ownership. In G. P. Prigatano (Ed.), *The study of anosognosia*. Oxford, UK: Oxford University Press.

Karnath, H.-O., & Dieterich, M. (2006). Spatial neglect—A vestibular disorder? *Brain, 129*(Pt. 2), 293–305. http://doi.org/10.1093/brain/awh698

Karnath, H.-O., Fruhmann Berger, M., Küker, W., & Rorden, C. (2004). The anatomy of spatial neglect based on voxelwise statistical analysis: A study of 140 patients. *Cerebral Cortex, 14*(10), 1164–1172. http://doi.org/10.1093/cercor/bhh076

Karnath, H.-O., Mandler, A., & Clavagnier, S. (2011). Object-based neglect varies with egocentric position. *Journal of Cognitive Neuroscience, 23*(10), 2983–2993. http://doi.org/10.1162/jocn_a_00005

Karnath, H.-O., & Rorden, C. (2012). The anatomy of spatial neglect. *Neuropsychologia, 50*(6), 1010–1017. http://doi.org/10.1016/j.neuropsychologia.2011.06.027

Karow, C. M., Marquardt, T. P., & Levitt, S. (2013). Processing of ambiguous emotional messages in brain injured patients with and without subcortical lesions. *Aphasiology*, 27(3), 344–363. http://doi.org/10.1080/026 87038.2012.727983

Kasparian, K. (2013). Hemispheric differences in figurative language processing: Contributions of neuroimaging methods and challenges in reconciling current empirical findings. *Journal of Neurolinguistics*, 26(1), 1–21. http://doi.org/10.1016/j.jneuroling .2012.07.001

Katz, N., Ring, H., Naveh, Y., Kizony, R., Feintuch, U., & Weiss, P. L. (2005). Interactive virtual environment training for safe street crossing of right hemisphere stroke patients with unilateral spatial neglect. *Disability and Rehabilitation*, 27(20), 1235–1243. http://doi .org/10.1080/09638280500076079

Kauranen, T., Laari, S., Turunen, K., Mustanoja, S., Baumann, P., & Poutiainen, E. (2014). The cognitive burden of stroke emerges even with an intact NIH Stroke Scale Score: A cohort study. *Journal of Neurology, Neurosurgery, and Psychiatry*, 85(3), 295–299. http://doi.org/10.1136/jnnp-2013-305585

Kempler, D., Van Lancker, D., Marchman, V., & Bates, E. (1999). Idiom comprehension in children and adults with unilateral brain damage. *Developmental Neuropsychology*, 15(3), 327–349.

Kennedy, M. R. T. (2000). Topic scenes in conversations with adults with right-hemisphere brain damage. *American Journal of Speech-Language Pathology*, 9, 72–86. http://doi .org/doi:10.1044/1058-0360.0901.72

Kerkhoff, G. (2001). Spatial hemineglect in humans. *Progress in Neurobiology*, 63, 1–27.

Kerkhoff, G., & Schenk, T. (2012). Rehabilitation of neglect: An update. *Neuropsychologia*, 50(6), 1072–1079. http://doi.org/10.1016/j .neuropsychologia.2012.01.024

Kessels, R. P., Van Zandvoort, M. J., Postma, A., Kappelle, L. J., & De Haan, E. H. (2000). The Corsi block-tapping task: Standardization and normative data. *Applied Neuropsychology*, 7(4), 252–258.

Khurshid, S., Trupe, L. A, Newhart, M., Davis, C., Molitoris, J. J., Medina, J., . . . Hillis, A. E. (2012). Reperfusion of specific cortical areas is associated with improvement in distinct forms of hemispatial neglect. *Cortex*, 48(5), 530–539. http://doi.org/10.1016/j .cortex.2011.01.003

Kiefer, M., Weisbrod, M., Kern, I., Maier, S., & Spitzer, M. (1998). Right hemisphere activation during indirect semantic priming: Evidence from event-related potentials. *Brain and Language*, 64(64), 377–408. http://doi .org/10.1006/brln.1998.1979

Kim, D. Y., Ku, J., Chang, W. H., Park, T. H., Lim, J. Y., Han, K., . . . Kim, S. I. (2010). Assessment of post-stroke extrapersonal neglect using a three-dimensional immersive virtual street crossing program. *Acta Neurologica Scandinavica*, 121(3), 171–177. http://doi.org/10.1111/j.1600-0404 .2009.01194.x

Kim, E.-J., Lee, B., Jo, M.-K., Jung, K., You, H., Lee, B. H., . . . Na, D. L. (2013). Directional and spatial motor intentional disorders in patients with right versus left hemisphere strokes. *Neuropsychology*, 27(4), 428–437. http://doi.org/10.1037/a0032824

Kim, H. J., Craik, F. I. M., Luo, L., & Ween, J. E. (2009). Impairments in prospective and retrospective memory following stroke. *Neurocase*, 15(2), 145–156. http://doi.org/ 10.1080/13554790802709039

Kim, K., Kim, J., Ku, J., Kim, D. Y., Chang, W. H., Shin, D. I., . . . Kim, S. I. (2004). A virtual reality assessment and training system for unilateral neglect. *Cyberpsychology & Behavior*, 7(6), 742–750.

Kimberg, D. Y., & Farah, M. J. (1993). A unified account of cognitive impairments following frontal lobe damage: The role of working memory in complex, organized behavior. *Journal of Experimental Psychology: General*, 122(4), 411–428. http://doi.org/ 10.1037/0096-3445.122.4.411

Kinsbourne, M. (1970). A model for the mechanism of unilateral neglect of space. *Transactions of the American Neurological Association*, 95, 143–146. PMID: 5514359

Kintsch, W. (1988). The role of knowledge in discourse comprehension: A Construction-

Integration Model. *Psychological Review, 95,* 163–182.

Kircher, T. T. J., Brammer, M., Andreu, N. T., Williams, S. C. R., & McGuire, P. K. (2001). Engagement of right temporal cortex during processing of linguistic context. *Neuropsychologia, 39*(8), 798–809. http://doi.org/10.1016/S0028-3932(01)00014-8

Klinke, M. E., Hjaltason, H., Hafsteinsdóttir, T. B., & Jónsdóttir, H. (2016). Spatial neglect in stroke patients after discharge from rehabilitation to own home: A mixed method study. *Disability and Rehabilitation, 8288*(January), 1–16. http://doi.org/10.3109/09638288.2015.1130176

Kluding, P. M., Tseng, B. Y., & Billinger, S. (2012). Exercise and executive function in individuals with chronic stroke: A pilot study. *Journal of Neurology and Physical Therapy, 35*(1), 11–17. http://doi.org/10.1097/NPT.0b013e318208ee6c.Exercise

Koivisto, M. (1998). Categorical priming in the cerebral hemispheres: Automatic in the left hemisphere, postlexical in the right hemisphere? *Neuropsychologia, 36*(7), 661–668. http://doi.org/10.1016/S0028-3932(97)00147-4

Kong, K.-H., Chua, K., & Tow, A. P. (1998). Clinical characteristics and functional outcome of stroke patients 75 years old and older. *Archives of Physical Medicine & Rehabilitation, 79*(12), 1535–1539.

Kortte, K., & Hillis, A. E. (2009). Recent advances in the understanding of neglect and anosognosia following right hemisphere stroke. *Current Neurology and Neuroscience Reports, 9,* 459–465.

Kortte, K. B., McWhorter, J. W., Pawlak, M. A., Slentz, J., Sur, S., & Hillis, A. E. (2015). Anosognosia for hemiplegia: The contributory role of right inferior frontal gyrus. *Neuropsychology, 29*(3), 421–432. http://doi.org/10.1037/neu0000135

Kotz, S. A., Kalberlah, C., Bahlmann, J., Friederici, A. D., & Haynes, J.-D. (2013). Predicting vocal emotion expressions from the human brain. *Human Brain Mapping, 34*(8), 1971–1981. http://doi.org/10.1002/hbm.22041

Kotz, S. A, Meyer, M., Alter, K., Besson, M., von Cramon, D. Y., & Friederici, A. D. (2003). On the lateralization of emotional prosody: An event-related functional MR investigation. *Brain and Language, 86*(3), 366–376. http://doi.org/10.1016/S0093-934X(02)00532-1

Krauss, R. M., & Chiu, Y. (1998). Language and social behavior. In D. Gilbert, S. Fiske, & G. Lindzey (Eds.), *The handbook of social psychology* (Vol. 2, 4th ed., pp. 41–88). New York, NY: McGraw-Hill.

Kristensen, L. B., Wang, L., Petersson, K. M., & Hagoort, P. (2013). The interface between language and attention: Prosodic focus marking recruits a general attention network in spoken language comprehension. *Cerebral Cortex, 23*(8), 1836–1848. http://doi.org/10.1093/cercor/bhs164

Kucharska-Pietura, K., Phillips, M. L., Gernand, W., & David, A. S. (2003). Perception of emotions from faces and voices following unilateral brain damage. *Neuropsychologia, 41*(8), 1082–1090. http://doi.org/10.1016/S0028-3932(02)00294-4

Kucyi, A., Moayedi, M., Weissman-Fogel, I., Hodaie, M., & Davis, K. D. (2012). Hemispheric asymmetry in white matter connectivity of the temporoparietal junction with the insula and prefrontal cortex. *PLoS ONE, 7*(4). http://doi.org/10.1371/journal.pone.0035589

Lai, V. T., van Dam, W., Conant, L. L., Binder, J. R., & Desai, R. H. (2015). Familiarity differentially affects right hemisphere contributions to processing metaphors and literals. *Frontiers in Human Neuroscience, 9*(February), 44. http://doi.org/10.3389/fnhum.2015.00044

Langer, K. G., & Levine, D. N. (2014). Babinski, J. (1914). Contribution to the study of the mental disorders in hemiplegia of organic cerebral origin (anosognosia). Translated by K. G. Langer & D. N. Levine, from the original Contribution à l'Étude des Troubles Mentaux dans l'Hémiplé. *Cortex, 61,*

5–8. http://doi.org/10.1016/j.cortex.2014.04.019

Langhorne, P., Bernhardt, J., & Kwakkel, G. (2011). Stroke rehabilitation. *The Lancet, 377,* 1693–1702. http://doi.org/10.1016/S0140-6736(11)60325-5

Laplane, D., & Degos, J. D. (1983). Motor neglect. *Journal of Neurology, Neurosurgery, and Psychiatry, 46*(2), 152–158. http://doi.org/10.1136/jnnp.46.2.152

LaPointe, L. L. (1991). Brain damage and humor: Not a laughing matter. In *Clinical Aphasiology Conference Proceedings* (pp. 53–60).

Lauro, L. J. R., Tettamanti, M., Cappa, S. F., & Papagno, C. (2007). Idiom comprehension: A prefrontal task? *Cerebral Cortex, 18*(1), 162–170. http://doi.org/10.1093/cercor/bhm042

Lawson, M. J., & Rice, D. N. (1989). Effects of training in use of executive strategies on a verbal memory problem resulting from closed head injury. *Journal of Clinical and Experimental Neuropsychology, 11*(6), 842–854. http://doi.org/10.1080/01688638908400939

Le, A., Stojanoski, B. B., Khan, S., Keough, M., & Niemeier, M. (2015). A toggle switch of visual awareness? *Cortex, 64,* 169–178. http://doi.org/10.1016/j.cortex.2014.09.015

Lê, K., Coelho, C., Mozeiko, J., & Grafman, J. (2011). Measuring goodness of story narratives. *Journal of Speech, Language, and Hearing Research: JSLHR, 54*(February), 118–126. http://doi.org/10.1080/02687038.2010.539696

Lee, B. H., Suh, M. K., Kim, E. J., Seo, S. W., Choi, K. M., Kim, G. M., . . . Na, D. L. (2009). Neglect dyslexia: Frequency, association with other hemispatial neglects, and lesion localization. *Neuropsychologia, 47*(3), 704–710. http://doi.org/10.1016/j.neuropsychologia.2008.11.027

Lee, S. S., & Dapretto, M. (2006). Metaphorical vs. literal word meanings: fMRI evidence against a selective role of the right hemisphere. *NeuroImage, 29*(2), 536–544. http://doi.org/10.1016/j.neuroimage.2005.08.003

Lehman, M. T., & Tompkins, C. A. (2000). Inferencing in adults with right hemisphere brain damage: An analysis of conflicting results. *Aphasiology, 14*(5-6), 485–499. http://doi.org/10.1080/026870300401261

Lehman-Blake, M. T., & Tompkins, C. A. (2001). Predictive inferencing in adults with right hemisphere brain damage. *Journal of Speech, Language, and Hearing Research, 44,* 639–654. http://doi.org/10.1044/1092-4388(2001/052)

Leigh, R., Oishi, K., Hsu, J., Lindquist, M., Gottesman, R. F., Jarso, S., . . . Hillis, A. E. (2013). Acute lesions that impair affective empathy. *Brain: A Journal of Neurology, 136*(Pt. 8), 2539–2549. http://doi.org/10.1093/brain/awt177

Lemoncello, R., & Ness, B. (2013). Evidence-based practice & practice-based evidence applied to adult, medical speech-language pathology. *SIG 15 Perspectives on Gerontology, 18*(1), 14–26.

Leon, S. A., Rosenbek, J. C., Crucian, G. P., Hieber, B., Holiway, B., Rodriguez, A. D., . . . Gonzalez-Rothi, L. (2004). Active treatments for aprosodia secondary to right hemisphere stroke. *The Journal of Rehabilitation Research and Development, 41*(1), 93. http://doi.org/10.1682/JRRD.2003.12.0182

Leonard, C. L., Waters, G. S., & Caplan, D. (1997a). The use of contextual information by right brain-damaged individuals in the resolution of ambiguous pronouns. *Brain and Language, 57*(3), 309–342.

Leonard, C. L., Waters, G. S., & Caplan, D. (1997b). The use of contextual information related to general world knowledge by right brain-damaged individuals in pronoun resolution. *Brain and Language, 57*(3), 343–359.

Levelt, W. J. M. (1989). *Speaking: From intention to articulation.* Cambridge, MA: MIT Press.

Levine, B., Dawson, D., Boutet, I., Schwartz, M. L., & Stuss, D. T. (2000). Assessment of strategic self-regulation in traumatic brain injury: Its relationship to injury severity and psychosocial outcome. *Neuropsychology,*

14(4), 491–500. http://doi.org/10.1037/0894-4105.14.4.491

Levine, B., Schweizer, T. A., O'Connor, C., Turner, G., Gillingham, S., Stuss, D. T., . . . Robertson, I. H. (2011). Rehabilitation of executive functioning in patients with frontal lobe brain damage with goal management training. *Frontiers Human Neuroscience, 5*(9), 1–9. http://doi.org/10.3389/fnhum.2011.00009

Levine, D. A., Galecki, A. T., Langa, K. M., Unverzagt, F. W., Kabeto, M. U., Giordani, B., & Wadley, V. G. (2015). Trajectory of cognitive decline after incident stroke. *Journal of the American Medical Association, 314*(1), 41–51. http://doi.org/10.1001/jama.2015.6968

Levine, J., Warrenburg, S., Kerns, R., Schwartz, G., Delaney, R., Fontana, A., . . . Cascione, R. (1987). The role of denial in recovery from coronary heart disease. *Psychosomatic Medicine, 49*(2), 109–117.

Lezak, M. D., Howieson, D. B., & Loring, D. W. (2004). *Neuropsychological evaluation.* Oxford, UK: Oxford University Press.

Li, M., Chen, H., Wang, J., Liu, F., Long, Z., Wang, Y., . . . Chen, H. (2014). Handedness- and hemisphere-related differences in small-world brain networks: A diffusion tensor imaging tractography study. *Brain Connect, 4*(2), 145–156. http://doi.org/10.1089/brain.2013.0211

Lim, C., & Alexander, M. P. (2009). Stroke and episodic memory disorders. *Neuropsychologia, 47*(14), 3045–3058. http://doi.org/10.1016/j.neuropsychologia.2009.08.002

Lindell, A. B., Jalas, M. J., Tenovuo, O., Brunila, T., Voeten, M. J. M., & Hämäläinen, H. (2007). Clinical assessment of hemispatial neglect: Evaluation of different measures and dimensions. *The Clinical Neuropsychologist, 21*(3), 479–497. http://doi.org/10.1080/13854040600630061

Linscott, R. J., Knight, R. G., & Godfrey, H. P. D. (1996). The Profile of Functional Impairment in Communication (PFIC): A measure of communication impairment for clinical use. *Brain Injury, 10*(6), 397–412. http://doi.org/10.1080/026990596124269

Liu-Ambrose, T., & Eng, J. J. (2014). Exercise training and recreational activities to promote executive functions in chronic stroke: A proof-of-concept study. *Journal of Stroke and Cerebrovascular Diseases: The Official Journal of National Stroke Association, 24*(1), 130–137. http://doi.org/10.1016/j.jstrokecerebrovasdis.2014.08.012

Long, D. L., & Baynes, K. (2002). Discourse representation in the two cerebral hemispheres. *Journal of Cognitive Neuroscience, 14*(2), 228–242. http://doi.org/10.1162/089892902317236867

Longo, M. R., Trippier, S., Vagnoni, E., & Lourenco, S. F. (2015). Right hemisphere control of visuospatial attention in near space. *Neuropsychologia, 70*, 350–357. http://doi.org/10.1016/j.neuropsychologia.2014.10.035

Lovseth, K., & Atchley, R. A. (2010). Examining lateralized semantic access using pictures. *Brain and Cognition, 72*(2), 202–209. http://doi.org/10.1016/j.bandc.2009.08.016

Luauté, J., Halligan, P., Rode, G., Rossetti, Y., & Boisson, D. (2006). Visuo-spatial neglect: A systematic review of current interventions and their effectiveness. *Neuroscience and Biobehavioral Reviews, 30*(7), 961–982. http://doi.org/10.1016/j.neubiorev.2006.03.001

Lucas, N., & Vuilleumier, P. (2008). Effects of emotional and non-emotional cues on visual search in neglect patients: Evidence for distinct sources of attentional guidance. *Neuropsychologia, 46*(5), 1401–1414. http://doi.org/10.1016/j.neuropsychologia.2007.12.027

Lundgren, K., & Brownell, H. H. (2010). Remediation of Theory of Mind impairments in brain-injured adults. In J. Guendouzi, F. Loncke, & M. J. Williams (Eds.), *Handbook of psycholinguistic and cognitive processes: Perspectives in communication disorders* (pp. 579–602). London, UK: Psychology Press.

Lundgren, K., Brownell, H. H., Cayer-Meade, C., Milione, J., & Kearns, K. (2011). Treating metaphor interpretation deficits subsequent to right hemisphere brain damage: Preliminary results. *Aphasiology, 25*(4), 456–474. http://doi.org/http://dx.doi.org/10.1080/02687038.2010.500809

Lundqvist, A., Grundstrom, K., Samuelsson, K., & Ronnberg, J. (2010). Computerized training of working memory in a group of patients suffering from acquired brain injury. *Brain Injury, 24*(10), 1173–1183. http://doi.org/10.3109/02699052.2010.498007

Luukkainen-Markkula, R., Tarkka, I. M., Pitkänen, K., Sivenius, J., & Hämäläinen, H. (2009). Rehabilitation of hemispatial neglect: A randomized study using either arm activation or visual scanning training. *Restorative Neurology and Neuroscience, 27*(6), 663–672. http://doi.org/10.3233/RNN-2009-0520

Luvizutto, J. G., Bazan, R., Braga, P. G., Resende, A. L., Bazan, G. S., & El Dib, R. (2015). Pharmacological interventions for unilateral spatial neglect after stroke. *Cochrane Database of Systematic Reviews* (11). http://doi.org/10.1002/14651858.CD010882.pub2.www.cochranelibrary.com

MacDonald, J. S. P., & Lavie, N. (2011). Visual perceptual load induces inattentional deafness. *Attention, Perception & Psychophysics, 73*(6), 1780–1789. http://doi.org/10.3758/s13414-011-0144-4

MacDonald, S. (2005). *Functional Assessment of Verbal Reasoning and Executive Strategies.* Guelph, Ontario: CCD Publishers.

MacDonald, S., & Wiseman-Hakes, C. (2010). Knowledge translation in ABI rehabilitation: A model for consolidating and applying the evidence for cognitive-communication interventions. *Brain Injury, 24*(3), 486–508. http://doi.org/10.3109/02699050903518118

Machner, B., Konemund, I., Sprenger, A., von der Gablentz, J., & Helmchen, C. (2014). Randomized controlled trial on hemifield eye patching and optokinetic stimulation in acute spatial neglect. *Stroke, 45*, 2465–2468.

Mackenzie, C., Begg, T., Brady, M., & Lees, K. R. (1997). The effects on verbal communication skills of right hemishere stroke in middle age. *Aphasiology, 11*(10), 929–945. http://doi.org/10.1080/02687039708249420

Mackenzie, C., Begg, T., Lees, K. R., & Brady, M. (1999). The communication effects of right brain damage on the very old and the not so old. *Journal of Neurolinguistics, 12,* 79–93.

Mackisack, E. L., Myers, P. S., & Duffy, J. R. (1987). Verbosity and labeling behavior: The performance of right hemisphere and non-brain-damaged adults on an inferential picture description task. In *Clinical Aphasiology Conference Proceedings* (pp. 143–151). Minneapolis, MN: BRK.

Majerus, S., Attout, L., D'Argembeau, A., Degueldre, C., Fias, W., Maquet, P., . . . Balteau, E. (2012). Attention supports verbal short-term memory via competition between dorsal and ventral attention networks. *Cerebral Cortex, 22*(5), 1086–1097. http://doi.org/10.1093/cercor/bhr174

Man, D. W. K., Fleming, J., Hohaus, L., & Shum, D. (2011). Development of the Brief Assessment of Prospective Memory (BAPM) for use with traumatic brain injury populations. *Neuropsychological Rehabilitation, 21*(6), 884–898. http://doi.org/10.1080/09602011.2011.627270

Maravita, A., McNeil, J., Malhotra, P., Greenwood, R., Husain, M., & Driver, J. (2003). Prism adaptation can improve contralesional tactile perception in neglect. *Neurology, 60*(11), 1829–1831. http://doi.org/10.1212/WNL.60.11.1829

Marcel, A. J., Tegnér, R., & Nimmo-Smith, I. (2004). Anosognosia for plegia: Specificity, extension, partiality and disunity of bodily unawareness. *Cortex, 40*(1), 19–40. http://doi.org/10.1016/S0010-9452(08)70919-5

Marini, A., Carlomagno, S., Caltagirone, C., & Nocentini, U. (2005). The role played by the right hemisphere in the organization of complex textual structures. *Brain and Language, 93*(1), 46–54. http://doi.org/10.1016/j.bandl.2004.08.002

Marinkovic, K., Baldwin, S., Courtney, M. G., Witzel, T., Dale, A. M., & Halgren, E. (2011). Right hemisphere has the last laugh: Neural dynamics of joke appreciation. *Cognitive, Affective & Behavioral Neuroscience*, *11*(1), 113–130. http://doi.org/10.3758/s13415-010-0017-7

Mark, V. W., Kooistra, C. A., & Heilman, K. M. (1988). Hemispatial neglect affected by nonneglected stimuli. *Neurology, 38*, 1207–1211.

Marschark, M., Katz, A. N., & Paivio, A. (1983). Dimensions of metaphor. *Journal of Psycholinguistic Research*, *12*(1), 17–40. http://doi.org/10.1007/BF01072712

Marsh, E. B., & Hillis, A. E. (2008). Dissociation between egocentric and allocentric visuospatial and tactile neglect in acute stroke. *Cortex*, *44*(9), 1215–1220. http://doi.org/10.1016/j.cortex.2006.02.002

Marsh, N. V., & Knight, R. G. (1991). Behavioral assessment of social competence following severe head injury. *Journal of Clinical and Experimental Neuropsychology*, *13*(5), 729–740. http://doi.org/10.1080/01688639108401086

Marshall, J. C., & Halligan, P. W. (1988). Blind-sight and insight in visuo-spatial neglect. *Nature, 336*, 766–767. http://dx.doi.org/10.1038/336766a0

Martelli, M., Arduino, L. S., & Daini, R. (2011). Two different mechanisms for omission and substitution errors in neglect dyslexia. *Neurocase*, *17*(2), 122–132. http://doi.org/10.1080/13554794.2010.498382

Martin, I., & McDonald, S. (2003). Weak coherence, no theory of mind, or executive dysfunction? Solving the puzzle of pragmatic language disorders. *Brain and Language*, *85*(3), 451–466. http://doi.org/10.1016/S0093-934X(03)00070-1

Martin, I., & McDonald, S. (2006). That can't be right! What causes pragmatic language impairment following right hemisphere damage? *Brain Impairment*, *7*(3), 202–211. http://doi.org/10.1375/brim.7.3.202

Martín-Rodríguez, J. F., & León-Carrión, J. (2010). Theory of mind deficits in patients with acquired brain injury: A quantitative review. *Neuropsychologia*, *48*(5), 1181–1191. http://doi.org/10.1016/j.neuropsychologia.2010.02.009

Marvel, C. L., & Desmond, J. E. (2010). Functional topography of the cerebellum in verbal working memory. *Neuropsychology Review*, *20*, 271–279. http://doi.org/10.1007/s11065-010-9137-7

Mashal, N., Faust, M., Hendler, T., & Jung-Beeman, M. (2007). An fMRI investigation of the neural correlates underlying the processing of novel metaphoric expressions. *Brain and Language*, *100*(2), 115–126. http://doi.org/10.1016/j.bandl.2005.10.005

Mashal, N., Faust, M., Hendler, T., & Jung-Beeman, M. (2008). Hemispheric differences in processing the literal interpretation of idioms: Converging evidence from behavioral and fMRI studies. *Cortex, 44*(7), 848–860. http://doi.org/10.1016/j.cortex.2007.04.004

Mashal, N., Faust, M., Hendler, T., & Jung-Beeman, M. (2009). An fMRI study of processing novel metaphoric sentences. *Laterality*, *14*(1), 30–54. http://doi.org/10.1080/13576500802049433

Matano, A., Iosa, M., Guariglia, C., Pizzamiglio, G., & Paolucci, S. (2015). Does outcome of neuropsychological treatment in patients with unilateral spatial neglect after stroke affect functional outcome? *European Journal of Physical Rehabilitation and Medicine*, *51*(737–743).

Mattingley, J. B., Driver, J., Beschin, N., & Robertson, I. H. (1997). Attentional competition between modalities: Extinction between touch and vision after right hemisphere damage. *Neuropsychologia*, *35*(6), 867–880. http://doi.org/10.1016/S0028-3932(97)00008-0

Maze, L. M., & Bakas, T. (2004). Factors associated with hospital arrival time for stroke patients. *Journal of Neuroscience Nursing*, *36*(3), 139–144. http://doi.org/10.1097/01376517-200406000-00005

McDonald, C. R., Bauer, R. M., Filoteo, J. V, Grande, L., Roper, S. N., Buchanan, R. J., & Gilmore, R. (2005). Semantic priming in patients with right frontal lobe lesions. *Journal of the International Neuropsychological Society, 11*(2), 132–143. Retrieved from http://www.ncbi.nlm.nih.gov/pub med/15962701

McDonald, S. (2000). Exploring the cognitive basis of right-hemisphere pragmatic language disorders. *Brain and Language, 75*(1), 82–107. http://doi.org/10.1006/brln .2000.2342

McDonald, S., & Wales, R. (1986). An investigation of the ability to process inferences in language following right hemisphere brain damage. *Brain and Language, 29*(1), 68–80. http://doi.org/10.1016/0093 -934X(86)90034-9

McFie, J., Piercy, M. F., & Zangwill, O. L. (1950). Visual-spatial agnosia associated with lesions of the right cerebral hemisphere. *Brain, 73*(2), 167–190.

McGann, W., Werven, G., & Douglas, M. M. (1997). Social competence and head injury: A practical approach. *Brain Injury, 11*(9), 621–628. Retrieved from http://www.ncbi .nlm.nih.gov/pubmed/9376830

McGlynn, S. M., & Schacter, D. L. (1989). Unawareness of deficits in neuropsychological syndromes. *Journal of Clinical and Experimental Neuropsychology, 11*(2), 143–205. http://doi.org/10.1080/01688638908400882

McKoon, G., & Ratcliff, R. (1990). Dimensions of inferences. In A. C. Graesser and G. H. Bower (Eds.), *Inferences and Text Comprehension*. San Diego, CA: Academic Press.

Medley, A. R., & Powell, T. (2010). Motivational Interviewing to promote self-awareness and engagement in rehabilitation following acquired brain injury: A conceptual review. *Neuropsychological Rehabilitation, 20*(4), 481–508. http://doi. org/10.1080/09602010903529610

Medvedev, A. V. (2014). Does the resting state connectivity have hemispheric asymmetry? A near-infrared spectroscopy study. *NeuroImage, 85* (Pt. 1), 400–407. http://doi.org/ 10.1016/j.neuroimage.2013.05.092

Meier, T. B., Naing, L., Thomas, L. E., Nair, V. A., Hillis, A. E., & Prabhakaran, V. (2011). Validating age-related functional imaging changes in verbal working memory with acute stroke. *Behavioural Neurology, 24*(3), 187–199. http://doi.org/10.3233/BEN-2011-0331

Meijer, R., VanLimbeek, L., Peusens, G., Rulkens, M., Dankoor, K., Vermeulen, M., & DeHaan, R. J. (2005). The Stroke Unit Discharge Guideline, a prognostic framework for the discharge outcome from the hospital stroke unit. A prospective cohort study. *Clinical Rehabilitation, 19*(1), 770–779.

Melby-Lervåg, M., & Hulme, C. (2013). Is working memory training effective? A meta-analytic review. *Developmental Psychology, 49*(2), 270–291. http://doi.org/10.1037/a00 28228

Menenti, L., Petersson, K. M., Scheeringa, R., & Hagoort, P. (2008). When elephants fly: Differential sensitivity of right and left inferior frontal gyri to discourse and world knowledge. *Journal of Cognitive Neuroscience, 21*(12), 2358–2368.

Menon-Nair, A., Korner-Bitensky, N., Wood-Dauphinee, S., & Robertson, E. (2006). Assessment of unilateral spatial neglect post stroke in Canadian acute care hospitals: Are we neglecting neglect ? *Clinical Rehabilitation, 20*, 623–634.

Mesulam, M.-M. (1981). A cortical network for directed attention and unilateral neglect. *Annals of Neurology, 10*, 309–325.

Mesulam, M.-M. (1985). Attention, confusional states, and neglect. In M. Mesulam (Ed.), *Principles of behavioral neurology* (pp. 125–168). Philadelphia, PA: F. A. Davis. ISSN: 1538-6899.

Mesulam, M.-M. (2002). The human frontal lobes: Transcending the default mode through contingent encoding. In D. T. Stuss & R. G. Knight (Eds.), *Principles of frontal lobe function* (pp. 8–30). New York, NY: Oxford University Press.

Middleton, L. E., Lam, B., Fahmi, H., Black, S. E., McIlroy, W. E., Stuss, D. T., . . . Turner, G.

R. (2014). Frequency of domain-specific cognitive impairment in sub-acute and chronic stroke. *NeuroRehabilitation, 34*(2), 305–312. http://doi.org/10.3233/NRE-131030

Milders, M., Fuchs, S., & Crawford, J. R. (2003). Neuropsychological impairments and changes in emotional and social behaviour following severe traumatic brain injury. *Journal of Clinical and Experimental Neuropsychology, 25*(2), 157–172. http://doi.org/10.1076/jcen.25.2.157.13642

Milders, M., Ietswaart, M., Crawford, J. R., & Currie, D. (2008). Social behavior following traumatic brain injury and its association with emotion recognition, understanding of intentions, and cognitive flexibility. *Journal of the International Neuropsychological Society, 14*(2), 318–326. http://doi.org/10.1017/S1355617708080351

Miller, L. A., & Radford, K. (2014). Testing the effectiveness of group-based memory rehabilitation in chronic stroke patients. *Neuropsychological Rehabilitation, 5*, 721–737. http://doi.org/10.1080/09602011.2014.894479

Miller, L. J., Myers, A., Prinzi, L., & Mittenberg, W. (2009). Changes in intellectual functioning associated with normal aging. *Archives of Clinical Neuropsychology, 24*(7), 681–688. http://doi.org/10.1093/arclin/acp072

Mograbi, D. C., & Morris, R. G. (2013). Discussion paper: Implicit awareness in anosognosia: Clinical observations, experimental evidence, and theoretical implications. *Cognitive Neuroscience, 4*(3-4), 181–209.

Monetta, L., Ouellet-Plamondon, C., & Joanette, Y. (2006). Simulating the pattern of right-hemisphere-damaged patients for the processing of the alternative metaphorical meanings of words: Evidence in favor of a cognitive resources hypothesis. *Brain and Language, 96*(2), 171–177. http://doi.org/10.1016/j.bandl.2004.10.014

Monrad-Krohn, G. H. (1947). Dysprosody or altered "melody of language." *Brain, 70*, 405–415.

Monti, A., Ferrucci, R., Fumagalli, M., Mameli, F., Cogiamanian, F., Ardolino, G., & Priori, A. (2013). Transcranial direct current stimulation (tDCS) and language. *Journal of Neurology, Neurosurgery, and Psychiatry, 84*(8), 832–842. http://doi.org/10.1136/jnnp-2012-302825

Moro, V., Pernigo, S., Zapparoli, P., Cordioli, Z., & Aglioti, S. M. (2011). Phenomenology and neural correlates of implicit and emergent motor awareness in patients with anosognosia for hemiplegia. *Behavioural Brain Research, 225*(1), 259–269. http://doi.org/10.1016/j.bbr.2011.07.010

Moya, K. L., Benowitz, L. I., Levine, D. N., & Finklestein, S. (1986). Covariant defects invisuospatial abilities and recall of verbal narrative after right hemisphere stroke. *Cortex, 22*(3), 381–397. http://doi.org/http://dx.doi.org.ezproxy.lib.uh.edu/10.1016/S0010-9452(86)80003-X

Murakami, T., Hama, S., Yamashita, H., Onoda, K., Hibino, S., Sato, H., . . . Kurisu, K. (2014). Neuroanatomic pathway associated with attentional deficits after stroke. *Brain Research, 1544*, 25–32. http://doi.org/10.1016/j.brainres.2013.11.029

Myers, J. E., & Myers, K. R. (1995). *Rey Complex Figure Test and Recognition Trial.* Lutz, FL: Psychological Assessment Resources.

Myers, P. S. (1979). Profiles of communication deficits in patients with right cerebral hemisphere damage: Implications for diagnosis and treatment. In *Clinical Aphasiology Conference Proceedings* (pp. 38–46).

Myers, P. S. (1991). Inference Failure: The underlying impairment in right-hemisphere communication disorders. In *Clinical Aphasiology Conference Proceedings* (pp. 167–180). Austin, TX: Pro-Ed.

Myers, P. S. (1999). Process-oriented treatment of right hemisphere communication disorders. *Seminars in Speech & Language, 20*(4), 319–333.

Myers, P. S. (1999). *Right hemisphere damage: Disorders of communication and cognition.* San Diego, CA: Singular.

Myers, P. S., & Brookshire, R. H. (1994). The effects of visual and inferential complexity on the picture descriptions of non-brain-damaged and right-hemisphere-damaged adults. *Clinical Aphasiology, 22,* 25–34.

Myers, P. S., & Linebaugh, C. W. (1981). Comprehension of idiomatic expressions by right-hemisphere-damaged adults. In R. Brookshire (Ed.), *Clinical Aphasiology Conference Proceedings* (pp. 254–261). Minneapolis, MN: BRK.

Myers, P. S., & Mackisack, E. L. (1986). Defining single versus dual definition idioms: The performance of right hemisphere and non-brain-damaged adults. In *Clinical Aphasiology Conference Proceedings* (pp. 267–274). Minneapoli, MN: BRK.

Nahemow, L., & Lawton, M. P. (2016). Toward an ecological theory of adaptation and aging. In W. Preiser (Ed.), *Environmental design research: Volume 1: Selected papers.* London, UK: Routledge.

Nardone, I. B., Ward, R., Fotopoulou, A., & Turnbull, O. H. (2007). Attention and emotion in anosognosia: Evidence of implicit awareness and repression? *Neurocase, 13*(5), 438–445. http://doi.org/10.1080/13554790701881749

Nasreddine, Z. S., Phillips, N. A., Bédirian, V., Charbonneau, S., Whitehead, V., Collin, I., . . . Chertkow, H. (2005). The Montreal Cognitive Assessment (MoCA): A brief screening tool for mild cognitive impairment. *Journal of the American Geriatrics Society, 53,* 695–699.

Nathanson, M., Bergman, P. S., & Gordon, G. G. (1952). Denial of illness: Its occurrence in one hundred consecutive cases of hemiplegia. *A.M.A. Archives of Neurology & Psychiatry, 68*(3), 380–387. http://doi.org/10.1001/archneurpsyc.1952.02320210090010

Navarro, M.-D., Alcañiz, M., Ferri, J., Lozano, J. A., Herrero, N., & Chirivella, J. (2009). Preliminary validation of Ecotrain-Cognitive: A virtual environment task for safe street crossing in acquired brain injury patients wtih and without unilateral spatial neglect. *Journal of CyberTherapy and Rehabilitation, 2*(3), 199–203.

Navarro, M.-D., Lloréns, R., Noé, E., Ferri, J., & Alcañiz, M. (2013). Validation of a low-cost virtual reality system for training street-crossing. A comparative study in healthy, neglected and non-neglected stroke individuals. *Neuropsychological Rehabilitation, 23*(4), 597–618. http://doi.org/10.1080/09602011.2013.806269

Newport, R., & Schenk, T. (2012). Prisms and neglect: What have we learned? *Neuropsychologia, 50*(6), 1080–1091. http://doi.org/10.1016/j.neuropsychologia.2012.01.023

Niemeier, J. P., Cifu, D. X., & Kishore, R. (2001). The lighthouse strategy: Improving the functional status of patients with unilateral neglect after stroke and brain injury using a visual imagery intervention. *Topics in Stroke Rehabilitation, 8,* 10–18.

Nijboer, T. C. W., & Jellema, T. (2012). Unequal impairment in the recognition of positive and negative emotions after right hemisphere lesions: A left hemisphere bias for happy faces. *Journal of Neuropsychology, 6*(1), 79–93. http://doi.org/10.1111/j.1748-6653.2011.02007.x

Noroozi, I., & Salehi, H. (2013). The effect of the etymological elaboration and rote memorization on learning idioms by Iranian EFL learners. *Journal of Language Teaching and Research, 4*(4), 845–851. http://doi.org/10.4304/jltr.4.4.845-851

Novakovic-Agopian, T., Chen, A. J.-W., Rome, S., Abrams, G., Castelli, H., Rossi, A., . . . Mckim, R. (2011). Rehabilitation of executive functioning with training in attention regulation applied to individually defined goals: A pilot study bridging theory, assessment, and treatment. *The Journal of Head Trauma Rehabilitation, 26*(5), 325–338. http://doi.org/10.1097/HTR.0b013e3181f1ead2

Nurmi, M. E., & Jehkonen, M. (2014). Assessing anosognosias after stroke: A review of the methods used and developed over the past 35 years. *Cortex, 61,* 43–63. http://doi.org/10.1016/j.cortex.2014.04.008

Nys, G. M. S., Van Zandvoort, M. J. E., De Kort, P. L. M., Jansen, B. P. W., Van Der Worp, H. B., Kappelle, L. J., & De Haan, E. H. F. (2005). Domain-specific cognitive recovery after first-ever stroke: A follow-up study of 111 cases. *Journal of the International Neuropsychological Society, 11*(07), 795–806. http://doi.org/10.1017/S1355617705050952

Oishi, K., Faria, A. V, Hsu, J., Tippett, D., Mori, S., & Hillis, A. E. (2015). Critical role of the right uncinate fasciculus in emotional empathy. *Annals of Neurology, 77*(1), 68–74. http://doi.org/10.1002/ana.24300

Oksala, N. K. J., Jokinen, H., Melkas, S., Oksala, A., Pohjasvaara, T., Hietanen, M., . . . Erkinjuntti, T. (2009). Cognitive impairment predicts poststroke death in long-term follow-up. *Journal of Neurology, Neurosurgery, and Psychiatry, 80*(11), 1230–1235. http://doi.org/10.1136/jnnp.2009.174573

Olesen, P. J., Westerberg, H., & Klingberg, T. (2004). Increased prefrontal and parietal activity after training of working memory. *Nature Neuroscience, 7*(1), 75–79. http://doi.org/10.1038/nn1165

Oliveri, M. (2011). Brain stimulation procedures for treatment of contralesional spatial neglect. *Restorative Neurology and Neuroscience, 29*(6), 421–425. http://doi.org/10.3233/RNN-2011-0613

Olswang, L. B., & Prelock, P. A. (2015). Bridging the gap between research and practice: Implementation science. *Journal of Speech, Language, and Hearing Research, 58,* S1818–S1826. http://doi.org/10.1044/2015_JSLHR-L-14-0305

Orbelo, D. M., Testa, J. A., & Ross, E. D. (2003). Age-related impairments in comprehending affective prosody with comparison to brain-damaged subjects. *Journal of Geriatric Psychiatry and Neurology, 16*(1), 44–52. http://doi.org/10.1177/0891988702250565

Orfei, M. D., Caltagirone, C., & Spalletta, G. (2009). The evaluation of anosognosia in stroke patients. *Cerebrovascular Diseases, 27*(3), 280–289. http://doi.org/10.1159/000199466

Orfei, M. D., Robinson, R. G., Prigatano, G. P., Starkstein, S., Rüsch, N., Bria, P., . . . Spalletta, G. (2007). Anosognosia for hemiplegia after stroke is a multifaceted phenomenon: A systematic review of the literature. *Brain: A Journal of Neurology, 130*(Pt 12), 3075–3090. http://doi.org/10.1093/brain/awm106

Osborne, C. L. (2000). *Over my head: A doctor's own story of head injury from the inside looking out.* Kansas City, MO: Andrews McMeel.

Osborne-Crowley, K., & McDonald, S. (2016). Hyposmia, not emotion perception, is associated with psychosocial outcome after severe traumatic brain injury. *Neuropsychology, 30*(7): 820–829.

Ota, H., Fujii, T., Suzuki, K., Fukatsu, R., & Yamadori, A. (2001). Dissociation of body-centered and stimulus-centered representations in unilateral neglect. *Neurology, 57*(11), 2064–2069. http://doi.org/10.1212/WNL.57.11.2064

Ownsworth, T. L., Fleming, J., Desbois, J., Strong, J., & Kuipers, P. (2006). A metacognitive contextual intervention to enhance error awareness and functional outcome following traumatic brain injury: A single-case experimental design. *Journal of the International Neuropsychological Society, 12*(1), 54–63.

Ownsworth, T., Fleming, J., Strong, J., Radel, M., Chan, W., & Clare, L. (2007). Awareness typologies, long-term emotional adjustment and psychosocial outcomes following acquired brain injury. *Neuropsychological Rehabilitation, 17*(2), 129–150. http://doi.org/10.1080/09602010600615506

Ownsworth, T., & Shum, D. (2008). Relationship between executive functions and productivity outcomes following stroke. *Disability and Rehabilitation, 30*(7), 531–540.

http://doi.org/779580111 [pii] 10.1080/09638280701355694 [doi]

Påhlman, U., Sävborg, M., & Tarkowski, E. (2012). Cognitive dysfunction and physical activity after stroke: The Gothenburg Cognitive Stroke Study in the Elderly. *Journal of Stroke and Cerebrovascular Diseases, 21*(8), 652–658. http://doi.org/10.1016/j.jstroke cerebrovasdis.2011.02.012

Pandian, J. D., Arora, R., Kaur, P., Sharma, D., Vishwambaran, D. K., & Arima, H. (2014). Mirror therapy in unilateral neglect after stroke (MUST trial): A randomized controlled trial. *Neurology, 83*(11), 1012–1017. http://doi.org/10.1212/WNL.0000000 000000773

Paolucci, S., Antonucci, G., Gialloreti, L. E., Traballesi, M., Lubich, S., Pratesi, L., & Palombi, L. (1996). Predicting stroke in-patient rehabilitation outcome: The prominent role of neuropsychological disorders. *European Journal of Neurology, 36*, 385–390.

Papagno, C., Curti, R., Rizzo, S., Crippa, F., & Colombo, M. R. (2006). Is the right hemisphere involved in idiom comprehension? A neuropsychological study. *Neuropsychology, 20*(5), 598–606. http://doi.org/10.1037/0894-4105.20.5.598

Park, N. W., & Ingles, J. L. (2001). Effectiveness of attention rehabilitation after an acquired brain injury: A meta-analysis. *Neuropsychology, 15*(2), 199–210. http://doi.org/10.1037//0894-4105.15.2.199

Park, Y. H., Jang, J.-W., Park, S. Y., Wang, M. J., Lim, J.-S., Baek, M. J., . . . Kim, S. (2015). Executive function as a strong predictor of recovery from disability in patients with acute stroke: A preliminary study. *Journal of Stroke and Cerebrovascular Diseases, 24*(3), 554–561. http://doi.org/10.1016/j.jstroke cerebrovasdis.2014.09.033

Parker, C., Power, M., Hamdy, S., Bowen, A., Tyrrell, P., & Thompson, D. G. (2004). Awareness of dysphagia by patients following stroke predicts swallowing performance. *Dysphagia, 19*(1), 28–35. http://doi.org/10.1007/s00455-003-0032-8

Passeri, A., Capotosto, P., & Di Matteo, R. (2015). The right hemisphere contribution to semantic categorization: A TMS study. *Cortex, 64*, 318–326. http://doi.org/10.1016/j.cortex.2014.11.014

Paulmann, S., & Pell, M. D. (2010). Contextual influences of emotional speech prosody on face processing: How much is enough? *Cognitive, Affective & Behavioral Neuroscience, 10*(2), 230–242. http://doi.org/10.3758/CA BN.10.2.230

Paulmann, S., Pell, M. D., & Kotz, S. A. (2008). Functional contributions of the basal ganglia to emotional prosody: Evidence from ERPs. *Brain Research, 1217*, 171–178. http://doi.org/10.1016/j.brainres.2008.04.032

Paulmann, S., Seifert, S., & Kotz, S. A. (2010). Orbito-frontal lesions cause impairment during late but not early emotional prosodic processing. *Social Neuroscience, 5*(1), 59–75. http://doi.org/10.1080/17470910903135668

Pavani, F., Husain, M., Ladavas, E., & Driver, J. (2004). Auditory deficits in visuospatial neglect patients. *Cortex, 40*, 347–365.

Pavani, F., Làdavas, E., & Driver, J. (2002). Selective deficit of auditory localisation in patients with visuospatial neglect. *Neuropsychologia, 40*(3), 291–301. http://doi.org/10.1016/S0028-3932(01)00091-4

Pearce, S. C., Stolwyk, R. J., New, P. W., & Anderson, C. (2016). Sleep disturbance and deficits of sustained attention following stroke. *Journal of Clinical and Experimental Neuropsychology, 38*(1), 1–11. http://doi.org/10.1080/13803395.2015.1078295

Pedersen, P. M., Jorgensen, H. S., Nakayama, H., Raaschou, H. O., & Olsen, T. S. (1996). General cognitive function in acute stroke: The Copenhagen Stroke Study. *Journal of Neurological Rehabilitation, 10*, 153–158.

Pedersen, P. M., Jorgensen, H. S., Nakayama, H., Raaschou, H. O., & Olsen, T. S. (1997). Hemineglect in acute stroke—incidence and prognostic implications: The Copenhagen Stroke Study. *American Journal of Physical Medicine and Rehabilitation, 76,* 122–127.

Pedroli, E., Serino, S., Cipresso, P., Pallavicini, F., & Riva, G. (2015). Assessment and rehabilitation of neglect using virtual reality: A systematic review. *Frontiers in Behavioral Neuroscience, 9*(August), 226. http://doi.org/10.3389/fnbeh.2015.00226

Peleg, O., & Eviatar, Z. (2017). Controlled semantic processes within and between the two cerebral hemispheres. *Laterality, 22*(1), 1–16. http://doi.org/10.1080/1357650X.2015.1092547

Peleg, O., Giora, R., & Fein, O. (2001). Salience and context effects: Two are better than one. *Metaphor and Symbol, 16*(3), 173–192. http://doi.org/10.1207/S15327868MS1603&4_4

Pell, M. D. (2005). Prosody–face interactions in emotional processing as revealed by the Facial Affect Decision Task. *Journal of Nonverbal Behavior, 29*(4), 193–215. http://doi.org/10.1007/s10919-005-7720-z

Pell, M. D. (2006). Cerebral mechanisms for understanding emotional prosody in speech. *Brain and Language, 96*(2), 221–234. http://doi.org/10.1016/j.bandl.2005.04.007

Pell, M. D. (2007). Reduced sensitivity to prosodic attitudes in adults with focal right hemisphere brain damage. *Brain and Language, 101*(1), 64–79. http://doi.org/10.1016/j.bandl.2006.10.003

Pell, M. D., Jaywant, A., Monetta, L., & Kotz, S. A. (2011). Emotional speech processing: Disentangling the effects of prosody and semantic cues. *Cognition & Emotion, 25*(5), 834–853. http://doi.org/10.1080/02699931.2010.516915

Pell, M. D., Monetta, L., Paulmann, S., & Kotz, S. A. (2009). Recognizing emotions in a foreign language. *Journal of Nonverbal Behavior, 33*(2), 107–120. http://doi.org/10.1007/s10919-008-0065-7

Perecman, E. (Ed.). (1983). *Cognitive processing in the right hemisphere.* New York, NY: Academic Press.

Pernet, L., Jughters, A., & Kerckhofs, E. (2013). The effectiveness of different treatment modalities for the rehabilitation of unilateral neglect in stroke patients: A systematic review. *NeuroRehabilitation, 33*(4), 611–620. http://doi.org/10.3233/NRE-130986

Philipose, L. E., Alphs, H., Prabhakaran, V., & Hillis, A. E. (2007). Testing conclusions from functional imaging of working memory with data from acute stroke. *Behavioural Neurology, 18*(1), 37–43.

Pia, L., Neppi-Modona, M., Ricci, R., & Berti, A. (2004). The anatomy of anosognosia for hemiplegia: A meta-analysis. *Cortex, 40*(2), 367–377. http://doi.org/10.1016/S0010-9452(08)70131-X

Pickens, S., Ostwald, S. K., Murphy-Pace, K., & Bergstrom, N. (2010). Systematic review of current executive function measures in adults with and without cognitive impairments. *International Journal of Evidence-Based Healthcare, 8*(3), 110–125. http://doi.org/10.1111/j.1744-1609.2010.00170.x

Pierce, S. R., & Buxbaum, L. J. (2002). Treatments of unilateral neglect: A review. *Archives of Physical Medicine and Rehabilitation, 83*(2), 256–268. http://doi.org/10.1053/apmr.2002.27333

Pitteri, M., Arcara, G., Passarini, L., Meneghello, F., & Priftis, K. (2013). Is two better than one? Limb activation treatment combined with contralesional arm vibration to ameliorate signs of left neglect. *Frontiers in Human Neuroscience, 7,* 1–10. http://doi.org/10.3389/fnhum.2013.00460

Pizzamiglio, L., Antonucci, G., Judica, A., Montenero, P., Razzanno, C., & Zoccolotti, P. (1992). Cognitive rehabilitation of the hemineglect disorder in chronic patients with unilateral right brain-damage. *Journal of Clinical and Experimental Neuropsychology, 14,* 901–923.

Plow, E. B., Cattaneo, Z., Carlson, T. A, Alvarez, G. A, Pascual-Leone, A., & Battelli, L. (2014). The compensatory dynamic of inter-hemispheric interactions in visuospatial attention revealed using rTMS and fMRI. *Frontiers in Human Neuroscience, 8*(April), 226. http://doi.org/10.3389/fnhum.2014.00226

Ponsford, J., & Kinsella, G. (1991). The use of a rating scale of attentional behaviour. *Neuropsychological Rehabilitation, 1*(4), 241–257. http://doi.org/http://dx.doi.org.ezproxy.lib.uh.edu/10.1080/09602019108402257

Posner, M. I. (1980). Orienting of attention. *Quarterly Journal of Experimental Psychology, 32*, 3–25. http://dx.doi.org/10.1080/00335558008248231

Posner, M. I., Walker, J. A., Friedrich, F. J., & Raphal, R. D. (1984). Effects of parietal lobe injury on convert orienting of visual attention. *Journal of Neuroscience, 4*, 1863–1864. PMID: 6737043

Poulin, V., Korner-Bitensky, N., Dawson, D. R., & Bherer, L. (2012). Efficacy of executive function interventions after stoke: A systematic review. *Topics in Stroke Rehabilitation, 19*(2), 158–171.

Powell, D., Kaplan, E., Whitla, D., Weintraub, S., Catlin, R., & Funkenstein, H. (2004). *MicroCog: Assessment of Cognitive Functioning.* San Antonio, TX: Pearson Assessment.

Price, C. J. (1998). The functional neuroanatomy of word comprehension and production. *Trends in Cognitive Sciences, 2*(8), 281–288. http://doi.org/http://dx.doi.org/10.1016/S1364-6613(98)01201-7

Priftis, K., Passarini, L., Pilosio, C., Meneghello, F., & Pitteri, M. (2013). Visual Scanning Training, Limb Activation Treatment, and Prism Adaptation for rehabilitating left neglect: Who is the winner? *Frontiers in Human Neuroscience, 7*(July), 1–12. http://doi.org/10.3389/fnhum.2013.00360

Prigatano, G. P. (1999). *Principles of neuropsychological rehabilitation.* New York. NY: Oxford University Press.

Prigatano, G. P. (2010a). Anosognosia after traumatic brain injury. In G. P. Prigatano (Ed.), *The study of anosognosia* (pp. 229–254). New York, NY: Oxford University Press.

Prigatano, G. P. (2010b). Historical observations relevant to the study of anosognosia. In G.P. Prigatano (Ed.), *The study of anosognosia* (pp. 3–14). New York, NY: Oxford University Press.

Prigatano, G. P. (2013). Denial, anosodiaphoria, and emotional reactivity in anosognosia: Commentary on Mograbi and Morris. *Cognitive Neuroscience, 4*(3-4), 201–202.

Prigatano, G. P., & Klonoff, P. S. (1998). A clinician's rating scale for evaluating impaired self-awareness and denial of disability after brain injury. *The Clinical Neuropsychologist, 12*(1), 56–67.

Prigatano, G. P., & Morrone-Strupinsky, J. (2010). Management and rehabilitation of persons with anosognosia and impaired self-awareness. In G. P. Prigatano (Ed.), *The study of anosognosia* (pp. 495–516). New York, NY: Oxford University Press.

Primativo, S., Arduino, L. S., De Luca, M., Daini, R., & Martelli, M. (2013). Neglect dyslexia: A matter of "good looking." *Neuropsychologia, 51*(11), 2109–2119. http://doi.org/10.1016/j.neuropsychologia.2013.07.002

Prutting, C. A., & Kirchner, D. M. (1987). A clinical appraisal of the pragmatic aspects of language. *The Journal of Speech and Hearing Disorders, 52*(2), 105–119. http://doi.org/10.1044/jshd.5202.105

Ptak, R., Di Pietro, M., & Schnider, A. (2012). The neural correlates of object-centered processing in reading: A lesion study of neglect dyslexia. *Neuropsychologia, 50*(6), 1142–1150. http://doi.org/10.1016/j.neuropsychologia.2011.09.036

Ptak, R., & Schnider, A. (2010). The dorsal attention network mediates orienting toward behaviorally relevant stimuli in spatial neglect. *Journal of Neuroscience, 30*(38), 12557–12565. http://doi.org/10.1523/JNEUROSCI.2722-10.2010

Ptak, R., & Schnider, A. (2011). The attention network of the human brain: Relating structural damage associated with spatial neglect to functional imaging correlates of spatial attention. *Neuropsychologia, 49*(11), 3063–3070. http://doi.org/10.1016/j.neuro psychologia.2011.07.008

Punt, T. D., & Riddoch, M. J. (2006). Motor neglect: Implications for movement and rehabilitation following stroke. *Disability and Rehabilitation, 28*(13-14), 857–864. http://doi.org/10.1080/09638280500535025

Qiang, W., Sonoda, S., Suzuki, M., Okamoto, S., & Saitoh, E. (2005). Reliability and validity of a wheelchair collision test for screening behavioral assessment of unilateral neglect after stroke. *American Journal of Physical Medicine and Rehabilitation, 84*(3), 161–166.

Rajah, M. N., & Esposito, M. D. (2005). Region-specific changes in prefrontal function with age: A review of PET and fMRI studies on working and episodic memory. *Brain, 128,* 1964–1983. http://doi.org/10.1093/brain/awh608

Rand, D., Eng, J. J., Liu-Ambrose, T., & Tawashy, A. E. (2010). Feasibility of a 6-month exercise and recreation program to improve executive functioning and memory of individuals with chronic stroke. *Neurorehabilitation and Neural Repair, 24*(8), 722–729. http://doi.org/10.1167/iovs.07-1072 .Complement-Associated

Randolph, C. (1998). *Repeatable Battery for the Assessment of Neuropsychological Status.* San Antonio, TX: The Psychological Corporation.

Raposo, A., & Marques, J. F. (2013). The contribution of fronto-parietal regions to sentence comprehension: Insights from the Moses illusion. *NeuroImage, 83,* 431–437. http://doi.org/10.1016/j.neuroimage.2013.06.052

Raskin, S., Buckheit, C., & Sherrod, C. (2010). *Memory for Intention Test.* Lutz, FL: Psychological Assessment Resources.

Rassafiani, M., & Sahaf, R. (2010). Single case experimental design: An overview. *International Journal of Therapy & Rehabilitation, 17*(6), 285–289. Retrieved from http://proxy .library.lincoln.ac.uk/login?url=http:// search.ebscohost.com/login.aspx?dire

ct=true&db=a9h&AN=51127712&site= eds-live&scope=site

Rath, J. F., Simon, D., Langenbahn, D. M., Sherr, R. L., & Diller, L. (2003). Group treatment of problem-solving deficits in outpatients with traumatic brain injury: A randomised outcome study. *Neuropsychological Rehabilitation, 13*(May 2015), 461–488. http://doi .org/10.1080/09602010343000039

Raz, N., Lindenberger, U., Rodrigue, K. M., Kennedy, K. M., Head, D., Williamson, A., . . . Acker, J. D. (2005). Regional brain changes in aging healthy adults: General trends, individual differences and modifiers. *Cerebral Cortex, 15*(11), 1676–1689. http://doi .org/10.1093/cercor/bhi044

Reilly, M., Machado, N., & Blumstein, S. E. (2015). Hemispheric lateralization of semantic feature distinctiveness. *Neuropsychologia, 75,* 99–108. http://doi.org/10.1016/j .neuropsychologia.2015.05.025

Reinhart, S., Schaadt, A. K., Adams, M., Leonhardt, E., & Kerkhoff, G. (2013). The frequency and significance of the word length effect in neglect dyslexia. *Neuropsychologia, 51*(7), 1273–1278. http://doi.org/10.1016/j .neuropsychologia.2013.03.006

Reinhart, S., Schindler, I., & Kerkhoff, G. (2011). Optokinetic stimulation affects word omissions but not stimulus-centered reading errors in paragraph reading in neglect dyslexia. *Neuropsychologia, 49*(9), 2728–2735. http://doi.org/10.1016/j.neuro psychologia.2011.05.022

Reinhart, S., Schunck, A., Schaadt, A. K., Adams, M., Simon, A., & Kerkhoff, G. (2016). Assessing neglect dyslexia with compound words. *Neuropsychology, August* (Advance online publication).

Reitan, R. M. (1958). Validity of the Trail Making test as an indicator of organic brain damage. *Perceptual and Motor Skills, 8,* 271–276.

Reyna, V. F., & Brainerd, J. (1995). Fuzzy-trace theory: An interim synthesis. *Learning and Individual Differences, 7*(1), 1–75. Retrieved from http://www.sciencedirect.com/science/article/pii/1041608095900314

Reynolds, C. R., & Voress, J. K. (2007). *Test of Memory and Learning* (2nd ed.). Austin, TX: Pro-Ed.

Richardson, C., & Blake, M. (June, 2017). *The effectiveness of gist reasoning training in an adult with right-hemiphere damage*. Presented at Clinical Aphasiology Conference, Snowbird, UT.

Rinaldi, M. C., Marangolo, P., & Baldassarri, F. (2004). Metaphor comprehension in right brain-damaged patients with visuo-verbal and verbal material: A dissociation (re)considered. *Cortex, 40*, 479–490. http://doi.org/http://dx.doi.org/10.1016/S0010-9452(08)70141-2

Robertson, I. H. (2001). Do we need the "lateral" in unilateral neglect? Spatially nonselective attention deficits in unilateral neglect and their implications for rehabilitation. *NeuroImage, 14*(1 Pt. 2), S85–S90. http://doi.org/10.1006/nimg.2001.0838

Robertson, I. H. (2014). Right hemisphere role in cognitive reserve. *Neurobiology of Aging, 35*(6), 1375–1385. http://doi.org/10.1016/j.neurobiolaging.2013.11.028

Robertson, I. H., Manly, T., Beschin, N., Daini, R., Haeske-Dewick, H., Homberg, V., . . . Weber, E. (1997). Auditory sustained attention is a marker of unilateral spatial neglect. *Neuropsychologia, 35*(12), 1257–1532.

Robertson, I. H., McMillan, T. M., MacLeod, E., Edgeworth, J., & Brock, D. (2002). Rehabilitation by limb activation training reduces left-sided motor impairment in unilateral neglect patients. *Neuropsychological Rehabilitation, 12*, 439–454.

Robertson, I. H., Tegnér, R., Tham, K., Lo, A., & Nimmo-Smith, I. (1995). Sustained attention training for unilateral neglect: Theoretical and rehabilitation implications. *Journal of Clinical and Experimental Neuropsychology, 17*, 416–430. http://doi.org/10.1080/01688639508405133

Robertson, I. H., Ward, T., Ridgeway, V., & Nimmo-Smith, I. (1994). *Test of Everyday Attention*. Oxford, UK: Pearson Assessment.

Robinson, F. P. (1970). *Effective study*. New York, NY: Harper and Row.

Robinson, R. G. (1997). Neuropsychiatric consequences of stroke. *Annual Review of Medicine, 48*, 217–219.

Rode, G., Pisella, L., Marsal, L., Mercier, S., Rossetti, Y., & Boisson, D. (2006). Prism adaptation improves spatial dysgraphia following right brain damage. *Neuropsychologia, 44*(12), 2487–2493. http://doi.org/10.1016/j.neuropsychologia.2006.04.002

Rode, G., Rossetti, Y., Boisson, D., Bernard, C., & Cedex, L. (2001). Prism adaptation improves representational neglect. *Neuropsychologia, 39*, 1250–1254.

Rogalski, Y., Altmann, L. J. P., Plummer-D'Amato, P., Behrman, A. L., & Marsiske, M. (2010). Discourse coherence and cognition after stroke: A dual task study. *Journal of Communication Disorders, 43*(3), 212–224. http://doi.org/10.1016/j.jcomdis.2010.02.001

Ronchi, R., Algeri, L., Chiapella, L., Gallucci, M., Spada, M. S., & Vallar, G. (2016). Left neglect dyslexia: Perseveration and reading error types. *Neuropsychologia, 89*, 453–464. http://doi.org/10.1016/j.neuropsychologia.2016.07.023

Ronchi, R., Rode, G., Cotton, F., Farnè, A., Rossetti, Y., & Jacquin-Courtois, S. (2013). Remission of anosognosia for right hemiplegia and neglect after caloric vestibular stimulation. *Restorative Neurology and Neuroscience, 31*(1), 19–24. http://doi.org/10.3233/RNN-120236

Rorden, C., Hjaltason, H., Fillmore, P., Fridriksson, J., Kjartansson, O., Magnusdottir, S., & Karnath, H.-O. (2012). Allocentric neglect strongly associated with egocentric neglect. *Neuropsychologia, 50*(6), 1151–1157. http://doi.org/10.1016/j.neuropsychologia.2012.03.031

Rorden, C., & Karnath, H.-O. (2010). A simple measure of neglect severity. *Neuropsychologia, 48*(9), 2758–2763. http://doi.org/10.1016/j.neuropsychologia.2010.04.018

Rosen, M. L., Stern, C. E., Michalka, S. W., Devaney, K. J., & Somers, D. C. (2015). Influences of long-term memory-guided attention and stimulus-guided attention on visuospatial representations within human intraparietal sulcus. *Journal of Neuroscience, 35*(32), 11358–11363. http://doi.org/10.1523/JNEURO SCI.1055-15.2015

Rosenbek, J. C., Crucian, G. P., Leon, S. A, Hieber, B., Rodriguez, A. D., Holiway, B., . . . Gonzalez-Rothi, L. (2004). Novel treatments for expressive aprosodia: A phase I investigation of cognitive linguistic and imitative interventions. *Journal of the International Neuropsychological Society, 10*, 786–793. http://doi.org/10.1017/S135561770410502X

Rosenbek, J. C., Rodriguez, A. D., Hieber, B., Leon, S. A., Crucian, G. P., Ketterson, T. U., . . . Gonzalez Rothi, L. J. (2006). Effects of two treatments for aprosodia secondary to acquired brain injury. *The Journal of Rehabilitation Research and Development, 43*(3), 379. http://doi.org/10.1682/JRRD.2005.01.0029

Ross, E. D. (1981). The aprosodias: Functional-anatomic organization of the affective components of language in the right hemisphere. *Archives of Neurology, 38*(9), 561–569. doi:10.1001/archneur.1981.00510090055006.

Ross, E. D. (1984). Right hemisphere's role in language, affective behavior and emotion. *Trends in Neurosciences, 7*(9), 342–346. http://doi.org/10.1016/S0166-2236(84)80085-5

Ross, E. D., & Monnot, M. (2011). Affective prosody: What do comprehension errors tell us about hemispheric lateralization of emotions, sex and aging effects, and the role of cognitive appraisal. *Neuropsychologia, 49*(5), 866–877. http://doi.org/10.1016/j.neuropsychologia.2010.12.024

Roth, R. M., Isquith, P. K., & Gioia, G. A. (2005). *Behavioural Regulation Index of Executive Function–Adult Version.* Lutz, FL: Psychological Assessment Resources.

Roussel, M., Dujardin, K., Hénon, H., & Godefroy, O. (2012). Is the frontal dysexecutive syndrome due to a working memory deficit? Evidence from patients with stroke. *Brain, 135*(7), 2192–2201. http://doi.org/10.1093/brain/aws132

Royle, J., & Lincoln, N. B. (2008). The Everyday Memory Questionnaire-revised: Development of a 13-item scale. *Disability and Rehabilitation, 30*(2), 114–121. http://doi.org/10.1080/09638280701223876

Rueckert, L., & Grafman, J. (1996). Sustained attention deficits in patients with right frontal lesions. *Neuropsychologia, 34*(10), 953–963. http://doi.org/10.1016/0028-3932(96)00016-4

Ruff, R. M. (1995). *Ruff 2 & 7 Selective Attention Test.* Lutz, FL: Psychological Assessment Resources.

Ruff, R. M., Light, R. H., & Evans, R. W. (1987). The ruff figural fluency test: A normative study with adults. *Developmental Neuropsychology, 3*, 37–51. http://doi.org/10.1080/87565648709540362

Rusconi, M. L., & Carelli, L. (2012). Long-term efficacy of prism adaptation on spatial neglect: Preliminary results on different spatial components. *The Scientific World Journal, 2012*, 1–8. http://doi.org/10.1100/2012/618528

Russell, C., Malhotra, P., Deidda, C., & Husain, M. (2013). Dynamic attentional modulation of vision across space and time after right hemisphere stroke and in ageing. *Cortex, 49*(7), 1874–1883. http://doi.org/10.1016/j.cortex.2012.10.005

Russowsky, A., & Vanderhasselt, M. (2014). Working memory improvement with non-invasive brain stimulation of the dorsolateral prefrontal cortex: A systematic review and meta-analysis. *Brain and Cognition, 86*, 1–9. http://doi.org/10.1016/j.bandc.2014.01.008

Rymarczyk, K., & Grabowska, A. (2007). Sex differences in brain control of prosody. *Neuropsychologia, 45*(5), 921–930. http://doi.org/10.1016/j.neuropsychologia.2006.08.021

Sackett, D. L., Straus, S. E., Richardson, W. S., Rosenberg, W., & Haynes, R. B. (Eds.).

(2000). *Evidence-based medicine: How to practice and teach EBM.* New York:, NY Churchill Livingstone.

Saevarsson, S., Halsband, U., & Kristjansson, A. (2011). Designing rehabilitation programs for neglect: Could 2 be more than 1+1? *Applied Neuropsychology, 18*(2), 95–106. http://doi.org/10.1080/09084282.2010.547774

Salas Riquelme, C. E., Radovic, D., Castro, O., & Turnbull, O. H. (2015). Internally and externally generated emotions in people with acquired brain injury: Preservation of emotional experience after right hemisphere lesions. *Frontiers in Psychology, 6*(February), 101. http://doi.org/10.3389/fpsyg.2015.00101

Salat, D. H., Buckner, R. L., Snyder, A. Z., Greve, D. N., Desikan, R. S. R., Busa, E., . . . Fischl, B. (2004). Thinning of the cerebral cortex in aging. *Cerebral Cortex, 14*(7), 721–730. http://doi.org/10.1093/cercor/bhh032

Saldert, C., & Ahlsén, E. (2007). Inference in right hemisphere damaged individuals' comprehension: The role of sustained attention. *Clinical Linguistics & Phonetics, 21*(8), 637–655. http://doi.org/10.1080/02699200701431056

Salvato, G., Sedda, A., & Bottini, G. (2014). In search of the disappeared half of it: 35 years of studies on representational neglect. *Neuropsychology, 28*(5), 1–11. http://doi.org/10.1037/neu0000062

Sampanis, D. S., & Riddoch, J. (2013). Motor neglect and future directions for research. *Frontiers in Human Neuroscience, 7*(March), 110. http://doi.org/10.3389/fnhum.2013.00110

Savazzi, S. (2003). Object-based versus object-centred neglect in reading words. *Neurocase, 9*(3), 203–212. http://doi.org/10.1076/neur.9.3.203.15560

Saxton, M. E., Younan, S. S., & Lah, S. (2013). Social behaviour following severe traumatic brain injury: Contribution of emotion perception deficits. *NeuroRehabilitation, 33*(2), 263–271. http://doi.org/10.3233/NRE-130954

Scandinavian Stroke Study Group. (1985). Research in progress: Multicenter trial of hemodilution in ischemic stroke background and study protocol. *Stroke, 16*(5), 885–890.

Schenkenberg, T., Bradford, D. C., & Ajax, E. T. (1980). Line bisection and unilateral visual neglect in patients with neurologic impairment. *Neurology, 30*(5), 509–517.

Schindler, I., Clavagnier, S., Karnath, H. O., Derex, L., & Perenin, M. T. (2006). A common basis for visual and tactile exploration deficits in spatial neglect? *Neuropsychologia, 44*(8), 1444–1451. http://doi.org/10.1016/j.neuropsychologia.2005.12.003

Schirmer, A., Alter, K., Kotz, S. A., & Friederici, A. D. (2001). Lateralization of prosody during language production: A lesion study. *Brain and Language, 76*(1), 1–17. http://doi.org/10.1006/brln.2000.2381

Schirmer, A., & Kotz, S. A. (2006). Beyond the right hemisphere: Brain mechanisms mediating vocal emotional processing. *Trends in Cognitive Sciences, 10*(1), 24–30. http://doi.org/10.1016/j.tics.2005.11.009

Schmidt, J., Lannin, N., Fleming, J., & Ownsworth, T. (2011). Feedback interventions for impaired self-awareness following brain injury: A systematic review. *Journal of Rehabilitation Medicine, 43*(8), 673–680. http://doi.org/10.2340/16501977-0846

Schmidt, M. (1996). *Rey Auditory Verbal Learning Test.* Torrance, CA: Western Psychological Services.

Schmolck, H., Buffalo, E. A., & Squire, L. R. (2000). Memory distortions develop over time: Recollections of the O.J. Simpson trial verdict after 15 and 32 months. *Psychological Science* (August 1998), 39–45.

Schneiderman, E. I., Murasugi, K. G., & Saddy, J. D. (1992). Story arrangement ability in right brain damaged patients. *Brain and Language, 43*, 107–120.

Schober, M.F. (1998). Different kinds of conversational perspective-taking. In S. R. Fussel & R. J. Kreuz (Eds.), *Social and cognitive approaches to interpersonal communica-*

tion (pp. 145–174). Mahwah, NJ: Lawrence Erlbaum.

Schoo, L. A., van Zandvoort, M. J. E., Reijmer, Y. D., Biessels, G. J., Kappelle, L. J., & Postma, A. (2014). Absolute and relative temporal order memory for performed activities following stroke. *Journal of Clinical and Experimental Neuropsychology, 36*(6), 648–658. http://doi.org/10.1080/13803395.2014.925093

Schretlen, D. (1997). *Brief Test of Attention*. Lutz, FL: Psychological Assessment Resources.

Schrijnemaekers, A.-C., Smeets, S. M. J., Ponds, R. W. H. M., van Heugten, C. M., & Rasquin, S. (2013). Treatment of unawareness of deficits in patients with acquired brain injury: A systematic review. *The Journal of Head Trauma Rehabilitation, 29*(June), 14–18. http://doi.org/10.1097/01.HTR.0000438117.63852.b4

Schwartz, M. F., Buxbaum, L. J., Ferraro, M., Veramonti, T., & Segal, M. (2002). *Naturalistic Action Test*. Oxford, UK: Pearson Assessment.

Scottish Intercollegiate Guidelines Network (SIGN). (2013). *Brain injury rehabilitation in adults*. Edinburgh: SIGN publication no. 130. Retrieved from http://www.sign.ac.uk

Searle, J. R. (1969). *Speech acts: An essay in the philosophy of language*. Cambridge, UK: Cambridge University Press.

Searleman, A. (1977). A review of right hemisphere linguistic capabilities. *Psychological Bulletin, 84*(3), 503–528. http://doi.org/10.1037/0033-2909.84.3.503

Shah-Basak, P. P., Norise, C., Garcia, G., Torres, J., Faseyitan, O., & Hamilton, R. H. (2015). Individualized treatment with transcranial direct current stimulation in patients with chronic non-fluent aphasia due to stroke. *Frontiers in Human Neuroscience, 9*(April), 201. http://doi.org/10.3389/fnhum.2015.00201

Shallice, T. (1982). Specific impairments in planning. *Philosophical Transactions of the Royal Society of London. Series B, Biological Sciences, 25*(298), 199–209.

Shallice, T., & Burgess, P. W. (1991). Deficits in strategy application following frontal lobe damage in man. *Brain, 114*, 727–741.

Shamay-Tsoory, S. G., Tomer, R., & Aharon-Peretz, J. (2005). The neuroanatomical basis of understanding sarcasm and its relationship to social cognition. *Neuropsychology, 19*(3), 288–300. http://doi.org/10.1037/0894-4105.19.3.288

Shamay-Tsoory, S. G., Tomer, R., Berger, B. D., Goldsher, D., & Aharon-Peretz, J. (2005). Impaired "affective theory of mind" is associated with right ventromedial prefrontal damage. *Cognitive and Behavioral Neurology, 18*(1), 55–67. http://doi.org/10.1097/01.wnn.0000152228.90129.99

Shamay-Tsoory, S. G., Tomer, R., Goldsher, D., Berger, B. D., & Aharon-Peretz, J. (2004). Impairment in cognitive and affective empathy in patients with brain lesions: Anatomical and cognitive correlates. *Journal of Clinical and Experimental Neuropsychology, 26*(8), 1113–1127. http://doi.org/10.1080/13803390490515531

Shammi, P., & Stuss, D. T. (1999). Humour appreciation: A role of the right frontal lobe. *Brain, 122*, 657–666. Retrieved from papers2://publication/uuid/BF7DE5B9-70CF-4A2A-B04F-FA2E301BCA9B

Shapiro, K. L., Arnell, K. M., & Raymond, J. E. (1997). The attentional blink. *Trends in Cognitive Science, 1*(8), 291–296. http://doi.org/10.1016/S1364-6613(97)01094-2

Sherer, M., Bergloff, P., Boake, C., High Jr, W., & Levin, E. (1998). The Awareness Questionnaire: Factor structure and internal consistency. *Brain Injury, 12*(1), 63–68. http://doi.org/10.1080/026990598122863

Sherer, M., Hart, T., & Nick, T. G. (2003). Measurement of impaired self-awareness after traumatic brain injury: A comparison of the Patient Competency Rating Scale and the Awareness Questionnaire. *Brain Injury, 17*(1), 25–37.

Sherratt, S. (2007). Right brain damage and the verbal expression of emotion: A preliminary investigation. *Aphasiology, 21*(3-4), 320–339.

http://doi.org/10.1080/026870306009
11401

Sherratt, S., & Bryan, K. (2012). Discourse production after right brain damage: Gaining a comprehensive picture using a multi-level processing model. *Journal of Neurolinguistics*, 25(4), 213–239. http://doi.org/10.1016/j.jneuroling.2012.01.001

Shulman, G. L., Pope, D. L. W., Astafiev, S. V., McAvoy, M. P., Snyder, A. Z., & Corbetta, M. (2010). Right hemisphere dominance during spatial selective attention and target detection occurs outside the dorsal frontoparietal network. *Journal of Neuroscience*, 30(10), 3640–3651. http://doi.org/10.1523/JNEUROSCI.4085-09.2010

Siegal, M., Carrington, J., & Radel, M. (1996). Theory of mind and pragmatic understanding following right hemisphere damage. *Brain and Language*, 53(1), 40–50. http://doi.org/10.1006/brln.1996.0035

Siéroff, E. (2015). Acquired spatial dyslexia. *Annals of Physical and Rehabilitation Medicine*. http://doi.org/10.1016/j.rehab.2015.07.004

Simons, D. J. (2000). Attentional capture and inattentional blindness. *Trends in Cognitive Science*, 4(4), 147–155. Retrieved from http://www.ncbi.nlm.nih.gov/pubmed/10740279

Simons, D. J., & Chabris, C. F. (1999). Gorillas in our midst: Sustained inattentional blindness for dynamic events. *Perception*, 28, 1059–1074.

Singer, M. (1994). Discourse inference processes. In M. A. Gernsbacher (Ed.), *Handbook of psycholinguistics*. San Diego, CA: Academic Press.

Sivan, A. B. (1992). *Bention Visual Retention Test* (5th ed.). San Antonio, TX: Psychological Corporation.

Sivan, M., Neumann, V., Kent, R., Stroud, A., & Bhakta, B. B. (2010). Pharmacotherapy for treatment of attention deficits after non-progressive acquired brain injury. A systematic review. *Clinical Rehabilitation*, 24(2), 110–121. http://doi.org/10.1177/0269215509343234

Skidmore, E. R., Dawson, D. R., Butters, M. A., Grattan, E. S., Juengst, S. B., Whyte, E. M., . . . Becker, J. T. (2015). Strategy training shows promise for addressing disability in the first 6 months after stroke. *Neurorehabilitation and Neural Repair*, 29(7), 668–676. http://doi.org/10.1177/1545968314562113

Smigasiewicz, K., Asanowicz, D., Westphal, N., & Verleger, R. (2014). Bias for the left visual field in rapid serial visual presentation: Effects of additional salient cues suggest a critical role of attention. *Journal of Cognitive Neuroscience*, 27(2), 266–279. http://doi.org/10.1162/jocn_a_00714

Smith, A. (1973). *Symbol Digit Modalities Test*. Torrance, CA: Western Psychological Services.

Smith, D. V, Clithero, J. A., Rorden, C., & Karnath, H.-O. (2013). Decoding the anatomical network of spatial attention. *Proceedings of the National Academy of Sciences*, 110(4), 1518–1523. http://doi.org/10.1073/pnas.1210126110

Smith, G., Della Sala, S., Logie, R. H., & Maylor, E. A. (2000). Prospective and retrospective memory in normal ageing and dementia: A questionnaire study. *Memory*, 8(5), 311–321.

Snaphaan, L., & De Leeuw, F. E. (2007). Poststroke memory function in nondemented patients: A systematic review on frequency and neuroimaging correlates. *Stroke*, 38(1), 198–203. http://doi.org/10.1161/01.STR.0000251842.34322.8f

Sohlberg, M. M., Avery, J., Kennedy, M., Ylvisaker, M., Coelho, C., Turkstra, L., & Yorkston, K. (2003). Practice guidelines for direct attention training. *Journal of Medical Speech-Language Pathology*, 11(3), xix–xxxix. http://doi.org/10.1037/t00741-000

Sohlberg, M. M., Kennedy, M., Avery, J., Coelho, C., Turkstra, L., Ylvisaker, M., & Yorkston, K. (2007). Evidence-based practice for the use of external aids as a memory compensation technique. *Journal of Medical Speech-Language Pathology*, 15(1), xv–li.

Sohlberg, M. M., & Mateer, C. A. (2001). *Cognitive rehabilitation: An integrative neuropsychological approach*. New York, NY: Guilford Press.

Sohlberg, M. M., & Mateer, C. (2011). *Attention Process Training-3*. Youngsville, NC: Lash & Associates.

Sohlberg, M. M., McLaughlin, K. A., Pavese, A., Heidrich, A., & Posner, M. I. (2000). Evaluation of Attention Process Training and brain injury education in persons with acquired brain injury. *Neuropsychology, 22*(5), 656–676. http://doi.org/10.1076/1380-3395(2000)22:5;1-9;FT656

Sohlberg, M. M., & Turkstra, L. S. (2011). *Optimizing cognitive rehabilitation: Effective instructional methods*. New York, NY: Guilford Press.

Soto, D., Rotshtein, P., & Kanai, R. (2014). Parietal structure and function explain human variation in working memory biases of visual attention. *NeuroImage, 89*, 289–296. http://doi.org/10.1016/j.neuroimage.2013.11.036

Spache G. D., & Berge P. C. (1966). *The arts of efficient reading*. New York, NY: Macmillan.

Sparing, R., Dafotakis, M., Meister, I. G., Thirugnanasambandam, N., & Fink, G. R. (2008). Enhancing language performance with non-invasive brain stimulation—A transcranial direct current stimulation study in healthy humans. *Neuropsychologia, 46*(1), 261–268. http://doi.org/10.1016/j.neuropsychologia.2007.07.009

Sperber, D., & Wilson, D. (1981). Irony and the use-mention distinction. In P. Cole (Ed.), *Radical pragmatics* (pp. 295–318). New York, NY: Academic Press.

Spikman, J. M., Boelen, D. H. E., Pijnenborg, G. H. M., Timmerman, M. E., van der Naalt, J., & Fasotti, L. (2013). Who benefits from treatment for executive dysfunction after brain injury? Negative effects of emotion recognition deficits. *Neuropsychological Rehabilitation, 23*(6), 824–845. http://doi.org/10.1080/09602011.2013.826138

Spinazzola, L., Pia, L., Folegatti, A., Marchetti, C., & Berti, A. (2008). Modular structure of awareness for sensorimotor disorders: Evidence from anosognosia for hemiplegia and anosognosia for hemianaesthesia.

Neuropsychologia, 46(3), 915–926. http://doi.org/10.1016/j.neuropsychologia.2007.12.015

Spotorno, S., & Faure, S. (2011). The right hemisphere advantage in visual change detection depends on temporal factors. *Brain and Cognition, 77*(3), 365–371. http://doi.org/10.1016/j.bandc.2011.09.003

Spreng, R. N., & Grady, C. L. (2010). Patterns of brain activity supporting autobiographical memory, prospection, and theory of mind, and their relationship to the default mode network. *Journal of Cognitive Neuroscience, 22*, 1112–1123. http://doi.org/10.1162/jocn.2009.21282

Srikanth, V. K., Thrift, A. G., Saling, M. M., Anderson, J. F. I., Dewey, H. M., MacDonell, R. A. L., & Donnan, G. A. (2003). Increased risk of cognitive impairment 3 months after mild to moderate first-ever stroke: A community-based prospective study of nonaphasic English-speaking survivors. *Stroke: A Journal of Cerebral Circulation, 34*(5), 1136–1143. http://doi.org/10.1161/01.STR.0000069161.35736.39

Starkstein, S. E., Jorge, R. E., & Robinson, R. G. (2010). The frequency, clinical correlates, and mechanism of anosognosia after stroke. *Canadian Journal of Psychiatry, 55*(6), 355–361.

Steinel, M. P., Hulstijn, J. H., & Steinel, W. (2007). Second language idiom learning in a paired-associate paradigm: Effects of direction of learning, direction of testing, idiom imageability, and idiom transparency. *Studies in Second Language Acquisition, 29*(03), 449–484. http://doi.org/10.1017/S0272263107070271

St. Jacques, P. L., & Schacter, D. L. (2013). Modifying memory: selectively enhancing and updating personal memories for a museum tour by reactivating them. *Psychological Science, 24*(4), 537–543. http://doi.org/10.1177/0956797612457377

Stone, S., Wilson, B., Wroot, A., Halligan, P. W., Lange, L. S., Marshall, J. C., & Greenwood, R. J. (1991). The assessment of visuo-spatial neglect after acute stroke. *Journal of Neurology, Neurosurgery & Psychiatry, 54*, 345–350.

Stroop, J. R. (1935) Studies of interference in serial verbal reactions. *Journal of Experimental Psychology, 18,* 643–662.

Sturm, W., Longoni, F., Weis, S., Specht, K., Herzog, H., Vohn, R., . . . Willmes, K. (2004) Functional reorganisation in patients with right hemisphere stroke after training of alertness: A longitudinal PET and fMRI study in eight cases. *Neuropsychologia, 42,* 434–450. doi:10.1016/j.neuropsychologia.2003.09.001

Sturm, W., Thimm, M., Kust, J., Karbe, H., & Fink, G. R. (2006). Alertness-training in neglect: Behavioral and imaging results. *Restorative Neurology and Neuroscience, 24,* 371–384.

Sturm, W., & Willmes, K. (1991). Efficacy of a reaction training on various attentional and cognitive functions in stroke patients. *Neuropsychological Rehabilitation, 1,* 259–280.

Sturm, W., Willmes, K., Orgass, B., & Hartje, W. (1997). Do specific attention deficits need specific training? *Neuropsychological Rehabilitation, 7,* 81–103.

Stuss, D. T., Alexander, M. P., Floden, D., Binns, M. A., Levine, B., McIntosh, . . . Hevenor, S. J. (2002). Fractionation and localization of distinct frontal lobe processes: Evidence from focal lesions in humans. In D. T. Stuss & R. T. Knight (Eds.), *Principles of frontal lobe function* (pp. 392–407). New York, NY: Oxford University Press.

Surian, L., & Siegal, M. (2001). Sources of performance on theory of mind tasks in right hemisphere-damaged patients. *Brain and Language, 78*(2), 224–232. http://doi.org/10.1006/brln.2001.2465

Tamietto, M., Geminiani, G., Genero, R., & de Gelder, B. (2007). Seeing fearful body language overcomes attentional deficits in patients with neglect. *Journal of Cognitive Neuroscience, 19,* 445–454. doi:10.1162/jocn.2007.19.3.445

Tate, R. L., McDonald, S., Perdices, M., Togher, L., Schultz, R., & Savage, S. (2008). Rating the methodological quality of single-subject designs and n-of-1 trials: Introducing the Single-Case Experimental Design (SCED) Scale. *Neuropsychological Rehabilitation, 18*(4), 385–401. http://doi.org/10.1080/09602010802009201

Thiebaut de Schotten, M., ffytche, D. H., Bizzi, A., Dell'Acqua, F., Allin, M., Walshe, M., . . . Catani, M. (2011). Atlasing location, asymmetry and inter-subject variability of white matter tracts in the human brain with MR diffusion tractography. *NeuroImage, 54*(1), 49–59. http://doi.org/10.1016/j.neuroimage.2010.07.055

Thimm, M., Fink, G. R., Küst, J., Karbe, H., Willmes, K., & Sturm, W. (2009). Recovery from hemineglect: Differential neurobiological effects of optokinetic stimulation and alertness training. *Cortex: A Journal Devoted to the Study of the Nervous System and Behavior, 45*(7), 850–862. http://doi.org/10.1016/j.cortex.2008.10.007

Thomas, N. A., Wignall, S. J., Loetscher, T., & Nicholls, M. E. R. (2014). Searching the expressive face: Evidence for both the right hemisphere and valence-specific hypotheses. *Emotion, 14*(5), 962–977.

Thompson, C. K. (2006). Single subject controlled experiments in aphasia: The science and the state of the science. *Journal of Communication Disorders, 39*(4), 266–291. http://doi.org/10.1016/j.jcomdis.2006.02.003

Tipper, S. P., & Behrmann, M. (1996). Object-centered not scene-based visual neglect. *Journal of Experimental Psychology: Human Perception and Performance, 22*(5), 1261–1278. http://doi.org/10.1037//0096-1523.22.5.1261

Titone, D. A., & Connine, C. M. (1994). Descriptive norms for 171 idiomatic expressions: familiarity, compositionality, predictability, and literality. *Metaphor and Symbolic Activity, 9*(4), 247–270.

Togher, L., Power, E., Rietdijk, R., McDonald, S., & Tate, R. (2012). An exploration of participant experience of a communication training program for people with traumatic brain injury and their communication partners. *Disability and Rehabilitation, 34*(18), 1562–1574. http://doi.org/10.3109/09638288.2012.656788

Togher, L., Power, E., Tate, R., McDonald, S., & Rietdijk, R. (2010). Measuring the social interactions of people with traumatic brain injury and their communication partners: The adapted Kagan scales. *Aphasiology, 24*(6–8), 914–927. http://doi.org/10.1080/02687030903422478

Togher, L., Taylor, C., Aird, V., & Grant, S. (2006). The impact of varied speaker role and communication partner on the communicative interactions of a person with traumatic brain injury: A single case study using systemic functional linguistics. *Brain Impairment, 7*(3), 190–201. http://doi.org/10.1375/brim.7.3.190

Toglia, J. P. (1993). *Contextual Memory Test*. San Antonio, TX: Pearson Assessment.

Toglia, J., Fitzgerald, K. A., O'Dell, M. W., Mastrogiovanni, A. R., & Lin, C. D. (2011). The Mini-Mental State Examination and Montreal Cognitive Assessment in persons with mild subacute stroke: Relationship to functional outcome. *Archives of Physical Medicine and Rehabilitation, 92*(5), 792–798. http://doi.org/10.1016/j.apmr.2010.12.034

Tompkins, C. A. (1991a). Automatic and effortful processing of emotional intonation after right or left hemisphere brain damage. *Journal of Speech and Hearing Research, 34*, 820–830.

Tompkins, C. A. (1991b). Redundancy enhances emotional inferencing by right- and left-hemisphere-damaged adults. *Journal of Speech and Hearing Research, 34*, 1142–1149.

Tompkins, C. A. (1995). *Right hemisphere communication disorders: Theory and management*. San Diego, CA: Singular.

Tompkins, C. A., Baumgaertner, A., Lehman, M. T., & Fassbinder, W. (2000). Mechanisms of discourse comprehension impairment after right hemisphere brain damage: Suppression in lexical ambiguity resolution. *Journal of Speech, Language, and Hearing Research, 43*, 62–78.

Tompkins, C. A., Blake, M. T., Scharp, V. L., Meigh, K. M., & Wambaugh, J. L. (May, 2013). *Implicit treatment of underlying comprehension processes improves narrative comprehension in right hemisphere brain damage*. Paper presented at Clinical Aphasiology Conference, Tucson, AZ.

Tompkins, C. A., Blake, M. T., Wambaugh, J., & Meigh, K. (2011). A novel, implicit treatment for language comprehension processes in right hemisphere brain damage: Phase I data. *Aphasiology, 25*(6-7), 789–799. http://doi.org/10.1080/02687038.2010.539784

Tompkins, C. A., Bloise, C. G. R., Timko, M. L., & Baumgaertner, A. (1994). Working memory and inference revision in brain-damaged and normally aging adults. *Journal of Speech and Hearing Research, 37*(4), 896–912. http://doi.org/10.1044/jshr.3704.896

Tompkins, C. A., Boada, R., & McGarry, K. (1992). The access and processing of familiar idioms by brain-damaged and normally aging adults. *Journal of Speech and Hearing Research, 35*, 626–637.

Tompkins, C. A., Boada, R., McGarry, K., Jones, J., Rahn, A. E., & Ranier, S. (1992). Connected speech characteristics of right-hemisphere-damaged adults: A re-examination. In *Clinical Aphasiology Conference Proceedings* (pp. 113–122). Austin, TX: Pro-Ed.

Tompkins, C. A., Fassbinder, W., Blake, M. L., Baumgaertner, A., & Jayaram, N. (2004). Inference generation during text comprehension by adults with right hemisphere brain damage: Activation failure versus multiple activation. *Journal of Speech, Language, and Hearing Research, 47*, 1308–1395.

Tompkins, C. A., Fassbinder, W., Scharp, V. L., & Meigh, K. M. (2008). Activation and maintenance of peripheral semantic features of unambiguous words after right hemisphere brain damage in adults. *Aphasiology, 22*(2), 119–138. http://doi.org/10.1080/02687030601040861

Tompkins, C. A., Lehman, M. T., & Baumgaert-ner, A. (1999). Suppression and infer-ence revision in right brain-damaged and non-brain-damaged adults. *Aphasi-ology, 13*(9-11), 725–742. http://doi.org/10.1080/026870399401830

Tompkins, C. A., Lehman-Blake, M. T., Baumgaertner, A., & Fassbinder, W. (2001). Mechanisms of discourse comprehen-sion after right hemisphere brain damage: Inferential ambiguity resolution. *Journal of Speech, Language, and Hearing Research, 44*, 400–415.

Tompkins, C. A., Scharp, V. L., Fassbinder, W., Meigh, K. M., & Armstrong, E. M. (2008). A different story on "Theory of Mind" deficit in adults with right hemisphere brain dam-age. *Aphasiology, 22*(1), 42–61. http://doi.org/10.1080/02687030600830999

Tompkins, C. A., Scharp, V. L., Meigh, K., Blake, M. L., & Wambaugh, J. (2012). Gen-eralization of a novel, implicit treatment for coarse coding deficit in right hemisphere brain damage: A single subject experiment. *Aphasiology, 26*(5), 689–708. http://doi.org/10.1080/02687038.2012.676869

Tompkins, C. A., Scharp, V. L., Meigh, K. M., & Fassbinder, W. (2008). Coarse coding and discourse comprehension in adults with right hemisphere brain damage. *Aphasiol-ogy, 22*(2), 204–223. http://doi.org/10.1080/02687030601125019

Tompkins, C. A., & Scott, A. G. (2013). Treat-ment of right hemisphere disorders. In I. Papathanasiou, P. Coppens, & C. Potagas (Eds.), *Aphasia and related neurogenic com-munication disorders* (1st ed., pp. 345–364). Burlington, MA: Jones & Bartlett.

Turan, T. N., Hertzberg, V., Weiss, P., McClel-lan, W., Presley, R., Krompf, K., . . . Fran-kel, M. R. (2005). Clinical characteristics of patients with early hospital arrival after stroke symptom onset. *Journal of Stroke and Cerebrovascular Diseases, 14*(6), 272–277. http://doi.org/10.1016/j.jstrokecerebro vasdis.2005.07.002

Turkstra, L. S., Brehm, S. E., & Montgomery, E. B. (2006). Analysing conversational dis-course after traumatic brain injury: Isn't it about time? *Brain Impairment, 7*(03), 234–245. http://doi.org/10.1375/brim.7.3.234

Turkstra, L., Ylvisaker, M., Coelho, C., Ken-nedy, M., Sohlberg, M. M., Avery, J., & Yorkston, K. (2005). Practice guidelines for standardized assessment for persons with traumatic brain injury. *Journal of Medical Speech-Language Pathology.* http://doi.org/10.1037/t05377-000

Turnbull, O. H., Fotopoulou, A., & Solms, M. (2014). Anosognosia as motivated unaware-ness: the "defense" hypothesis revisited. *Cortex; a Journal Devoted to the Study of the Nervous System and Behavior, 61*, 18–29. http://doi.org/10.1016/j.cortex.2014.10.008

Turner, C. E., & Kellogg, R. T. (2016). Category membership and semantic coding in the cerebral hemispheres. *The American Journal of Psychology, 129*(2), 135–148.

Trahan, D. E., & Larrabee, G. (1988). *Continuous Visual Memory Test: Professional Manual.* Lutz, FL: Psychological Assessment Resources.

Tranel, D., Rudrauf, D., Vianna, E. P. M., & Damasio, H. (2008). Does the clock drawing test have focal neuroanatomical correlates? *Neuropsychology, 22*(5), 553–562. http://doi .org/10.1037/0894-4105.22.5.553.DOES

Treisman, A. (2009). Attention: Theoretical and psychological perspectives. In M. S. Gazzan-iga (Ed.), *The cognitive neurosciences* (4th ed., pp. 189–204). Cambridge, MA: MIT Press.

Trupe, E. H., & Hillis, A. E. (1985). Paucity vs. verbosity: Another analysis of right hemi-sphere communication deficits. In *Clinical Aphasiology* (pp. 83–96). Rockville, MD: BRK.

Tsirlin, I., Dupierrix, E., Chokron, S., Coquil-lart, S., & Ohlmann, T. (2009). Uses of vir-tual reality for diagnosis, rehabilitation and study of unilateral spatial neglect: Review and analysis. *Cyberpsychology & Behavior, 12*(2), 175–181. http://doi.org/10.1089/cpb .2008.0208

Tulving, E. (2002). Episodic memory: From mind to brain. *Annual Review of Psychology, 53*, 1–25.

Tulving, E., & Craik, F. I. M. (Eds.). (2000). *The Oxford handbook of memory.* New York, NY: Oxford University Press.

Turunen, K. E. A., Laari, S. P. K., Kauranen, T. V, Mustanoja, S., Tatlisumak, T., & Poutiainen, E. (2016). Executive impairment is associated with impaired memory performance in working-aged stroke patients. *Journal of the International Neuropsychological Society,* 1–10. http://doi.org/10.1017/S1355617716000205

Tyler, S. C., Dasgupta, S., Agosta, S., Battelli, L., & Grossman, E. D. (2015). Functional connectivity of parietal cortex during temporal selective attention. *Cortex, 65*, 195–207. http://doi.org/10.1016/j.cortex.2015.01.015

Uddin, L. Q., Kelly, A. M. C., Biswal, B. B., Castellanos, F. X., & Milham, M. P. (2009). Functional connectivity of default mode network components: Correlation, autocorrelation, and causality. *Human Brain Mapping, 30*(2). http://doi.org/doi:10.1002/hbm.20531

Umarova, R. M., Reisert, M., Beier, T. U., Kiselev, V. G., Kloppel, S., Kaller, C. P., . . . Weiller, C. (2014). Attention-network specific alterations of structural connectivity in the undamaged white matter in acute neglect. *Human Brain Mapping, 35*(9), 4678–4692. http://doi.org/10.1002/hbm.22503

Vallar, G. (1993). The anatomical basis of spatial hemi-neglect in humans. In I. H. Robertson & J. C. Marshall (Eds.), *Unilateral neglect: Clinical and experimental studies.* Hillsdale, NJ: Lawrence Erlbaum. ISBN: 0-86377-218-8

Vallar, G., Burani, C., & Arduino, L. S. (2010). Neglect dyslexia: A review of the neuropsychological literature. *Experimental Brain Research, 206*(2), 219–235. http://doi.org/10.1007/s00221-010-2386-0

Vallar, G., & Perani, D. (1986). The anatomy of unilateral neglect after right-hemisphere stroke lesions: A clinical/CT-scan correlation study in man. *Neuropsychologia, 24*, 609–622. DOI 10.1016/0028-3932(86)90001-1

Vallar, G., Rusconi, M. L., Geminiani, G., & Berti, A. (1991). Visual and nonvisual neglect after unilateral brain lesions: Modulation by visual input. *International Journal of Neuroscience, 61*(3–4), 229–239.

van den Broek, P. (1994). Comprehension and memory of narrative texts: Inferences and coherence. In M. A. Gernsbacher (Ed.), *Handbook of psycholinguistics.* San Diego, CA: Academic Press.

van Ettinger-Veenstra, H. M., Ragnehed, M., Hällgren, M., Karlsson, T., Landtblom, A.-M., Lundberg, P., & Engström, M. (2010). Right-hemispheric brain activation correlates to language performance. *NeuroImage, 49*(4), 3481–3488. http://doi.org/10.1016/j.neuroimage.2009.10.041

Vanhalle, C., Lemieux, S., Joubert, S., Goulet, P., Ska, B., & Joanettee, Y. (2000). Processing of speech acts by right hemisphere brain-damaged patients: An ecological approach. *Aphasiology, 14*(July 2015), 1127–1141. http://doi.org/10.1080/02687030050174665

Van Lancker, D. R., & Kempler, D. (1987). Comprehension of familiar phrases by left- but not by right-hemisphere damaged patients. *Brain and Language, 32*, 265–277.

Van Lancker Sidtis, D., Pachana, N., Cummings, J. L., & Sidtis, J. J. (2006). Dysprosodic speech following basal ganglia insult: Toward a conceptual framework for the study of the cerebral representation of prosody. *Brain and Language, 97*(2), 135–153. http://doi.org/10.1016/j.bandl.2005.09.001

Van Lancker Sidtis, D., & Postman, W. A. (2006). Formulaic expressions in spontaneous speech of left- and right-hemisphere–damaged subjects. *Aphasiology, 20*(5), 411–426. http://doi.org/10.1080/02687030500538148

van Zandvoort, M. J. E., Kessels, R. P. C., Nys, G. M. S., de Haan, E. H. F., & Kappelle, L. J. (2005). Early neuropsychological evaluation in patients with ischaemic stroke provides valid information. *Clinical Neurology and Neurosurgery, 107*(5), 385–392. http://doi.org/10.1016/j.clineuro.2004.10.012

Vertosick, F. (1996). *When the air hits your brain: Tales of neurosurgery* (pp. 213–214). New York, NY: Fawcett Crest.

Vigneau, M., Beaucousin, V., Hervé, P. Y., Jobard, G., Petit, L., Crivello, F., . . . Tzourio-Mazoyer, N. (2011). What is right-hemisphere contribution to phonological, lexico-semantic, and sentence processing? Insights from a meta-analysis. *NeuroImage, 54*(1), 577–593. http://doi.org/10.1016/j.neuroimage.2010.07.036

Viorst, J. (1972). *Alexander and the terrible, horrible, no good, very bad day.* New York, NY: Simon & Schuster.

Virk, S., Williams, T., Brunsdon, R., Suh, F., & Morrow, A. (2015). Cognitive remediation of attention deficits following acquired brain injury: A systematic review and meta-analysis. *NeuroRehabilitation, 36*(3), 367–377. http://doi.org/10.3233/NRE-151225

Viscogliosi, C., Belleville, S., Desrosiers, J., Caron, C. D., & Ska, B. (2011). Participation after a stroke: Changes over time as a function of cognitive deficits. *Archives of Gerontology and Geriatrics, 52*(3), 336–343. http://doi.org/10.1016/j.archger.2010.04.020

Visser-Keizer, A. C., Meyboom-deJong, B., Deelman, B. G., Berg, I. J., & Gerritsen, M. J. J. (2002). Subjective changes in emotion, cognition and behavior after stroke: Factors affecting the perception of patients and partners. *Journal of Clinical and Experimental Neuropsychology, 24*(8), 1032–1045.

Vocat, R., Staub, F., Stroppini, T., & Vuilleumier, P. (2010). Anosognosia for hemiplegia: A clinical-anatomical prospective study. *Brain: A Journal of Neurology, 133*(Pt. 12), 3578–3597. http://doi.org/10.1093/brain/awq297

Vocat, R., & Vuilleumier, P. (2010). Neuroanatomy of impaired body awareness in anosognosia and hysteria: A multi-component account. In G. P. Prigatano (Ed.), *The study of anosognosia.* New York, NY: Oxford University Press.

Vossel, S., Weiss, P. H., Eschenbeck, P., & Fink, G. R. (2012). Anosognosia, neglect, extinction and lesion site predict impairment of daily living after right-hemispheric stroke. *Cortex, 49*(7), 1782–1789. http://doi.org/10.1016/j.cortex.2012.12.011

Vromen, A., Verbunt, J. A., Rasquin, S., & Wade, D. T. (2011). Motor imagery in patients with a right hemisphere stroke and unilateral neglect. *Brain Injury, 25*(4), 387–393. http://doi.org/10.3109/02699052.2011.558041

Vuilleumier, P., Schwartz, S., Clarke, K., Husain, M., & Driver, J. (2002). Testing memory for unseen visual stimuli in patients with extinction and spatial neglect. *Journal of Cognitive Neuroscience, 14,* 875–886. http://doi.org/10.1162/089892902760191108

Vuilleumier, P., Schwartz, S., Husain, M., Clarke, K., & Driver, J. (2001). Implicit processing and learning of visual stimuli in parietal extinction and neglect. *Cortex, 37*(5), 741–744. http://doi.org/10.1016/S0010-9452(08)70629-4

Wagner, A. D., Shannon, B. J., Kahn, I., & Buckner, R. L. (2005). Parietal lobe contributions to episodic memory retrieval. *Trends in Cognitive Sciences, 9*(9), 445–453. http://doi.org/10.1016/j.tics.2005.07.001

Walker, J. P., Daigle, T., & Buzzard, M. (2002). Hemispheric specialisation in processing prosodic structures: Revisited. *Aphasiology, 16*(12), 1155–1172. http://doi.org/10.1080/02687030244000392

Walker, J. P., Pelletier, R., & Reif, L. (2004). The production of linguistic prosodic structures in subjects with right hemisphere damage. *Clinical Linguistics & Phonetics, 18*(2), 85–106. http://doi.org/10.1080/02699200310001596179

Wallander, J. L., Conger, A. J., & Conger, J. C. (1985). Development and evaluation of a behaviorally referenced rating system for heterosocial skills. *Behavioral Assessment, 7,* 137–153.

Wambaugh, J. L. (2007). The evidence-based practice and practice-based evidence nexus. *Perspectives on Neurophysiology and Neurogenic Speech and Language Disorders, 14,* 14–18. Retrieved from http://sig2perspectives.pubs.asha.org

Wapner, W., Hamby, S., & Gardner, H. (1981). The role of the right hemisphere in the apprehension of complex linguistic materials. *Brain and Language, 14,* 15–33. http://doi.org/http://dx.doi.org/10.1016/0093-934X(81)90061-4

Warden, D. L., Gordon, B., McAllister, T. W., Silver, J. M., Barth, J. T., Bruns, J., . . . Zitnay, G. (2006). Guidelines for the pharmacologic treatment of neurobehavioral sequelae of traumatic brain injury. *Journal of Neurotrauma, 23*(10), 1468–1501. http://doi.org/10.1089/neu.2006.23.1468

Warrington, E. K. (1984). *Recognition Memory Test.* Torrance, CA: Western Psychological Services.

Watkins, C. L., Auton, M. F., Deans, C. F., Dickinson, H. A., Jack, C. E., Lightbody, C. E., . . . Leathley, M. J. (2007). Motivational interviewing early after acute stroke: A randomized, controlled trial. *Stroke, 38*(3), 1004–1009.

Wechsler, D. (2009). *Wechsler Memory Scale, Fourth Edition.* San Antonio, TX: Pearson Assessment.

Wee, J. Y. M., & Hopman, W. M. (2005). Stroke impairment predictors of discharge function, length of stay, and discharge destination in stroke rehabilitation. *American Journal of Physical Medicine and Rehabilitation, 84,* 604–612. http://doi.org/10.1097/01.phm.0000171005.08744.ab

Weed, E., McGregor, W., Feldbaek Nielsen, J., Roepstorff, A., & Frith, U. (2010). Theory of Mind in adults with right hemisphere damage: What's the story? *Brain and Language, 113*(2), 65–72. http://doi.org/10.1016/j.bandl.2010.01.009

Weingarten, S., Garb, C. T., Blumenthal, D., Boren, S. A., & Brown, G. D. (2000). Improving preventive care by prompting physicians. *Archives of Internal Medicine, 160,* 301–308.

Weinstein, E. A. (1994). Hemineglect and extinction. *Neuropsychological Rehabilitation, 4*(2), 221–224. http://doi.org/10.1080/09602019408402288

Weinstein, E. A., & Kahn, R. L. (1955). Denial of illness: Symbolic and physiological aspects. In *Denial of illness: Symbolic and physiological aspects.* Springfield, IL: Charles C.Thomas. http://doi.org/http://dx.doi.org/10.1037/11516-000

Weissman, D. H., & Prado, J. (2012). Heightened activity in a key region of the ventral attention network is linked to reduced activity in a key region of the dorsal attention network during unexpected shifts of covert visual spatial attention. *NeuroImage, 61*(4), 798–804. http://doi.org/10.1016/j.neuroimage.2012.03.032

Wen, X., Yao, L., Liu, Y., & Ding, M. (2012). Causal interactions in attention networks predict behavioral performance. *Journal of Neuroscience, 32*(4), 1284–1292. http://doi.org/10.1523/JNEUROSCI.2817-11.2012

Westerberg, H., Jacobaeus, H., Hirvikoski, T., Clevberger, P., Ostensson, M.-L., Bartfai, A., & Klingberg, T. (2007). Computerized working memory training after stroke—A pilot study. *Brain Injury: [BI], 21*(1), 21–29. http://doi.org/10.1080/02699050601148726

Weylman, S. T., & Brownell, H. H. (1989). Appreciation of indirect requests by left- and right- brain-damaged patients: The effects of verbal context and conventionality of wording. *Brain and Language, 36,* 580–591. http://doi.org/http://dx.doi.org/10.1016/0093-934X(89)90087-4

Wild, B., Rodden, F. A., Grodd, W., & Ruch, W. (2003). Neural correlates of laughter and humour. *Brain, 126*(10), 2121–2138. http://doi.org/10.1093/brain/awg226

Wildgruber, D., Ethofer, T., Grandjean, D., & Kreifelts, B. (2009). A cerebral network model of speech prosody comprehension. *International Journal of Speech-Language Pathology, 11*(4), 277–281. http://doi.org/10.1080/17549500902943043

Wildgruber, D., Hertrich, I., Riecker, A., Erb, M., Anders, S., Grodd, W., & Ackermann, H. (2004). Distinct frontal regions subserve evaluation of linguistic and emotional aspects of speech intonation. *Cerebral Cortex, 14*(12), 1384–1389. http://doi.org/10.1093/cercor/bhh099

Wildgruber, D., Riecker, A., Hertrich, I., Erb, M., Grodd, W., Ethofer, T., & Ackermann, H. (2005). Identification of emotional intonation evaluated by fMRI. *NeuroImage*, 24(4), 1233–1241. http://doi.org/10.1016/j.neuroimage.2004.10.034

Wilkinson, D., Sakel, M., & Milberg, W. (2011). The practical constraints of developing new therapies for hemi-spatial neglect in the US and UK. *NeuroRehabilitation*, 28(2), 163–165. http://doi.org/10.3233/NRE-2011-0645

Wilson, B. A., Cockburn, J., Baddeley, A. D., Ivani-Chalian, R., & Aldrich, F. (2003). *Rivermead Behavioural Memory Test* (2nd ed.). Oxford, UK: Pearson Assessment.

Wilson, B. A., Cockburn, J., & Halligan, P. W. (1987). *Behavioural Inattention Test*. Oxford, UK: Pearson Assessment.

Wilson, B. A., Emslie, H., Evans, J. J., Alderman, N., & Burgess, P. W. (1996) *Behavioural Assessment of the Dysexecutive Syndrome (BADS)*. Oxford, UK: Pearson Assessment.

Wilson, B. A., Evans, J. J., Emslie, H., Foley, J., Shiel, A., Watson, P., . . . Groot, Y. (2005). *Cambridge Prospective Memory Test (CAM-PROMPT)*. Oxford, UK: Pearson Assessment.

Winner, E., Brownell, H. H., Happe, F., Blum, A., & Pincus, D. (1998). Distinguishing lies from jokes: Theory of Mind deficits and discourse interpretation in right hemisphere brain-damaged patients. *Brain and Language*, 62(62), 89–106. http://doi.org/ http://dx.doi.org/10.1006/brln.1997.1889

Witteman, J., van Ijzendoorn, M. H., van de Velde, D., van Heuven, V. J. J. P., & Schiller, N. O. (2011). The nature of hemispheric specialization for linguistic and emotional prosodic perception: A meta-analysis of the lesion literature. *Neuropsychologia*, 49(13), 3722–3738. http://doi.org/10.1016/j.neuropsychologia.2011.09.028

Wolfe, J., & Robertson, L. (Eds.). (2012). *From perception to consciousness: Searching with Anne Treisman*. New York, NY: Oxford University Press.

Wolpert, D. M., Ghahramani, Z., & Jordan, M. I. (1995). An internal model for senso-rimotor integration. *Science*, 269, 1880–1882. http://doi.org/10.1126/science.7569931

World Health Organization. (2002). Towards a common language for functioning, disability and health: ICF, 1–22. http://doi.org/WHO/EIP/GPE/CAS/01.3

Xu, J., Kemeny, S., Park, G., Frattali, C., & Braun, A. (2005). Language in context: Emergent features of word, sentence, and narrative comprehension. *NeuroImage*, 25(3), 1002–1015. http://doi.org/10.1016/j.neuroimage.2004.12.013

Xuan, B., Mackie, M. A., Spagna, A., Wu, T., Tian, Y., Hof, P. R., & Fan, J. (2016). The activation of interactive attentional networks. *NeuroImage*, 129, 308–319. http://doi.org/10.1016/j.neuroimage.2016.01.017

Yan, L.-R., Wu, Y.-B., Hu, D.-W., Qin, S.-Z., Xu, G.-Z., Zeng, X.-H., & Song, H. (2012). Network asymmetry of motor areas revealed by resting-state functional magnetic resonance imaging. *Behavioural Brain Research*, 227(1), 125–133. http://doi.org/10.1016/j.bbr.2011.11.012

Yang, J. (2014). The role of the right hemisphere in metaphor comprehension: A meta-analysis of functional magnetic resonance imaging studies. *Human Brain Mapping*, 35(1), 107–122. http://doi.org/10.1002/hbm.22160

Yang, N. Y. H., Zhou, D., Chung, R. C. K., Li-Tsang, C. W. P., & Fong, K. N. K. (2013). Rehabilitation interventions for unilateral neglect after stroke: A systematic review from 1997–2012. *Frontiers in Human Neuroscience*, 7, 1–11.

Yeh, Z.-T., & Tsai, C.-F. (2014). Impairment on theory of mind and empathy in patients with stroke. *Psychiatry and Clinical Neurosciences*, 68(8), 612–620. http://doi.org/10.1111/pcn.12173

Ylvisaker, M., & Feeney, T. J. (1998). *Collaborative brain injury intervention: Positive everyday routines*. San Diego, CA: Singular

Ylvisaker, M., Szekeres, S. F., & Feeney, T. J. (2008). Communication disorders associated with traumatic brain injury. In R. Chapey (Ed.), *Language intervention strategies in apha-*

sia and related neurogenic communication disorders (5th ed., pp. 879–962). Philadelphia, PA: Lippincott Williams & Wilkins.

Yochim, B. P., Kender, R., Abeare, C., Gustafson, A., & Whitman, R. D. (2005). Semantic activation within and across the cerebral hemispheres: What's left isn't right. *Laterality, 10*(2), 131–148. http://doi.org/10.1080/13576500342000356

Yokoyama, O., Miura, N., Watanabe, J., Takemoto, A., Uchida, S., Sugiura, M., . . . Nakamura, K. (2010). Right frontopolar cortex activity correlates with reliability of retrospective rating of confidence in short-term recognition memory performance. *Neuroscience Research, 68*(3), 199–206. http://doi.org/10.1016/j.neures.2010.07.2041

Yonelinas, A. P. (2002). The nature of recollection and familiarity: A review of 30 years of research. *Journal of Memory and Language, 517,* 441–517. http://doi.org/10.1006/jmla.2002.2864

Yorkston, K. M., & Beukelman, D. R. (1980). An analysis of connected speech samples of aphasic and normal speakers. *Journal of Speech and Hearing Disorders, 45,* 27–36. http://doi.org/doi:10.1044/jshd.4501.27

You, D. S., Kim, D. Y., Chun, M. H., Jung, S. E., & Park, S. J. (2011). Cathodal transcranial direct current stimulation of the right Wernicke's area improves comprehension in subacute stroke patients. *Brain and Language, 119*(1), 1–5. http://doi.org/10.1016/j.bandl.2011.05.002

Youngjohn, J. R., & Altman, I. M. (1989). A performance-based group approach to the treatment of anosognosia and denial. *Rehabilitation Psychology, 34*(3), 217–222.

Zickefoose, S., Hux, K., Brown, J., & Wulf, K. (2013). Let the games begin: A preliminary study using Attention Process Training-3 and Lumosity™ brain games to remediate attention deficits following traumatic brain injury. *Brain Injury, 27*(6), 707–716. http://doi.org/10.3109/02699052.2013.775484

Zientz, J., Rackley, A., Chapman, S. B., Hopper, T., Mahendra, N., Kim, E. S., & Cleary, S. (2007). Evidence-based practice recommendations for dementia: Educating caregivers on Alzheimer's disease and training communication strategies. *Journal of Medical Speech-Language Pathology, 15*(1), liii–lxiv.

Zimmer, U., Lewald, J., & Karnath, H. (2003). Disturbed sound lateralization in patients with spatial neglect. *Journal of Cognitive Neuroscience, 15*(5), 694–703.

Zimmermann, N., Gindri, G., de Oliveira, C. R., & Fonseca, R. P. (2011). Pragmatic and executive functions in traumatic brain injury and right brain damage: An exploratory comparative study. *Dementia Neuropsychology, 5*(4), 337–345.

Zinn, S., Bosworth, H. B., Hoenig, H. M., & Swartzwelder, H. S. (2007). Executive function deficits in acute stroke. *Archives of Physical Medicine and Rehabilitation, 88*(2), 173–180. http://doi.org/10.1016/j.apmr.2006.11.015

Zucchella, C., Capone, A., Codella, V., Vecchione, C., Buccino, G., Sandrini, G., . . . Bartolo, M. (2014). Assessing and restoring cognitive functions early after stroke. *Functional Neurology, 29*(4), 255–262.

Index

Note: Page numbers in **bold** reference non-text material.